Surgical Management of Low Back Pain

Surgical Management of Low Back Pain

EDITED BY

DANIEL K. RESNICK, M.D.
Department of Neurosurgery
University of Wisconsin Medical School
Madison, Wisconsin

REGIS W. HAID, JR., MD
Department of Neurological Surgery
Emory University School of Medicine
Atlanta, Georgia

American
Association of
Neurological
Surgeons

American Association of Neurological Surgeons • Rolling Meadows

Surgical Management of Low Back Pain
Daniel K. Resnick and Regis W. Haid, Jr., Editors

Library of Congress Cataloging-in-Publication Data

Surgical management of low back pain / [edited by] Daniel K. Resnick.
     p. ; cm — (Neurosurgical topics)
   ISBN 1-879284-78-2
    1. Backache—Surgery. 2. Backache—Treatment. I. Resnick, Daniel K.
  II. American Association of Neurological Surgeons. III. Series.
    [DNLM: 1. Low Back Pain—surgery. WE 755 S961 2001]
RD771.B217 S874 2001
617.5′64059—dc21   2001022265

This publication is written under the auspices of the Publications Committee of the
American Association or Neurological Surgeons (AANS). However, this should not
be construed as indicating endorsement or approval of the views presented, by the
AANS or by its committees, commissions, affiliates, or staff.

Warren R. Selman, MD, Chairman
AANS Publications Committee

Kristine Rynne Mednansky, Publisher

Contributors

Bryan Barnes, M.D.
Department of Neurosurgery
Emory University
Atlanta, Georgia

Edward C. Benzel, M.D., F.A.C.S.
Department of Neurosurgery
The Cleveland Clinic Foundation
Cleveland, Ohio

Regis W. Haid, Jr. M.D.
Department of Neurological Surgery
Emory University School of Medicine
Atlanta, Georgia

Victor Haughton, M.D.
Department of Radiology
University of Wisconsin
Madison, Wisconsin

Robert F. Heary, M.D.
Department of Neurological Surgery
UMDNJ–New Jersey Medical School
Newark, New Jersey

Jorge J. Lastra, M.D.
Department of Neurosurgery
The Cleveland Clinic Foundation
Cleveland, Ohio

Mark McLaughlin, M.D.
Neurosurgical and Neurological Group
Springfield, Massachusetts

Peter H. Nguyen M.D.
Department of Neurological Surgery
University of Wisconsin
Madison, Wisconsin

Richard B. North, M.D.
Department of Neurological Surgery
John Hopkins University
Baltimore, Maryland

Thomas M. Reilly, M.D.
Indianapolis Neurosurgical Group
Indianapolis, Indiana

Daniel K. Resnick, M.D., M.S.
Department of Neurological Surgery
University of Wisconsin Medical School
Madison, Wisconsin

Gerald Rodts, M.D.
Department of Neurological Surgery
Emory University School of Medicine
Atlanta, Georgia

Rick C. Sasso, M.D.
Department of Orthopaedic Surgery
Indiana University School of Medicine
Indianapolis Neurosurgical Group
Indianapolis, Indiana

Gordon Tang, M.D.
Department of Neurological Surgery
Emory University School of Medicine
Atlanta, Georgia

Clifford B. Tribus, M.D.
Division of Orthopedics
University of Wisconsin–Madison
Madison, Wisconsin

Gregory R. Trost M.D.
Department of Neurological Surgery
University of Wisconsin
Madison, Wisconsin

Ceslovas Vaicys, M.D.
Department of Neurological Surgery
UMDNJ–New Jersey Medical School
Newark, New Jersey

Byron H. Willis, M.D.
Department of Neurosurgery
The Cleveland Clinic Foundation
Cleveland, Ohio

Brian P. Witwer, M.D.
Department of Neurological Surgery
University of Wisconsin Medical School
Madison, Wisconsin

Seth M. Zeidman, M.D.
Department of Neurosurgery
University of Rochester
Rochester, New York

Foreword

Low back pain is extremely common, with approximately 80% of adults suffering a memorable episode of low back pain. The vast majority of patients are treated successfully with physical therapy, nonsteroidal anti-inflammatory medications, and encouragement. Because of the magnitude of the problem, however, the minority of patients who fail to respond to these measures still represent a large number of patients. These patients, with back pain recalcitrant to conservative therapy for a period of months to years, are appropriately referred to spinal surgeons. The spine surgeon of the 21st century is faced with a dizzying array of options for the treatment of a patient with low back pain. Each new treatment is purported to be the latest and greatest cure for low back pain. As we have learned from our experience with pedicle screws and with interbody cage technology, nothing is as good as the industry sponsored initial studies seem to indicate. Furthermore, because of the rapid pace with which new devices and techniques are appearing on the market, the ability of the practicing physician to learn the particular indications for a particular treatment strategy is limited. The lack of reliable information regarding a new technology at its introduction into widespread use in combination with the large number of competing techniques/devices/companies as well as variability and bias in physician training (neurosurgeon, orthopedic surgeon, anesthesiologist, rehabilitation physician) contribute to the confusion.

The text is intended to serve as an overview of new techniques for the diagnosis and management of medically refractory low back pain. Discussions of the pathophysiology and biomechanics of low back pain and its treatment serve as a rationale for later discussions of various fusion techniques, intradiscal electrothermy, spinal cord stimulation and facet rhizotomy. This information is useful for answering the real life questions that we encounter every day, such as: Which fusion technique, if any, is best for a 40-year-old athletic man with a collapsed L4/5 disc space? How about the 30-year old-laborer with a well-preserved disc space but a positive discogram? How about the 70-year-old man with stenosis and low grade spondylolisthesis? How does intradiscal electrothermy work and who are good candidates? How can I help patients with failed back surgery syndrome? How do we tell facet derived pain from discogenic pain and does it matter? It is hoped that this text will help provide a better understanding of the pathophysiology, biomechanics, and natural history of low back pain and the available treatments.

Contents

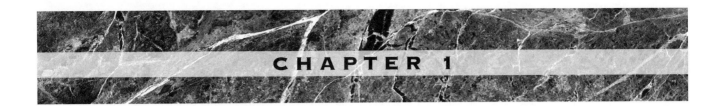

CHAPTER 1

The Pathophysiology of Low Back Pain and Its Treatment

Daniel K. Resnick, M.D., M.S.

Brian P. Witwer, M.D.

INTRODUCTION

Low back pain is a very common disorder. It is estimated that 50 to 80% of the adult population suffers from at least one memorable episode of low back pain per year.[26] In a 1985 study, 3% of the population reported severe low back pain that lasted for 31 days or more within the previous year.[37] Between 2 to 5% of adults (in the United States) will visit a physician or lose time from work because of low back pain each year. Low back pain is the single largest cause of lost workdays in the United States and is the fifth most common reason for a visit to a primary care physician's office.[26]

The vast majority of people with low back pain improve spontaneously. There exists a subgroup of patients, however, whose pain does not improve with "conservative measures." The definition of *conservative measures* is subject to interpretation. Whereas most surgeons would probably define *conservative measures* as a several month trial of physical therapy and nonsteroidal antiinflammatory medications, there has been a huge expansion in the nonoperative treatment of low back pain. Because of the large number of people who suffer from low back pain, new procedures, products, and philosophies have found an ever-expanding niche in the health care market. Whereas many of these treatments are innocuous (magneto-therapy, acupuncture, herbal medications), most are costly, and some are certainly invasive (facet rhizotomy, epidural steroid injections).

In addition to the advent of many new nonoperative treatment modalities, nonfusion procedures for low back pain, including intradiscal electrothermy and dorsal column stimulation, have been developed and will likely play an increasing role in the management of patients with low back pain. Finally, new fusion techniques have led to a significant increase in the spine surgeon's ability to treat low back pain. Better understanding of the biomechanics of the spine, the natural history of degenerative disc disease, and diagnostic imaging techniques have led to a rapid evolution of fusion techniques. Interbody fusion techniques, first described in the early part of the 20th century and buoyed by new technology, are increasingly popular. Anterior approaches, posterior approaches, and lateral approaches for fusion, as well as titanium, steel, and carbon fiber implants, are now routinely employed by orthopaedic and neurosurgical spine surgeons.

The emergence of competing new technologies for the operative and nonoperative treatment of low back pain is both exciting and frustrating. The majority of these new techniques have not been subject to randomized, controlled clinical trials. Patient selection criteria as well as outcome measures vary between various surgical and nonsurgical series. Finally, as soon as relatively concrete clinical data are gathered regarding one methodology, another "new and improved" methodology is aggressively marketed. This situation has re-emphasized the need for the physician treating patients with low back pain to have a clear understanding of the anatomy, pathophysiology, and natural history of low back pain. The only way that a physician can make an informed judgment regarding the need for and appropriateness of a given treatment modality (be it magnetism or instrumented fusion) is with a firm grasp of these basic principles. The purpose of this chapter is to review the anatomical substrate and basic pathophysiology of low back pain.

NOCICEPTION IN THE LUMBAR SPINE

Nociceptors are neural sensory organs that transmit information regarding potentially harmful stimuli to the central nervous system. Nociceptors are located in joint capsules and ligaments, perivascular sites, periosteum, muscles, and tendons. The afferent fibers of nociceptors consist of thin myelinated A (fast) and unmyelinated C (slow) fibers. The quality of pain sensation depends on the nociceptor being stimulated; stimulation of A fibers leads to pricking pain, whereas stimulation of cutaneous C nociceptors results in a burning, dull sensation.[32] Nociceptors are not among the large sensory fibers (A, A, or Groups I and II); these fibers subserve the mechano-sensitive functions of proprioception and motor control. Motivational affective circuits can also mimic pain states, most notably in patients with anxiety, neurotic depression, or hysteria.[6]

Most nociceptors from pain afferents are found in a "silent" or "sleeping" state. Certain inflammatory stimuli lead to sensitization of the nociceptor, producing an activated nerve ending. Primary hyperalgesia is believed to result in the sensitization of nociceptors during the process of inflammation. Sensitization of nociceptors depends on the release of inflammatory mediators, such as bradykinin, prostaglandins, serotonin, and histamine, in the damaged tissue.[36]

Sensory pain impulses arising from the lumbar spine are projected to the bipolar nerve cell body located within the dorsal root ganglion (DRG). Lindblum implicated the DRG as a modulator of low back pain.[24] Howe demonstrated that chronic injury to the dorsal root produces a marked increase in sensitivity to mechanical stimulation.[20]. Sensory afferent information is processed by the dorsal root ganglion and then transmitted to the central nervous system.

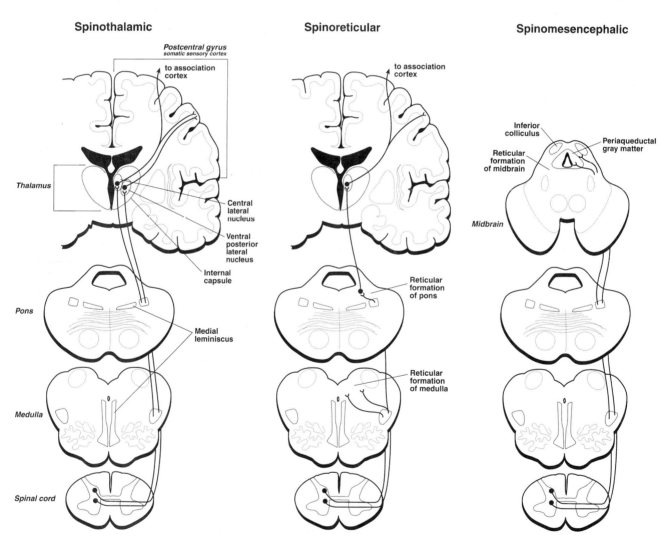

FIGURE 1-1 ■ The three major ascending pain pathways (spinothalamic, spinoreticular, spinomesencephalic) are illustrated in a schematic format. In addition to the well-described thalamic projections, these tracts project to other brainstem nuclei. These include the nucleus raphe magnus (NRM), nucleus magnocellularis (NMC), nucleus reticularis gigantocellularis (NRC), and periaqueductal gray (PAG). Other fibers simultaneously project to the reticular formation of the medulla and pons, as well as to the nucleus raphe dorsalis (NRD). At each relay point, information can be modified by descending pathways from the cortex.

The cells in the DRG are divided into two classes according to their diameters, large unmyelinated fibers, small unmyelinated (C), and finely myelinated (A) fibers. The central terminations of these primary afferent fibers, derived from the small cells, end mainly in Rexed's lamina II (the substantia gelatinosa) of the spinal cord. Several peptides, including calcitonin gene-related protein (CGRP) and substance P, have been localized to the small DRG cells. CGRP has been shown to be the most abundant peptide in the DRG.[15] Several groups have demonstrated increases in the concentrations of substance P and vasoactive intestinal polypeptide (VIP) following stimulation of the DRG.[42,45]

Nociceptive information terminates primarily on small interneurons within Rexed's laminae I and II. These interneurons produce both excitatory and inhibitory neurotransmitters and project to the dendrites of multiple dorsal horn cells within several adjacent levels of the spinal cord.[8] These interneurons are responsible for modulation of the stimulus that is ultimately projected centrally. Immunohistochemical studies demonstrate that these interneurons synthesize a wide variety of neurotransmitters, including excitatory amino acids (particularly glutamate) and multiple neuropeptides, such as substance P, CGRP, VIP, Somatostatin, and others.[9] These transmitters function as both excitatory and inhibitory modulators of nociceptive input.

Damage to a peripheral nerve can cause the upregulation of several neuropeptides, including galanin and VIP, as well as the downregulation of others such as substance P, somatostatin, and CGRP. In addition to this change in the neurotransmitter milieu, damage to the supporting structures of the nerve can lead to alterations in the anatomy of the pain system. Damage to Schwann cells can result in the upregulation of neurotrophins responsible for nerve regeneration.[11] It has been postulated that these growth factors may promote aberrant forms of regeneration and abnormal pain states. Woolf showed that large myelinated afferents, supplying mechanoreceptors, grew into lamina II after a peripheral nerve injury.[44] Abnormal connections of these large afferents to nociceptive processing circuits of the dorsal horn may contribute to allodynia, a sensation of pain that is provoked in pathologic circumstances by innocuous stimuli.

Nociceptive projection neurons in the spinal cord transmit information to numerous regions of the brainstem and diencephalon, including the thalamus, periaqueductal gray, parabrachial region, reticular formation, and limbic structures.

There is a high level of redundancy in nociceptive projections to higher processing centers (Figure 1-1). The spinothalamic tract mediates the sensations of pain, cold, warmth, and touch. These neuron cell bodies are located primarily in lamina I, and lamina IV to lamina VI. The axons cross in anterior white commissure, ascend in the lateral funiculus, and terminate on the posterior part of the ventral medial nucleus, ventral posterior lateral nucleus, and medial dorsal nucleus. Nociceptive information is also transmitted to multiple spinal cord relay nuclei via the spinomesencephalic and spinoreticular tracts. A multisynaptic pathway carries information about noxious inputs to the medial thalamus, where it is relayed to the nucleus accumbens, septal nuclei, and amygdala of the limbic system. This pathway is relevant to the motivational aspects of pain.[4]

Multiple higher centers can directly modulate nociception at the spinal level through descending projections (Figure 1-2). Reynolds demonstrated that

Descending Endongenous Pain System

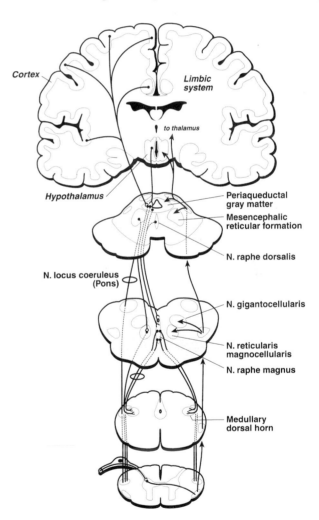

FIGURE 1-2 ■ The diagram depicts the endogenous descending pain inhibitory systems. Cortical projections, as well as projections from the hypothalamus, terminate in the periaqueductal gray matter. Axons from the periaqueductal gray then project to the dorsal horn of the spinal cord. Some mesencephalic neurons (containing the neurotransmitters enkephalin, dynorphin, serotonin, and neurotensin) project directly to the dorsal lateral funiculus of the spinal cord.

stimulation of the midbrain periaqueductal gray (PAG) inhibits the perception of noxious stimuli during surgical manipulations on rats.[35] The PAG neurons project to the nucleus raphe magnus (NRM) and adjacent reticular formations and to the spinal cord.[2] These pathways utilize several different neurotransmitters, including opioids, serotonin, and catecholamines. These descending inputs, largely from the cortex and thalamus, alter the perception of pain.[7] Cortical areas most prominently involved in this process include the SI and SII somatosensory cortex, the anterior insula, and the cingulate gyrus.[5, 34] The lentiform nucleus and cerebellum also provide descending input to the pain pathway. This activity is thought to allow for processing of reflexive motor responses to painful stimuli. Ventrally directed tactile processing from S1 to the temporal lobe limbic structures via relays in S2 and the insula may subserve tactile learning and memory.[12]

PAIN GENERATORS IN THE SPINE

The low back contains several potential anatomical sources of low back pain. The paraspinal musculature, facet joints, and ligaments of the intervertebral disc complex are innervated by nociceptive fibers and can all play a role in the pathogenesis of low back pain. Various authors have tried to characterize pain patterns thought to be produced by abnormalities of these structures. Persistent pain from a primarily muscular origin is often referred to as a *myofascial pain syndrome*. Pain syndromes thought to occur as the result of facet arthropathy have been referred to as *facet syndromes*. Finally, there has been much written about the nature and cause of *discogenic* low back pain. Each of these pain syndromes is felt to respond to therapy directed towards the presumed source of pain.

There is significant controversy regarding the existence of a "facet syndrome," and differentiating pain derived from facet arthropathy versus degenerative changes in the intervertebral disc may be impossible and, in the case of fusion, irrelevant. Muscle derived pain may present as a distinct syndrome, the "myofascial pain syndrome," which is distinct from pain derived from the axial spine. The majority of this discussion focuses on axial back pain, or pain derived from the axial spine. Because persistent low back pain of muscular origin is relatively common, a brief discussion of its nature, pathophysiology, and treatment follows.

Myofascial pain syndrome is characterized by nonaxial low back pain, that is, pain in the paraspinal or gluteal musculature. This pain is mediated by visceral nociceptive fibers found within the muscles themselves. There are invariably one or more local trigger points. These trigger points are characterized by local tenderness, an associated taut contracted muscle band (often palpable in the spine), a local twitch response, referred pain, and autonomic phenomena. The pain is usually caused by a stress or injury to the muscle and is perpetuated by mechanical factors such as structural inadequacies of the skeleton (short leg syndrome, long second metatarsal syndrome) or postural stresses. Referred pain develops as visceral and somatic afferents converge on the same dorsal horn cells, causing referred pain in "nondermatomal" or "bizarre" patterns. These patterns, however, are generally reproducible in the individual patient. There are currently no diagnostic tests for myofascial pain syndrome. Treatment options include spray and stretch, trigger point injection with local anesthetics, and various manipulation techniques.[13]

The facet joint represents another potential source of low back pain. "Facet syndrome," introduced by Ghormley in 1933, purports to describe pain of facet origin. The syndrome is characterized by hip and buttock pain, cramping leg pain (primarily above the knee), low back stiffness, and the absence of paresthesias. Patients usually exhibit local paraspinal tenderness; pain on spine hyperextension; hip, buttock, or back pain with straight leg raising; and no neurological deficit.[14,25]

The facet joints are innervated by the dorsal rami of the local nerve root and by dorsal rami of neighboring roots (Figure 1-3).[33,46] In one study, Ashton and colleagues found nociceptive fibers within the capsule of the facet and were unable to locate similar fibers in the annulus.[1] Also, injections into the facets caused back, hip, and buttock pain in six normal human volunteers.[29] Mooney and Robertson, who injected facets in patients with radicular symptoms, found that they could reproduce many symptoms of radiculopathy.[31] Unfortunately, therapy directed specifically at the facet joint (facet rhizotomy and facet injection) has not been successful in alleviating back pain in the majority of patients.[10,25]

Axial back pain is usually thought to arise from abnormalities involving the vertebral bodies and intervertebral discs. *Axial back pain* is generally described as deep, midline, aching pain. There may be some radiation of pain into the buttocks or upper thighs, and the pain is often positional in nature, worse when upright as opposed to supine. This type of pain is thought to be produced by the visceral afferents that innervate the intervertebral disc. The innervation of the intervertebral disc is via the sinuvertebral nerves, which were first described by Luschka in the mid 1800s. He showed that this nerve was derived mainly from the spinal nerve, with contribution from the sympathetic system (Figure 1-4).[27] Malinsky, in 1959, demonstrated multiple types of nerve endings in the outer portion of the annulus fibrosis, and this finding has been repeatedly corroborated and further defined by others.[3,28,33,47]

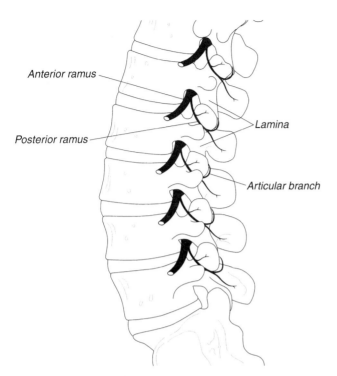

FIGURE 1-3 ■ Facet Joint Innervation. A lateral view of the lumbar vertebral column demonstrating lumbar spinal nerves exiting from the neural foramina. The dorsal ramus of the lumbar spinal nerve divides into several branches that innervate the superior facet of one joint and the inferior facet of the adjacent joint.

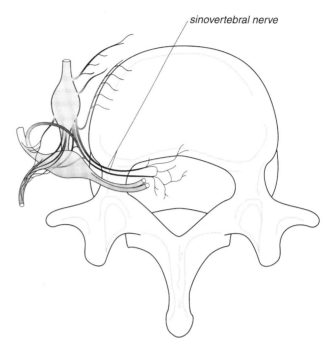

FIGURE 1-4 ■ Innervation of the spinal canal. The sinuvertebral nerve (SVN) is composed of two primary inputs. The diagram depicts the SVN contributions from the ventral primary ramus and the ramus communicans. The nerve enters the spinal canal through the neural foramina crossing the vertebral body caudal to the pedicle. The SVN then ramifies rostrally and caudally along the posterior longitudinal ligament. The nerve innervates the intervertebral disc at the level of the parent nerve and one level rostrally.

The sinuvertebral nerves (SVN) arise from two roots, one from the ventral primary ramus and the other from the ramus communicans. The SVN enters the neural canal through the intervertebral foramen. Within the canal the nerve ramifies into two branches. The major branch ascends rostrally along the lateral border of the posterior longitudinal ligament. A second division passes medially and dorsally to innervate the intervertebral disc at the level of origin of the parent nerve. Bogduk demonstrated through anatomical studies that a SVN, through its two primary branches, innervates two separate intervertebral levels. The inferior branch innervates the superior aspect of the disc at the level of entry, and the rostral branch provides innervation to the disc one level above.[3] The sinuvertebral nerve therefore provides the majority of innervation of the spinal canal. This network of nerve endings provides innervation of dura matter, ligaments, and blood vessels, including the posterior longitudinal ligament and the posterior aspect of the annulus fibrosis.

The nucleus pulposis of the intervertebral disc is composed of collagen, mucopolysaccharides, and water. Normal aging leads to degenerative changes in the chemical and physical structure of the disc. The concentration of keratosulfates increases over time, whereas the water content of the disc decreases,

changing the elastic properties of the disc. The degeneration of the proteoglycans results in changes in the local pH and the accumulation of prostaglandins and other inflammatory mediators. The annulus fibrosis also undergoes changes over time, with microscopic and then macroscopic tears developing. Fragmentation of fibers leads to concentric cracks and cavities, allowing for the aggregation of collagen. This type of degeneration leads to various types of annular tears.[39,40] Degeneration of the annulus is associated with circumferential clefts forming between fibrous layers. Minor trauma from aging may induce these clefts to enlarge and coalesce, most commonly in the posterolateral aspect of the annulus, forming radial tears.[21] Radial lesions are macroscopic deformities that extend radially from the nucleus to the periphery. They are seen in increasing frequency after age thirty.[18] These tears extend into the outer portion of the annulus that has a vascular supply, thus allowing for the ingrowth of vascular granulation tissue along the edges of the radial rupture.[39] Small tears may bridge the defect by forming fibrotic scar tissue. Large tears, subject to continuous movement, may be prevented from healing. Studies of experimental injuries to the annulus fibrosis of dogs demonstrate the limited healing potential of the annular fibers to radial tears.[17]

The nucleus pulposis and inner two thirds of the annulus are void of nerve endings. A rich network of nerve fibers innervates the supporting structures of the intervertebral disc. The lateral aspect of the vertebral column and the posterior longitudinal ligament are invested with a rich plexus of nerves derived from the SVN and the gray rami of the lumbar sympathetic trunks.[16] Nerve fibers extend beyond the longitudinal ligament deep into the outer third of the annulus fibrosis.[19] It is postulated that the intervertebral disc may become a pain producer when the outer third of the annulus is exposed to a painful stimulus.

The normal intact lumbar intervertebral disc does not produce pain. This is supported by discography studies that were unable to elicit a painful stimulus upon injection of the normal disc space.[41] This is explained by the fact that injection into the nucleus pulposus of a healthy disc does not aggravate the outer portion of the disc, which is protected by a healthy annulus. The annulus is designed to withstand high pressures within the nucleus pulposus. Disc degeneration produces injuries in the form of radial tears to the inner third of the annulus. Provocation discography of a diseased disc space produces a painful response when increased intra-disc pressure is communicated via the injured annular channels to the nerve endings in the outer third of the annulus.[30,38]

Several authors have provided direct in vivo studies that provide substantial evidence pointing towards the intervertebral disc as the source of pain for the majority of patients with low back pain. As discussed previously, numerous authors have identified nociceptive fibers within the outer annulus, posterior longitudinal ligament, and in granulation tissue associated with radial tears. Wiberg reported selective reproduction of back pain with stimulation of the intervertebral disc (posterior annulus) in a series of patients undergoing awake lumbar diskectomy.[43] Kuslich also noted the pain generating potential of the annulus fibrosis in awake humans. Kuslich used local anesthetic to perform lumbar discectomies in awake patients. He stimulated various structures, including the facet capsule, ligamentum flavum, and annulus fibrosis. Patients reliably reported the occurrence of axial back pain with stimulation of the annulus fibrosis. Stimulation of the other structures did not reliably result in the reproduction of low back pain.[22,23] Information derived from these studies, as well as the evidence presented previously, provides strong evidence for the hypothesis that the intervertebral disc is an important generator of pain in a substantial number of patients with low back pain.

SURGERY FOR LOW BACK PAIN

In cases of neurological deficit or structural instability of the spine, decompression of neural elements and reconstruction of the spine may result in restoration of function and the elimination of severe pain. The vast majority of patients who present with low back pain will have no neurological deficit and no evidence of acute instability of the spine. Most will have some evidence of degenerative disc disease, and many will display evidence of chronic or glacial instability (modic changes, disc space collapse, low grade spondylolisthesis). The major purpose of medical or surgical intervention in these patients is to relieve their low back pain. Theoretically, any interruption of the pain pathway, from the low back to the cerebral cortex, has the potential to relieve low back pain.

Spinal fusion is designed to eliminate the lumbar pain generator. It is hypothesized that stimuli for pain-generating afferents within the annulus (or facet joint) are eliminated with the removal of the disc and the elimination of motion at the fusion site. Conflicting reports in the literature exist concerning the efficacy of fusion for low back pain. Different diagnostic tests, surgical approaches, the use or nonuse of rigid, semi-rigid, or interbody instrumentation, and varying patient selection criteria and outcome measures make global statements difficult. It does appear certain, however, that there does exist a population of patients with degenerative disc disease and low back pain who respond very well to surgical fusion. Description of this patient population as it relates to a number of different fusion techniques follows in ensuing chapters.

Intradiscal electrothermy is a recently developed method used to denature the collagen of the annulus fibrosis. Exposure of the collagen to temperatures of 60° C leads to shortening of the collagen strands, which apparently leads to a "sealing" of annular tears. Passive heat spread leads to exposure of the outer annulus to temperatures in the range of 42° C, hot enough to coagulate local nociceptors. This technology would therefore (at least temporarily) destroy pain-generating structures in the annulus fibrosis but would not affect the facet capsule. A discussion of this novel technique to eliminate back pain follows in the text.

Another means by which pain generated at the level of the low back can be alleviated is by interruption of the pain signal. Dorsal column stimulation employs an electrical current to create a localized electromagnetic field around the spinal cord. This electromagnetic field causes tonic stimulation of large fibers in the dorsal column, causing a sensation of "buzzing" or "tingling" in the region of the body served by the particular group of fibers stimulated. This stimulation overrides the transmittal of information to higher centers from smaller diameter nociceptive tracts, thus eliminating the sensation of pain. A detailed description of the use of this modality for the treatment of low back pain and leg pain is included in the text.

SUMMARY

Low back pain is very common. The vast majority of patients with low back pain improve spontaneously. There exists a population of patients whose pain does not improve over time and with noninvasive therapy. Clearly, the capsule of the facet joint and the annulus of the intervertebral disc are potential pain generators. Regardless of the pain generator, once a painful stimulus is generated, several pathways exist for the transmittal of painful sensation to the central nervous system. The source of low back pain may be difficult to identify in an individual patient. There exist a large number of diagnostic tests and therapeutic modalities that are designed to identify and/or eliminate specific pain generators in the lumbar spine (e.g., anterior lumbar interbody fusion [ALIF], facet rhizotomy, intradiscal electrotherapy [IDET]). The patient selection criteria and the technical aspects of, and success rates of, many of these procedures are discussed in ensuing chapters. Other methodologies nonselectively eliminate several potential pain generators (consider the effect of PLIF on the facet joint and the intervertebral disc) or interrupt the pathways responsible for the perception of pain (dorsal column stimulation). This text reviews these various tests and therapies to clarify the rationale behind, the patient selection criteria for, the technical aspects of, and the expected outcomes of each of these therapies.

REFERENCES

———————————————■———————————————

1. Ashton I, Ashton B, Gibson S, et al: Morphological basis for back pain: the demonstration of nerve fibers and neuropeptides in the lumbar facet joint capsule but not in the ligamentum flavum. **J Orthop Res** 10:72-78, 1992.
2. Besson JM, Chaouch A: Peripheral and spinal mechanisms of nociception. **Physiol Rev** 67:67-186, 1987.
3. Bogduk N, Tynan W, Wilson AS: The nerve supply to the human lumbar intervertebral discs. **J Anat** 132:39-56, 1981.
4. Burstein R, Giesler GJ, Jr: Retrograde labeling of neurons in spinal cord that project directly to nucleus accumbens or the septal nuclei in the rat. **Brain Res** 497:149-54, 1989.
5. Casey KL, Minoshima S, Berger KL, et al: Positron emission tomographic analysis of cerebral structures activated specifically by repetitive noxious heat stimuli. **J Neurophysiol** 71:802-7, 1994.
6. Chaturvedi SK: Prevalence of chronic pain in psychiatric patients. **Pain** 29:231-7, 1987.
7. Chudler EH, Anton F, Dubner R, et al: Responses of nociceptive SI neurons in monkeys and pain sensation in humans elicited by noxious thermal stimulation: effect of interstimulus interval. **J Neurophysiol** 63:559-69, 1990.
8. Cruz F, Lima D, Zieglgansberger W, et al: Fine structure and synaptic architecture of HRP-labeled primary afferent terminations in lamina IIi of the rat dorsal horn. **J Comp Neurol** 305:3-16, 1991.
9. De Biasi S, Rustioni A: Glutamate and substance P coexist in primary afferent terminals in the superficial laminae of spinal cord. **Proceedings of the National Academy of Sciences of the United States of America** 85:7820-4, 1988.
10. Destout J, Gilula L, Murphy W, et al: Lumbar facet injection: indication, technique, clinical correlation, and preliminary results. **Radiology** 145:321-25, 1982.
11. Ernfors P, Rosario CM, Merlio JP, et al: Expression of mRNAs for neurotrophin receptors in the dorsal root ganglion and spinal cord during development and following peripheral or central axotomy. **Brain Res Mol Brain Res** 17:217-26, 1993.
12. Friedman DP, Murray EA, O'Neill JB, et al: Cortical connections of the somatosensory fields of the lateral sulcus of macaques: evidence for a corticolimbic pathway for touch. **J Comp Neurol** 252:323-47, 1986.
13. Gerwin R: Myofascial aspects of low back pain. **Neurosurg Clin N Am** 4:761-84, 1991.
14. Ghormley R: Low back pain with special reference to the articular facets with presentation of an operative procedure. **JAMA** 101:1773-77, 1933.
15. Gibson SJ, Polak JM, Bloom SR, et al: The distribution of nine peptides in rat spinal cord with special emphasis on the substantia gelatinosa and on the area around the central canal (lamina X). **J Comp Neurol** 201:65-79, 1981.
16. Groen GJ, Baljet B, Drukker J: Nerves and nerve plexuses of the human vertebral column. **Am J Anat** 188:282-96, 1990.
17. Hampton D, Laros G, McCarron R, et al: Healing potential of the anulus fibrosus. **Spine** 14:398-401, 1989.
18. Hilton RC, Ball J: Vertebral rim lesions in the dorsolumbar spine. **Ann Rheum Dis** 43:302-7, 1984.
19. Hirsch C, Ingelmark B, Miller M: The anatomical basis for low back pain. **Acta Orthop Scand** 33:1-17, 1963.
20. Howe JF, Loeser JD, Calvin WH: Mechanosensitivity of dorsal root ganglia and chronically injured axons: a physiological basis for the radicular pain of nerve root compression. **Pain** 3:25-41, 1977.
21. Kirkaldy-Willis WH, Wedge JH, Yong-Hing K, et al: Pathology and pathogenesis of lumbar spondylosis and stenosis. **Spine** 3:319-28, 1978.
22. Kuslich S, Ahern J, Garner M: An in-vivo, prospective analysis of tissue sensitivity of lumbar spinal tissues. New York: 12th Annual Meeting of the North American Spine Society, 1997.
23. Kuslich S, Ulstrom C, Michael C: The tissue of origin of low back pain and sciatica. **Orthop Clin North Am** 22:181-87, 1991.
24. Lindblum K, Rexed B: Spinal nerve injury in dorso-lateral protrusions of lumbar disks. **J Neurosurg** 5, 1948.

25. Lippitt A: The facet joint and its role in spine pain. **Spine** 9:746-50, 1984.
26. Loeser J, Volinn E: Epidemiology of low back pain. **Neurosurg Clin N Am** 4:713-18, 1991.
27. Luschka V, Hubert: **Die Nerven des menshlichen Wirbelkanales.** Tubingen: Laub, 1850.
28. Malinsky J: The ontogenetic development of nerve terminations in the intervertebral discs of man. **Acta Anat** 38:96, 1959.
29. McCall I, Park W, O'Brien J: Induced pain referral from posterior elements in normal subjects. **Spine** 4:441-46, 1979.
30. Mooney V: Where is the lumbar pain coming from? **Ann Med** 21:373-79, 1989.
31. Mooney V, Robertson J: The facet syndrome. **Clin Orthop** 115:149-56, 1976.
32. Ochoa J, Torebjork E: Sensations evoked by intraneural microstimulation of C nociceptor fibres in human skin nerves. **J Physiol** 415:583-99, 1989.
33. Pederson H, Blunck C, Gardner E: Anatomy of lumbosacral posterior rami and meningeal branches of the spinal nerves (sinu-vertebral nerves) with experimental study of their functions. **J Bone Joint Surg** 38:377-91, 1955.
34. Rainville P, Duncan GH, Price DD, et al: Pain affect encoded in human anterior cingulate but not somatosensory cortex. **Science** 277:968-71, 1997.
35. Reynolds DV: Surgery in the rat during electrical analgesia induced by focal brain stimulation. **Science** 164:444-45, 1969.
36. Schaible HG, Schmidt RF: Time course of mechanosensitivity changes in articular afferents during a developing experimental arthritis. **J Neurophysiol** 60:2180-95, 1988.
37. Taylor H, Curran N: **The Nuprin Pain Report.** New York: Louis Harris and Associates, 1985.
38. Vanharanta H, Sachs BL, Spivey MA, et al: The relationship of pain provocation to lumbar disc deterioration as seen by CT/discography. **Spine** 12:295-98, 1987.
39. Vernon-Roberts B, Pirie CJ: Degenerative changes in the intervertebral discs of the lumbar spine and their sequelae. **Rheumatology & Rehabilitation** 16:13-21, 1977.
40. Vernon-Roberts B, Pirie CJ: Healing trabecular microfractures in the bodies of lumbar vertebrae. **Ann Rheum Dis** 32:406-12, 1973.
41. Walsh TR, Weinstein JN, Spratt KF, et al: Lumbar discography in normal subjects. A controlled, prospective study. **J Bone Joint Surg—American Volume** 72:1081-8, 1990.
42. Weinstein J, Pope M, Schmidt R, et al: Neuropharmacologic effects of vibration on the dorsal root ganglion. An animal model. **Spine** 13:521-25, 1988.
43. Wiberg G: Back pain in relation to the nerve supply of the intervertebral disc. **Acta Orthop Scand** 19:211-21, 1950.
44. Woolf CJ, Shortland P, Reynolds M, et al: Reorganization of central terminals of myelinated primary afferents in the rat dorsal horn following peripheral axotomy. **J Comp Neurol** 360:121-34, 1995.
45. Yaksh TL, Jessell TM, Gamse R, et al: Intrathecal morphine inhibits substance P release from mammalian spinal cord in vivo. **Nature** 286:155-57, 1980.
46. Yamashita T, Cavanaugh J, El-Bohy A, et al: Mechanosensitive afferent units in the lumbar facet joints. **J Bone Joint Surg** 72-A:865-70, 1990.
47. Yoshizawa H, O'Brien J, Thomas-Smith W, et al: The neuropathology of intervertebral discs removed for low back pain. **J Pathol** 132:95-104, 1980.

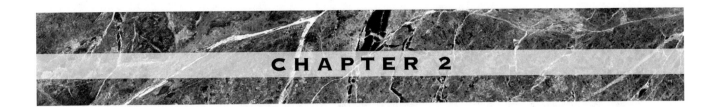

CHAPTER 2

Patient Selection in Lumbar Arthrodesis for Low Back Pain

GORDON TANG, M.D.

GERALD RODTS, M.D.

REGIS W. HAID, JR., M.D.

INTRODUCTION

Lumbar arthrodesis originated as a treatment for spinal tuberculosis in 1911 and later evolved to include the management of spinal deformity and traumatic injuries. Increasing familiarity extended the use of fusion for degenerative instability. With advancements in operative techniques, new spinal implants, and widespread education of fusion procedures, the indications for lumbar arthrodesis have broadened to include the treatment of low back pain.

In the environment of expanded indications and increasing population age, the rate of lumbar arthrodesis increased twofold between 1979 and 1987, then doubled again between 1990 and 1993, far exceeding the rates for laminectomy or discectomy. In patients with a diagnosis of spinal stenosis, the frequency of fusion procedures rose from 0.1 to 2.3 cases per 100,000 adults over the same period of time. More frequent use of diagnostic tests such as computed tomography (CT) and magnetic resonance imaging (MRI) have also contributed to a rise in operative procedures.

The concept of arthrodesis for the treatment of a painful joint arises from orthopedic experience elsewhere in the body. By analogy, treatment of low back pain by eliminating abnormal motion between adjacent vertebrae has conceptual appeal. However, its practical adaptation has been debated because of conflicting reports of postoperative results and the lack of appropriate outcome studies. Uncertainty of its indications has given rise to wide variations in lumbar arthrodesis rates. There is a greater than twofold variation in rates of lumbar arthrodesis from the West and the South, and as high as a 10-fold variation has been reported in communities fewer than 100 miles apart in the Northeast.[36]

It is generally acknowledged that in spite of all the advances in fusion procedures over the past 50 years, the critical factor in outcome following fusion procedures remains patient selection. Specific guidelines for lumbar arthrodesis in the management of low back pain remain elusive. Patient selection is currently as much of an art as it is a science, in which factors ranging from the patient's history, physical exam, response to conservative measures, psychosocial profile, and diagnostic tests, and the surgeon's self-knowledge are each weighed and considered in order to render a final decision.

GENERAL CONSIDERATIONS

Concepts of Spinal Instability

It is a basic medical tenet that, prior to instituting any therapy, the specific pathoanatomical diagnosis responsible for the majority of symptoms must be established. The selection of treatment alternatives relies on an understanding of the natural history, as well as on nonoperative and operative options. The ideal course of action should meet the goals of minimal tissue disruption, with restoration of normal biomechanics in a manner that is of minimal risk and greatest cost-effectiveness.

Arthrodesis for low back pain relies on the fact that abnormal movement in the lumbar spine contributes to the majority of a patient's symptoms. However, what is considered "abnormal" is an open question. Classically, the term *instability* has also been reserved for the interpretation of radiographs, with the criteria being greater than 4mm of translation and 10° of angulation between adjacent levels on flexion/extension films when com-

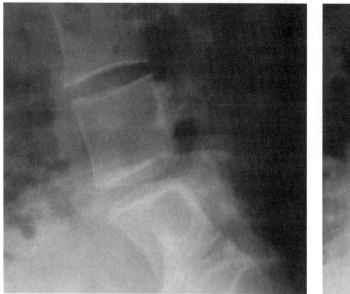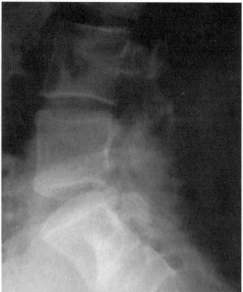

FIGURE 2-1 ■ Fusion CHP. Dynamic films illustrate instability at L4/5. The patient's symptoms were relieved by posterior segmental fixation.

pared with the adjacent levels (Figure 2-1). These radiographic criteria apply to only a minority of degenerative lumbar spine disease cases. Other definitions of instability provide no easy guidelines for usage. White

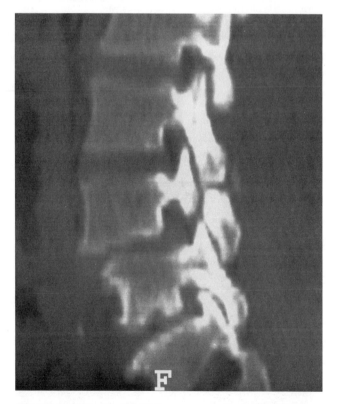

FIGURE 2-2 ■ Sagittal reconstruction of a CT of the lumbar spine illustrates a pars defect and accompanying spondylolisthesis.

and Panjabi offer the following definition of spinal instability: the inability of the spine to prevent initial or additional damage to the neural elements, deformity, or pain from structural changes (Figure 2-2).[69] Kirkaldy-Willis and Farfan provide a pathoanatomical definition of degeneration as a process that begins with the dysfunctional phase characterized by nuclear degeneration, annular tears, and facet arthritis, followed by the instability phase characterized by a reduction of disc height, laxity of the ligaments and facet capsules, degeneration of the facet joints and increased motion (Figure 2-3). This phase is followed by a restabilization phase with osteophyte formation, facet hypertrophy, and desiccation of the disc with an increase in intradiscal collagen.[37] On the other hand, pathologic changes such as these are often found on asymptomatic volunteers. Frymoyer has defined segmental instability as a "loss of motion stiffness such that force application to the motion segment produces greater displacement than would be seen in normal structures resulting in a painful condition that has the potential for progressive deformity and neurologic damage."[24]

Nonoperative Therapy and Pre-operative Management

Irrespective of diagnosis, the first step toward considering a fusion procedure is to ensure that the patient has truly failed the best conservative management for a minimum of three to four months. In addition to verifying the lack of alternatives, such a waiting period serves to illustrate the severity of the condition and affords an evaluation of the patient's commitment

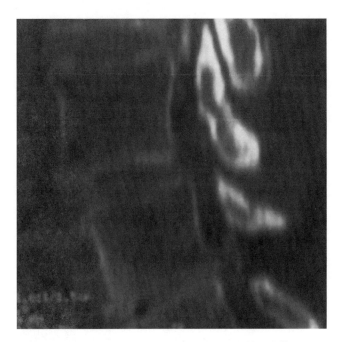

FIGURE 2-3 ■ CT sagittal reconstruction illustrates disc collapse and minimal anterolisthesis of L4 and L5. Patient improved following posterior segmental fixation.

toward the recovery. Maximizing function and minimizing illness behavior are the main goals of nonoperative therapy. An emphasis on smoking cessation for at least two to three months, minimizing chronic narcotic use, and optimizing nutritional status not only improve the chances that nonoperative therapy will be successful, but also enhance outcome if surgery proves to be necessary.

The literature provides little guidance on the form that nonoperative interventions should take. Twenty-eight randomized, controlled trials on the nonoperative treatment of low back pain have been recently reviewed.[64] For acute low back pain, nonsteroidal anti-inflammatories and muscle relaxants were strongly supported, whereas exercise did not appear to be substantially beneficial. For chronic low back pain, short-term improvement was reported following exercise, back school, and manipulation. No more than a brief (two days) of bed rest should be prescribed, with further inactivity possibly leading to deconditioning and the development of illness-related behavior.[22,71] Many exercise programs, including those involving extension, flexion, a combination of flexion and extension, aerobic conditioning, and stretching, have been advocated for the treatment of low back pain, although there is no strong evidence to support one type of therapy over other types.[18,26,48] The use of traction for the treatment of low back pain has not been supported in at least seven randomized trials. Similarly, no evidence could be found in support of acupuncture, transcuta-

neous electrical nerve stimulation, braces, or biofeedback.[59] Whereas ineffective for long-term control, such modalities may provide temporary relief to allow one to participate in exercises that are often precluded by the patient's painful state. In the same manner, corticosteroid injections in the form of nerve root blocks, facet injections, and epidural steroid injections may be of considerable value in the arsenal of conservative management.

In addition to attempts at alleviating pain, presurgical patients should also begin a program of functional restoration and work-hardening that focuses on behavioral modification in order to reduce future episodes of back pain. There should be an emphasis on rehabilitation for the purposes of returning to work and improving function despite continued pain. Such programs combine education, behavioral training, endurance training, and work simulation. Most authors have found back school to be beneficial for those patients with chronic back pain, although proper outcome studies have yet to justify the high cost.[16,30,52,64] A trial of immobilization with the use of a brace has often been used as a means of predicting which patients might benefit from intersegmental arthrodesis. However, biomechanical and radiographic studies have shown that lumbar orthoses have little effect on motion between vertebrae even when a thigh extension is added. Along with most clinicians, we have abandoned this approach as a diagnostic measure.[2,3,20,57] A trial of short-term external fixation has shown some promise in helping to determine which patients will benefit from arthrodesis, although we feel that this technique is impractical in most situations.[38]

Psychological Factors

The principal goal of lumbar arthrodesis in patients with low back pain is to relieve disability. However, psychological factors often dictate the relationship between disability and pathology. In selecting appropriate candidates for lumbar arthrodesis, an understanding of psychological factors and their relationship to low back pain cannot be overemphasized. In multiple studies, patients' perceptions of their degrees of disability provide the strongest predictor of outcome. In one study, patients who rated their health as poor before surgery had two- to threefold worse outcome at follow-up than those who rated their health as excellent. The patients' own rating of health was the most powerful predictor of symptom severity and walking capacity (P 0.0002) and satisfaction (p 0.001), even after control for comorbidity, physical functional capacity, depression, and age. In comparison, more objective measures such as preoperative walking capacity, noninstrumented fusion, and higher income had borderline significance (0.01 < 0.05).[45]

TABLE 2-1 ■ Negative Factors Associated
with Pain Relief

Older age
Prior history of low back pain
Normal gait
Maximum pain on extension following forward flexion in the
 standing position
Absence of leg pain, muscle spasm
Pain not worsened when rising from forward flexion
Pain well relieved by recumbency
Pain not worsened by extension-rotation
Lack of pain aggravation by Valsalva

Secondary gain by sick-role related psychological gain or by way of disability insurance or Workers' Compensation may limit the degree of success irrespective of treatment. Discrepancies between nociceptive stimuli and the behavioral and affective component should lead one to hesitate to recommend lumbar fusion. This desynchrony on exam has been outlined by Waddell and others (Table 2-1).[40,45,65] The presence of psychological stress that may aggravate or cause back pain should be screened for and addressed prior to any major operative intervention. Several validated psychometric instruments have been developed for this purpose.[44,75] Preoperative referral to trained professionals and community resources, including counselors and self-help groups, may optimize operative outcome or provide options in those cases in which clear operative indications are lacking.[58]

Psychological issues and patients' perceptions of their own health should be incorporated into discussions of expectations concerning the outcomes of fusion and decisions to elect surgery. Despite substantial improvement, one should counsel patients, especially those with a degenerative condition, that their conditions will not return to normal and that only a small percentage of patients have complete pain relief or a complete return to premorbid function.

General Diagnostic Tests

When considering patients for arthrodesis for low back pain, it must be understood that the majority of the patients' symptoms cannot be attributable to some other diagnosis in which arthrodesis alone is unlikely to be helpful. These include arachnoiditis, epidural fibrosis, and nerve root compression from unappreciated lateral recess stenosis. Other nonspinal causes of low back pain such as postherpetic neuralgia, sacroiliac disease, hip arthritis, referred retroperitoneal pain, or vascular pain must be sought out and excluded.

The initial diagnostic test remains the plain radiograph. Information regarding alignment, past surgical procedures, degree of degeneration, and status of a past fusion are quickly obtained. In addition, plain radiographs screen for unappreciated pathology such as infection, a malignant lesion, fracture, and inflammatory conditions. Indirect radiographic signs such as osteophytes, facet hypertrophy, and disc space narrowing may require further diagnostic investigation.[43] Meanwhile, negative results may help to reassure the patient that no major pathological condition is present.[35] In patients with some degree of deformity, lateral full-length spine radiographic films may be critical. Standing scoliosis radiographs (14–36 in.) (35.6–91.4 cm) fully assess the primary curvature as well as compensatory curves. Standing radiographic films also allow evaluation of both coronal and sagittal plane balance.

In patients considered for arthrodesis, dynamic radiographs, both standing and nonweight-bearing, are requisite. Lateral supine-bending films can also be obtained to assess the flexibility of the curvatures. Flexion and extension views are helpful to determine lumbar spine flexibility and the presence of sagittal plane instability. These views have been sufficient for preoperative planning in the vast majority of cases. Traction views may be helpful for severe deformities over 60°.

Because of the limitations of MRI in evaluating osseous anatomy, CT is often an adjunct in any patient for whom arthrodesis is considered. In instances of prior surgery, CT with multiplanar reconstruction is indispensable in evaluating the degree of fusion. Computerized tomography with myelography is helpful in evaluating the neural elements in cases of severe rotational deformity and in cases in which metal implants may obscure the neural elements in MR imaging. New advances in MR imaging that attenuate the signal loss from orthopaedic implants, along with the use of titanium implants, may, in the future, obviate the need for CT myelography. However, the clarity of these images depends upon the proximity of the metal to the area being investigated and may not provide enough data in all cases. Despite the merits of CT, magnetic resonance imaging continues to be invaluable for imaging the intervertebral disc and nerve roots. Unsuspected tumors, infections, and inflammatory processes can also be ruled out. In combination with gadolinium, MRI helps to eliminate cases of arachnoiditis and epidural fibrosis (Figure 2-4).

SPECIFIC CONDITIONS

Lumbar arthrodesis may be indicated for the treatment of low back pain in the following six conditions:

1. Iatrogenic instability.
2. Lumbar stenosis.
3. Degenerative spondylolisthesis.
4. Progressive scoliosis.

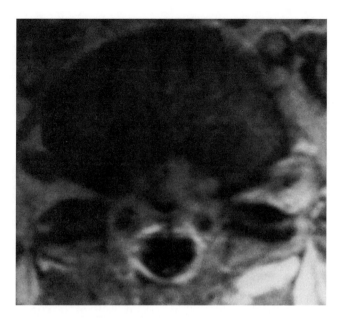

FIGURE 2-4 ■ MRI with gadolinium with the lumbar spine illustrates extensive epidural scarring.

5. Degenerative disc disease.
6. Facet syndrome.
7. Pseudoarthrosis.

Iatrogenic Instability

Instability is an infrequent sequelae of laminectomy for discectomy or foraminal decompression. In the absence of spinal deformity or instability, concomitant spinal arthrodesis generally does not provide additional clinical benefit.[28,55] Instability caused by the resection of facets at the time of the operation may be an indication for arthrodesis to prevent persistent instability and pain. It is generally accepted that spinal stability will be maintained if a total of at least one facet joint is preserved.[36] However, biomechanical evidence has suggested that instability (as indicated by markedly increased segmental motion) occurs after unilateral total facetectomy, even if the remaining facet has been left intact.[1] Unilateral or bilateral medial partial facetectomy has been shown to have little effect on segmental motion.[1] Abumi and associates performed a biomechanical analysis of anatomical specimens subjected to cyclic loading after progressive facetectomies.[1] They concluded that greater than 50% resection of each facet joint at the same level leads to unacceptable segmental instability. In addition to injury to the facet joint, resection of the pars or radical disruption of the intervertebral disc may also result in iatrogenic instability. Radical disc excision involves removal of as much of the disc material and end-plates as possible. This degree of removal destabilizes the anterior column and may lead to iatrogenic spondylolisthesis, especially in the presence of a posterior laminectomy.

Spinal Stenosis

Arthrodesis is rarely indicated in the management of spinal stenosis. Two meta-analyses have examined the surgical management of spinal stenosis.[56] These reviews suggest that decompression without arthrodesis is the safest procedure and provides better results in elderly patients and in patients with fewer than eight years of clinical history. These studies also suggest that decompression combined with instrumented fusion may provide some benefit to patients with degenerative spondylolisthesis or to those with more than 15 years of symptoms. However, these reviews were based mainly on uncontrolled, retrospective case series that reported widely varying results and thus do not permit firm conclusions. In general, we do not recommend arthrodesis in the treatment of spinal stenosis unless adequate decompression is likely to create iatrogenic instability.

Degenerative Spondylolisthesis

After more than 80 years, the role of a lumbar fusion in the management of degenerative spondylolisthesis continues to be debated. Wide variations in surgical technique, outcome measures, and indications have precluded any clear answers. With reported satisfactory clinical outcomes ranging from 16% to 95%, attempts at meta-analysis do not provide reliable conclusions.[17] Randomized controlled trials of fusion with instrumentation have appeared only in the past six years, and the results have yet to be thoroughly collated and evaluated.

At least one prospective randomized study by Fischgrund and associates reported no significant differences in clinical outcome when comparing spinal fusions for degenerative spondylolisthesis either with or without spinal instrumentation.[21] Similarly, a meta-analysis of published case series of degenerative spondylolisthesis suggested that fusion with pedicle screws produced a higher fusion rate (93% vs. 86%) than fusion without instrumentation, although the difference was not statistically significant and produced no difference in clinical outcomes (86% vs. 90%).[46] Three trials considered whether some form of posterolateral fusion, with or without instrumentation, was a useful adjunct to decompression alone.[10] These trials provided data on a total of 139 patients with 99% follow-up at two to three years. Meta-analysis showed no difference in outcomes between fusion of any type and laminectomy (OR, 0.80; 95% CI, 0.31, 2.10) as rated by the surgeon at 18 to 24 months.

In contrast, a prospective trial comparing decompressive laminectomy with intertransverse arthrodesis in 50 patients with spinal stenosis and degenerative spondylolisthesis demonstrated that patients who underwent arthrodesis had a statistically significantly better outcome with respect to relief of pain in the back and lower limbs when compared to patients who did not undergo fusion (96% vs. 44%).[25] Spondylolisthesis progressed in 96% of patients who were not fused as opposed to 28% in the fused group. Interestingly, pseudoarthrosis occurred in 36% of the 25 fused patients, although this had no impact on clinical outcome. Similarly, Bolesta and Bohlman compared the results of 24 patients who underwent decompression and 18 patients who underwent decompression and fusion for degenerative spondylolisthesis.[7] Good to excellent results were 100% in 24 patients with fusion compared with 50% in 18 patients without fusion.

Zdeblick reported on a prospective study of 124 patients who underwent lumbar fusion for degenerative disorders.[74] Patients were prospectively randomized into the following three groups: Group I, posterolateral fusion without instrumentation; Group II, posterolateral fusion with semirigid instrumentation; and Group III, posterolateral fusion with rigid pedicle screw instrumentation. The overall fusion rate (for the patients with degenerative spondylolisthesis) was 86% in patients with rigid instrumentation and 65% in patients with noninstrumented fusion. The group that had rigid instrumentation had 95% good to excellent results compared with 71% good to excellent results in the group that had noninstrumented fusion. The rate of revision surgery was 8% in the group that had noninstrumented fusion and 0% in the group that had instrumented fusion. The author recommended the use of rigid pedicle screw fixation in patients undergoing fusion for degenerative spondylolisthesis.

Bridwell and associates analyzed the role of fusion and instrumentation in patients with degenerative spondylolisthesis and spinal stenosis.[8] Forty-four patients with the above diagnosis were prospectively divided into the following three groups: no fusion, fusion without instrumentation, and posterolateral fusion with instrumentation. The group that had instrumentation experienced a statistically significantly higher fusion rate and lesser progression of spondylolisthesis than the other two groups. The authors recommended instrumentation and fusion in patients who undergo decompression for stenosis associated with degenerative spondylolisthesis.

Although definitive proof for the role of fusion in degenerative spondylolisthesis has yet to be provided, the preponderance of studies currently favors improved outcomes following fusion. Our practice has been to recommend instrumented short segment arthrodesis in the majority of patients with degenerative spondylolisthesis who are refractory to conservative measures. We avoid surgery in patients who are elderly, patients who are totally disabled, or patients with a complete collapse of the L4/5 disc space with osteophyte formation.

Scoliosis

Curve progression or lateral listhesis in degenerative lumbar scoliosis may imply relative instability, which may worsen after a posterior decompression. Excessive segmental or junctional kyphosis may also be an indicator of segmental instability at that motion segment. In scoliosis, curve progression in the sagittal plane and coronal imbalance may cause unrelenting back and leg pain. In evaluating patients with degenerative scoliosis for fusion, the following six factors should be considered as relative indications:

1. Curve flexibility, that is, curve does not correct with side-bending.
2. Curve progression, which carries an increased likelihood of continued or accelerated progression after decompression.
3. Radiculopathy within the concavity of the curve may be resistant to partial facetectomy alone and may require the use of instrumentation with distraction and neutralization to unload the compression on the nerve root.
4. Loss of lumbar lordosis, which places the patient in sagittal imbalance and kyphosis and may increase back pain.
5. Lateral listhesis with side-bending hypermobility.
6. Extent of decompression, a radical discectomy or excessive resection of the facet joints or the pars may lead to iatrogenic instability.

Decompression may result in an increase in rotatory and sagittal plane deformity. In general, if a patient has a more pronounced deformity (e.g., greater than 30°) with any degree of lateral translation, a fusion should be performed.

Degenerative Disc Disease

The role of fusion for low back pain is most controversial in the setting of degenerative disc disease. It is agreed by most authors that a degenerated disc can be a source of chronic, disabling low back pain.[14,23] The intervertebral disc is innervated by the (sinuvertebral) nerve, which supplies the posterior longitudinal ligament and the outer layers of the annulus fibrosus.[5,13,19,73] The end-plates and underlying cancellous bone have an increased density of sensory nerves and neuropeptides in patients who have degenerative disc disease.[28,73] Clinically, tissue stimulation experiments during lumbar spine procedures in awake patients suggest that direct stimulation of muscle and ligamentous tissue does not produce typical low back pain.[32,39,53,57,63,66,70] Instead, the outer layer of the annulus fibrosus has most often been implicated as the tissue causing axial low back pain.[53] Stimulation of the central and lateral portions of the annulus fibrosus also produced typical symptoms in more than two thirds of patients. The findings for the posterior longitudinal ligament were similar to those for the annulus fibrosus. The vertebral end-plate was sensitive to stimulation in 61% of patients, and the facet-joint capsule was sensitive in 30%. Pain in the buttocks could be reproduced by simultaneous stimulation of the annulus fibrosus and the nerve root. Indirect evidence of a discogenic source of pain is supported by reports that continuing pain after successful posterior lumbar spinal arthrodesis can be relieved by excision of the disc and interbody arthrodesis.[6] We believe, however, that these phenomena may also be explained by the greater biomechanical stiffness of the interbody graft as compared to a posterior fusion.

Although a degenerative disc may be a source of low back pain, identifying a patient in whom discogenic pain is the principal source of disability remains challenging. In most instances, imaging characteristics consistent with a degenerative disc are not associated with discogenic pain.[15] Boden and associates studied the findings on magnetic resonance imaging in 67 asymptomatic patients and found abnormalities in approximately one third.[4]

In order to correlate imaging characteristics of a degenerative disc with the clinical syndrome of discogenic pain, provocative discography is often used. It is unclear how injection of the disc provokes pain, although various theories have been postulated. One such theory is that stimulation of nociceptive fibers in the innervated part of the annulus fibrosus[29,72] or the vertebral end-plate or body[9,31] causes pain as the injection increases intradiscal pressure. Another theory is that injection leads to chemical stimulation that produces pain.[67]

Since its introduction by Hirsch in 1948, provocative discography has undergone continuous attack.[39] Even today, most opponents of discography often cite a study reported in 1968 by Holt.[33] He found a 37% rate of false positive results with regard to an association between the production of symptoms and abnormal morphological characteristics of the disc in 30 asymptomatic inmates at a correctional institution. Some studies have also reported poor outcomes of patients who underwent arthrodesis on the basis of discography.[68] As with most studies on discography, a number of critical flaws hinder their interpretation. As a retrospective study, it is uncertain whether the result from discography was the critical factor in the decision for fusion, thereby opening up the study to significant selection bias. Furthermore, the number of levels of fusion was not limited to the levels found to be positive on discography.

Numerous studies also support the use of discography. Simmons and associates re-analyzed Holt's data

and concluded that Holt's study "should no longer be used as scientific or authoritative evidence against the use of discography."[62] Major flaws that they identified included use of a study whose reliability may be questionable, the high rate of failure of needle placement, and use of a contrast agent that is a neuro irritant. Colhoun and associates reviewed the outcomes for 137 patients with low back pain who had undergone spinal arthrodesis at levels for which discography demonstrated abnormal morphological characteristics and produced symptoms.[12] At a mean of 3.6 years, 121 patients (88%) had a successful result compared with only 13 (52%) of 25 who had arthrodesis without reproduction of the typical symptom. Simmons and Segil found discography to be accurate for the localization and planning of arthrodesis of symptomatic levels in 89% of 272 patients who had discogenic disease of the spine.[61]

The authors agree with the North American Spine Society Diagnostic and Therapeutic Committee that the use of lumbar discography is supported by recent literature in select circumstances. Patients with intractable axial pain with disc space narrowing, and end-plate sclerosis, and who are otherwise excellent candidates for fusion, may benefit from discography to confirm the diagnosis. We have found that discography is most valuable for its negative predictive value and thereby identifies patients who should not undergo operative procedures. Patients with multiple levels of typical pain raise our concern about the ability of a fusion to relieve them from disability. Multi-level fusion for discogenic low back pain has a high failure rate, and the inability to limit the level of a fusion bodes poorly. Analogously, patients with even classic findings of degenerative disc disease on MRI with a negative discogram are strongly reconsidered prior to surgical intervention. The discogram is similar to a physical exam, and its validity is often based on the experience and skill of the operator. All discograms should be performed with negative blinded controls. Needle placement should be rapid and cause only a brief moment of discomfort. An injection into a morphologically normal disc should be nearly pain free.

Facet Syndrome

The role of the facet joint in the generation of low back pain is discussed elsewhere in this book. As with degenerative disc disease, few outcome studies have examined the role of surgery for the treatment of low back pain from a facet source. The natural history is unknown, and as with degenerative disc disease, identifying suitable candidates for lumbar fusion is uncertain.

Degeneration of facet joints as a cause of low back pain was first postulated in 1933 and remains controversial. As with degenerative disc disease, anatomical studies strongly favor the facet joints as a source of low back pain. Nociceptive nerve fibers have been identified in facet-joint capsules, and in synovial and pericapsular tissue.[11,27,49] Biomechanically, it is hypothesized that hypermobility and instability of the motion segments lead to overstress of the facet joint capsule resulting in changes that ultimately produce pain.

In the facet syndrome, pain worsens with extension and diminishes with flexion. Pain may radiate posterolaterally into lateral buttock and may occasionally radiate into the upper thigh. Pain radiating below the knee and neurologic findings are not expected. History of pain with movement and palpable tenderness over a joint has been suggested by some. Others have suggested that pain provocation by coughing, sneezing, or Valsalva can occur with facet pain. Radiological findings can also be nonspecific. Hypertrophied facet joints, accompanying disc space narrowing and subtle signs of long-standing hypermobility such as osteophytes may be found (Figure 2-5). A radionuclide scan may also be helpful for diagnosis.

The orthopaedic literature contains a number of studies addressing the use of facet blocks.[41,47,50,51,54,60,67] Most studies have been unable to correlate physical and historical findings with relief from a facet block. As a therapeutic modality, facet joint injections have met with disappointing results.[11] The use of a facet block to select patients for lumbar fusion has been incompletely evaluated. In a recent small, prospective study, 28 of 91 patients with chronic low back pain who had at least 70% relief of symptoms after facet blocks were subsequently managed with a posterolat-

eral spinal arthrodesis.[42] The symptoms resolved in more than two thirds of the patients postoperatively. However, other retrospective studies have not confirmed the predictive value of facet blocks for the success of lumbar arthrodesis.[17,34]

In the authors' experience, facet blocks have been useful both as a therapeutic and a diagnostic tool. We consider facet blocks as a part of the conservative regimen. In patients free of other potential etiologies for low back pain, dramatic relief following a low volume facet injection provides a strong basis for lumbar fusion. As facet arthropathy frequently accompanies degenerative disc disease, work-up should include a discogram to rule out accompanying discogenic pain. In the circumstance of concurrent disease, a posterior interbody fusion along with posterior segmental fixation can be combined with a facetectomy and possibly an adjuvant intertransverse fusion.

Pseudoarthrosis

Nonunion following lumbar fusions is not uncommon. For in situ single level arthrodesis, a 10% to 15% nonunion rate is acceptable. The pseudarthrosis rate may approach 30% to 40% for three level arthrodesis. As nonunion does not always create symptoms, its presence should be suspected as the etiology for intractable back pain in a patient in whom surgery was initially successful followed by a gradual worsening. Radiographically, lucency and movement at the fusion site generally alert one to pseudoarthrosis in most patients (Figure 2-6). However, in other patients, multiplanar computed tomography, bone scans, and even operative exploration can be the only way of confirming the presence of pseudoarthrosis. As patient selection for the surgical management of pseudoarthrosis can be challenging, the same algorithm of nonopera-

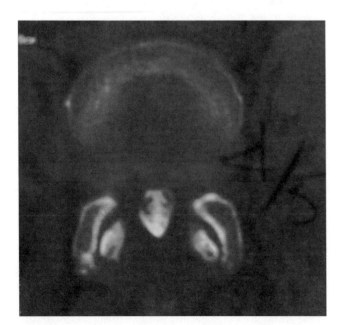

FIGURE 2-5 ■ Axial CT of the lumbar spine demonstrates marked degenerative changes of the facets.

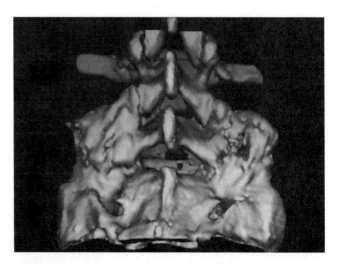

FIGURE 2-6 ■ CT reconstruction demonstrates pseudoarthrosis in the fusion mass on the right.

tive management, including aggressive physical therapy and judicious pharmacological management, should be exhausted prior to considering arthrodesis. In cases of doubt, diagnostic injection of the pseudo-joint may be helpful.

CONCLUSION

Patient heterogeneity and the lack of appropriate outcome studies make patient selection for lumbar arthrodesis a complicated task that requires consideration of a broad range of details. Factors that affect fusion success, such as comorbidities, tobacco abuse, psychosocial factors, and pre-existing narcotic use, can generally be optimized during a course of conservative management rather than used as a justification to refuse consideration for fusion procedures. In cases of degenerative spondylolisthesis, iatrogenic instability, and scoliosis, where the literature for lumbar fusion is clearer, a less stringent approach to patient selection is warranted. Patients with presumed discogenic pain from degenerative disc disease or facet arthropathy will generally require a longer period of conservative management in addition to ancillary tests to verify their likelihood of benefiting from lumbar fusion.

REFERENCES

1. Abumi K, Panjabi MM, Kramer KM, et al: Biomechanical evaluation of lumbar spinal stability after graded facetectomies. **Spine** 15:1142-7.
2. Axelsson P, Johnsson R, Stromqvist B: Lumbar orthosis with unilateral hip immobilization. Effect on intervertebral mobility determined by roentgen stereophotogrammetric analysis. **Spine** 18:876-79, 1993.
3. Axelsson P, Johnsson R, Stromqvist B: Effect of lumbar orthosis on intervertebral mobility. A roentgen stereophotogrammetric analysis. **Spine** 17:678-81, 1992.
4. Boden SD, Davis DO, Dina TS, et al: Abnormal magnetic-resonance scans of the lumbar spine in asymptomatic subjects. A prospective investigation. **J Bone Joint Surg** 72-A:403-8, March 1990.
5. Bogduk N: The innervation of the lumbar spine. **Spine** 8:286-93, 1983.
6. Bogduk N, Tynan W, Wilson AS: The nerve supply to the human lumbar intervertebral discs. **J Anat** 132:39-56, 1981.
7. Bolesta MJ, Bohlman HH: Degenerative spondylolisthesis. [Instructional Course Lectures.] 38:157-65, 1989.
8. Bridwell KH, Sedgewick TA, O'Brien MF, et al: The role of fusion and instrumentation in the treatment of degenerative spondylolisthesis with spinal stenosis. **J Spinal Disord** 6:461-72, 1993.
9. Brinckmann P, Horst M: The influence of vertebral body fracture, intradiscal injection, and partial discectomy on the radial bulge and height of human lumbar discs. **Spine** 10:138-45, 1985.
10. Brown MF, Hukkanen MVJ, McCarthy ID, et al: Sensory and sympathetic innervation of the vertebral endplate in patients with degenerative disc disease. **J Bone Joint Surg** 79-B(1):147-53, 1997.
11. Carette S, Marcoux S, Truchon R, et al: A controlled trial of corticosteroid injections into facet joints for chronic low back pain. **New Engl J Med** 325:1002-7, 1991.
12. Colhoun E, McCall IW, Williams L, et al: Provocation discography as a guide to planning operations on the spine. **J Bone Joint Surg** 70-B(2):267-71, 1988.
13. Coppes MH, Marani E, Thomeer RT, et al: Innervation of "painful" lumbar discs. **Spine** 22:2342-9, 1997.
14. Crock HV: Internal disc disruption. A challenge to disc prolapse fifty years on. **Spine** 11:650-53, 1986.
15. Deyo RA, Cherkin D, Conrad D, et al: Cost, controversy, crisis: low back pain and the health of the public. **Ann Rev Pub Health** 12:141-56, 1991.
16. Donelson R, Aprill C, Medcalf R, et al: A prospective study of centralization of lumbar and referred pain. A predictor of symptomatic discs and anular competence. **Spine** 22:1115-22, 1997.
17. Esses SI, Moro JK: The value of facet joint blocks in patient selection for lumbar fusion. **Spine** 18:185-90, 1993.
18. Faas A, Chavannes AW, van Eijk JT, et al: A randomized, placebo-controlled trial of exercise therapy in patients with acute low back pain. **Spine** 18:1388-95, 1993.
19. Falconer MA, McGeorge M, Begg AC: Observations on the cause and mechanism of symptom-production in sciatica and low-back pain. **J Neurol Neurosurg Psychiat** 11:13-26, 1948.
20. Fidler MW, Plasmans CMT: The effect of four types of support on the segmental mobility of the lumbosacral spine. **J Bone Joint Surg** 65-A:943-47, Sept. 1983.
21. Fischgrund JS, Mackay M, Herkowitz HN, et al: Degenerative lumbar spondylolisthesis with spinal stenosis: a prospective, randomized study comparing decompressive laminectomy and arthrodesis with and without spinal instrumentation. **Spine** 22(24):2807-12, Dec 15, 1997.
22. Fordyce WE, Brockway JA, Bergman JA, et al: Acute back pain: a control-group comparison of behavioral vs. traditional management methods. **J Behav Med** 9:127-40, 1986.
23. Fraser RD: Interbody, Posterior, and combined lumbar fusions. **Spine** 20(Supp 24):S167-77, 1995.
24. Frymoyer JW: Back pain and sciatica. **New Engl J Med** 318:291, 1988.
25. Ghormley RK: Low back pain. With special reference to the articular facets, with presentation of an operative procedure. **JAMA** 101:1773-7, 1933.
26. Gilbert JR, Taylor DW, Hildebrand A, et al: Clinical trial of common treatments for low back pain in family practice. **Br Med J** 291:791-94, 1985.
27. Giles LG, Harvey AR: Immunohistochemical demonstration of nociceptors in the capsule and synovial folds of human zygapophyseal joints. **Brit J Rheumatol** 26:362-64, 1987.
28. Grob D, Humke T, Dvorak J: Degenerative lumbar spinal stenosis: Decompression with and without arthrodesis. **J Bone Joint Surg** [Am] 77:1036-41, 1995.

29. Gunzburg R, Parkinson R, Moore R, et al: A cadaveric study comparing discography, magnetic resonance imaging, histology, and mechanical behavior of the human lumbar disc. **Spine** 17:417-26, 1992.

30. Hazard RG, Fenwick JW, Kalisch SM, et al: Functional restoration with behavioral support. A one-year prospective study of patients with chronic low-back pain. **Spine** 14:157-61, 1989.

31. Heggeness MH, Doherty BJ: Discography causes end plate deflection. **Spine** 18:1050-3, 1993.

32. Hirsch C: An attempt to diagnose the level of a disc lesion clinically by disc puncture. **Acta Orthop Scandinavica** 18:132-40, 1948.

33. Holt EP, Jr: The question of lumbar discography. **J Bone Joint Surg** 50-A:720-26, June 1968.

34. Jackson RP: The facet syndrome. Myth or reality? **Clin Orthop** 279:110-21, 1992

35. Kaplan DM, Knapp M, Romm FJ, et al: Low back pain and x-ray films of the lumbar spine: a prospective study in primary care. **South Med J** 79:811-14, 1986.

36. Katz JN, Lipson SJ, Lew RA, et al: Lumbar laminectomy alone or with instrumented or noninstrumented arthrodesis in degenerative lumbar spinal stenosis: patient selection, costs, and surgical outcomes. **Spine** 22:1123-31, 1997.

37. Kirkaldy-Willis WH, Farfan HF: Instability of the lumbar spine. **Clin Orthop** 165:110, 1982.

38. Kostuik JP, Harrington I, Alexander D, et al: Cauda equina syndrome and lumbar disc herniation. **J Bone Joint Surg** 68-A:386-91, March 1986.

39. Kuslich SD, Ulstrom CL, Michael CJ: The tissue origin of low back pain and sciatica: a report of pain response to tissue stimulation during operations on the lumbar spine using local anesthesia. **Orthop Clin NA** 22:181-87, 1991.

40. Lethem J, Slade PD, Troup JD, et al: Outline of a fear-avoidance model of exaggerated pain perception - I. **Behav Res Ther** 21:401-08, 1983.

41. Lilius G, Harilainen A, Laasonen EM, et al: Chronic unilateral low-back pain. Predictors of outcome of facet joint injections. **Spine** 15:780-82, 1990.

42. Lovely TJ, Rastogi P: The value of provocative facet blocking as a predictor of success in lumbar spine fusion. **J Spinal Disord** 10:512-17, 1997.

43. Macnab I: The traction spur. An indicator of segmental instability. **J Bone Joint Surg** 53-A:663-70, June 1971.

44. Main CJ: The modified somatic perception questionnaire (MSPQ). **J Psychosom Res** 27:503-14, 1983.

45. Main CJ, Wood PLR, Hollis S, et al: The distress and risk assessment method: a simple patient classification to identify distress and evaluate the risk of poor outcome. **Spine** 17:42-52, 1992.

46. Mardjetko SM, Connolly PJ, Shott S: Degenerative lumbar spondylosis: a meta-analysis of literature 1970–1993. **Spine**; 20(Supp l):S2256-65, 1994.

47. Marks RC, Houston T, Thulbourne T: Facet joint injection and facet nerve block: a randomized comparison in 86 patients with chronic low back pain. **Pain** 49:325-28, 1992.

48. McKenzie RA: Prophylaxis in recurrent low back pain. **N Z Med J** 89:22-23, 1979.

49. McLain RF: Mechanoreceptor endings in human cervical facet joints. **Spine** 19:495-501, 1994.

50. Mooney V, Robertson J: The facet syndrome. **Clin Orthop** 115:149-56, 1976.

51. Moran R, O'Connell D, Walsh MG: The diagnostic value of facet joint injections. **Spine** 13:1407-10, 1988.

52. Mossey JM, Shapiro E: Self-rated health: a predictor of mortality among the elderly. **Am J Public Health** 72:800-8, 1982.

53. Murphey F: Chapter 1. Experience with lumbar disc surgery. **Clin Neurosurg** 20:1-8, 1973.

54. Murtagh FR: Computed tomography and fluoroscopy guided anesthesia and steroid injection in facet syndrome. **Spine** 13:686-89, 1988.

55. Nasca RJ: Rationale for spinal fusion in lumbar spinal stenosis. **Spine** 14:451-54, 1989.

56. Niggemeyer O, Strauss JM, Schulitz KP: Comparison of surgical procedures for degenerative lumbar spinal stenosis: A meta-analysis of the literature from 1975 to 1995. **Eur Spine J** 6:423-29, 1997.

57. Norton PL, Brown T: The immobilizing efficiency of back braces. Their effect on the posture and motion of the lumbosacral spine. **J Bone Joint Surg** 39-A:111-38, Jan. 1957.

58. Polatin PB, Gatchel RJ: Point of view. **Spine** 22:2252-3, 1997.

59. Quebec Task Force on Spinal Disorders: Scientific approach to the assessment and management of activity-related spinal disorders. A monograph for clinicians. Report of the Quebec Task Force on Spinal Disorders. **Spine** 12(Supp 7), 1987.

60. Raymond J, Dumas JM: Intraarticular facet block: diagnostic test or therapeutic procedure? **Radiology** 151:333-36, 1984.

61. Simmons EH, Segil CM: An evaluation of discography in the localization of symptomatic levels in discogenic disease of the spine. **Clin Orthop** 108:57-69, 1975.

62. Simmons JW, Aprill CN, Dwyer AP, et al: A reassessment of Holt's data on: "the question of lumbar discography." **Clin Orthop** 237:120-24, 1988.

63. Spurling RG, Grantham EG: Neurologic picture of herniations of the nucleus pulposus in the lower part of the lumbar region. **Arch Surg** 40:375-88, 1940.

64. van Tulder MW, Koes BW, Bouter LM: Conservative treatment of acute and chronic nonspecific low back pain. A systematic review of randomized controlled trials of the most common interventions. **Spine** 22:2128-56, 1997.

65. Waddell G, Bircher M, Finlayson D, et al: Symptoms and signs: physical disease or illness behavior? **Br Med J** 289:739-741, 1984.

66. Weatherley CR, Prickett CF, O'Brien JP: Discogenic pain persisting despite solid posterior fusion. **J Bone Joint Surg** 68-B(1):142-43, 1986.

67. Weinstein J, Claverie W, Gibson S: The pain of discography. **Spine** 13:1344-8, 1988.

68. Wetzel FT, LaRocca SH, Lowery GL, et al: The treatment of lumbar spinal pain syndromes diagnosed by discography. Lumbar arthrodesis. **Spine** 19:792-800, 1994.

69. White AA, Panjabi MM: **Clinical biomechanics of the spine.** 2nd. Edition. Philadelphia: J.B. Lippincott Co., 1990.

70. Wiberg G: Back pain in relation to the nerve supply of the intervertebral disc. **Acta Orthop Scandinavica** 19:211-21, 1950.
71. Wiesel SW, Cuckler JM, Deluca F, et al: Acute low-back pain. An objective analysis of conservative therapy. **Spine** 5:324-30, 1980.
72. Wiley JJ, Macnab I, Wortzman G: Lumbar discography and its clinical applications. **Can J Surg** 11:280-89, 1968.
73. Yoshizawa H, O'Brien JP, Smith WT, et al: The neuropathology of intervertebral discs removed for low-back pain. **J Pathol** 132:95-104, 1980.
74. Zdeblick TA: A prospective, randomized study of lumbar fusion. Preliminary results. **Spine** 18:983-91, 1993.
75. Zung WWK: A self-rating depression scale. **Arch Gen Psychiat** 12:63-70, 1965.

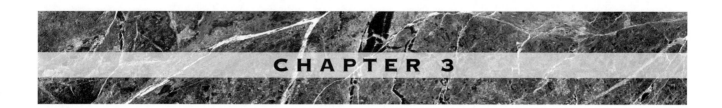

CHAPTER 3

Magnetic Resonance Imaging in Low Back Pain

Victor Haughton, M.D.

INTRODUCTION

Low back pain presently ranks among the most significant of public health problems. The incidence of back pain is 70% to 85% and the annual prevalence of back pain ranges from 15% to 45%. Surgical procedures for back pain continue to increase in frequency. From 1979 to 1987, U.S. rates of back surgery increased 49% to 55%, whereas the rate of nonsurgical hospitalization decreased 33%. Surgical fusions increased 100% from 1979 to 1990. Marked geographic variation has been reported in the rate of back surgery.

Clinical experience has suggested that lesions in the intervertebral disc far out-number all other causes of low back and sciatic pain, but the relationship of disc degeneration to back pain is not well understood. Intervertebral disc degeneration is common in patients with back pain and is also present in subjects who are asymptomatic. Tears in the annulus fibrosus of the intervertebral disc in symptomatic subjects are blamed for many cases of low back and sciatic pain, yet a radial tear of the annulus fibrosus occurs in 14% of asymptomatic individuals.[16]

Both magnetic resonance imaging (MRI) and computerized tomography (CT) provide diagnostically useful images of the spine noninvasively and without risk as long as selection criteria are followed. For CT, a small ionizing radiation dose is delivered, comparable to that of one or of several plain radiographs. Iodinated contrast media, used infrequently in CT examinations of the spine, may result in severe and life-threatening reactions in 0.01 % of patients after intravenous administration. MRI, safe in most patients, is possibly dangerous or contraindicated in patients with cardiac pacemakers, implanted wires, or ferromagnetic objects. Claustrophobic patients may not be able to undergo MRI without sedation. The intravenous contrast medium used for MRI does not have serious side effects or complications, but some caution is advised in administering it to patients with asthma.

The purpose of this chapter is to review the imaging of degenerative changes in the spine. Selection of patients for imaging studies is addressed. Since the disc is considered to be a major source of pain in patients with back pain, the anatomy of the disc, its age-related changes and its degenerative changes are reviewed. The spinal facet joints may also produce pain either in the back or radiating in the distribution of a spinal nerve. The anatomy of the facet joint and the degenerative and inflammatory processes that affect it will be reviewed.

SELECTION OF PATIENTS FOR IMAGING

In most cases of acute back pain, MRI and CT are not indicated. Exceptions in which emergency CT or MRI may be indicated include spinal trauma, infection, suspected tumor, cauda equina syndrome, and unexplained progressive neurological deterioration.

In back pain persisting more than six weeks, MRI and CT may be used to confirm findings in the history and physical examination. They are used appropriately to select between surgical and other treatment options but are inappropriately used as screening examinations. Imaging detects abnormalities in the spine effectively but fails to distinguish between symptomatic and incidental changes. Because of the high frequency of asymptomatic degenerative changes in the spine, inappropriate imaging may lead to unnecessary costs for the patient and to incorrect diagnoses based on incidental degenerative changes that are confused with significant lesions by the physicians.

MRI is useful in patients with chronic radiculopathy. With its capability to produce images in multiple planes, MRI effectively demonstrates the relationship of a nerve root, facet joint degenerative changes, or a herniated disc. The sagittal images are especially useful in some cases, such as spondylolisthesis, which may distort the anatomy of the neural foramen severely. CT, which demonstrates osseous anatomy effectively, is useful for imaging the vertebral body, facet joint, pedicle, and bony spurs. In cases in which intradiscal therapy is considered, MRI may be used to distinguish whether the disc herniation is sequestered, contained, or subligamentous. MRI may distinguish disc fragments that are contiguous with the disc from those that are not.

In myelopathy, MRI is indicated to distinguish intrinsic processes within the cord from processes that compress the spinal cord or cauda equina. MRI shows the relationship of the spinal cord and spinal nerve roots in the cauda equina and in the neural foramina to the spinal canal. The myelogram may provide additional information in selected cases because it demonstrates the relative degree of obstruction to the flow of contrast medium through a narrowed region of spine. The demonstration that cerebrospinal flow is impeded or blocked may be helpful in determining the severity of spinal stenosis.

In patients with suspected spinal instability or internal disc disruption, MRI may correctly predict the symptomatic level. MRI in these patients detects facet joint or disc degeneration, which may not produce nerve root compression. The demonstration of some degenerative changes, such as a radial tear of the annulus fibrosus, has a highly predictive value for a positive discogram at that level. In discs with a radial tear of the annulus fibrosus, MRI demonstrates diminished signal intensity from the fibrocartilagenous portion of the disc.[38] In these discs, MRI may also show bulging of the annulus fibrosus.[39] A curvilinear high signal intensity zone (HIZ) in the peripheral, normally low-signal annulus fibrosus is a reliable sign of a radial tear, but it is not found in all cases of a radial tear (Figure 3-1).[3] When intravenous contrast media are administered, MRI may show abnormal contrast enhancement in the radial tear in the annulus fibrosus.[29]

The capability of MRI to determine the symptomatic level in patients with back pain has been evaluated by comparing MRI and discography findings. In general, MRI findings have correlated well with disco-

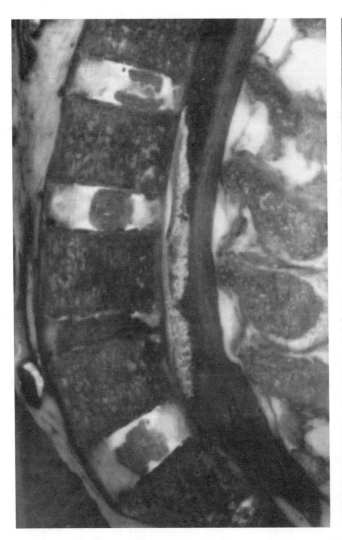 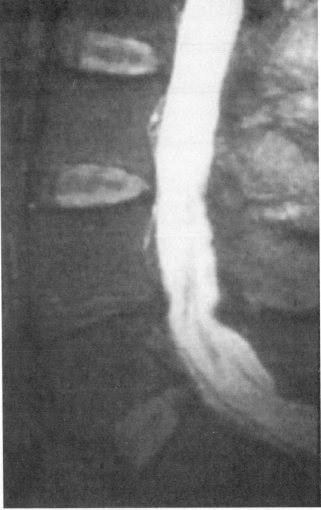

FIGURE 3-1 ■ Radial tear of the L4-L5 disc, anatomical *(left)* and MRI sections *(right)*.

graphic findings.[7] In a patient meeting certain clinical criteria, if an HIZ is present, it is highly likely that the patient has a painful disc.[3] Loss of signal in the disc correlates highly with positive discogram.[26, 37] In a patient with back pain and MRI evidence of a degenerated disc, some investigators suggest that it can be assumed that the abnormal disc on MRI is the source of pain.[14] According to one study, discography may be obviated in a patient with discogenic pain and torn outer annulus on T2-weighted MRI.[14] MRI is not considered by other investigators to be effective in determining the symptomatic disc.[8]

MRI TECHNIQUES

To minimize artifact and maximize spatial and contrast resolution in spine imaging, specialized MRI techniques are required. Localized or surface coils are used in place of the conventional body coils to improve the signal from the spine tissues. The coil's sensitive volume can be matched to the structures to be imaged, improving the resolution in the region of interest by eliminating the signal from tissues anterior and lateral to the spine, maximizing the image quality. Technical parameters such as short repetition time (TR), short echo time (TE), field of view, matrix, and number of excitation are cho-

sen to achieve optimal spatial and contrast resolution. Cardiac gating may be used to minimize the artifacts from pulsations in the cerebrospinal fluid.

Multiple planes are required for imaging the spine. Sagittal images are acquired, usually with T1- and T2-weighting and with 3 to 5 mm slice thickness. Axial images are acquired, preferably with the plane of sectioning parallel to the adjacent vertebral end-plate to minimize geometric distortion. Three dimensional volume acquisitions can be obtained to permit reconstruction in any selected plane or presentation as a pseudo-3D image.

Standard Sequences

T1- and T2-weighted images and, in some cases, other sequences are acquired for spine imaging. Images obtained with TR and TE provide T1-weighting and high signal-to-noise ratio (SNR). These images are characterized by high signal intensity from lipid-containing tissues such as epidural fat and bone marrow, intermediate signal intensity from the spinal cord, low signal intensity from cerebrospinal fluid, and no signal from cortical bone (Figure 3-2). These images demonstrate the vertebrae, neural foramina, facet joints and epidural space effectively. T1-weighted images also

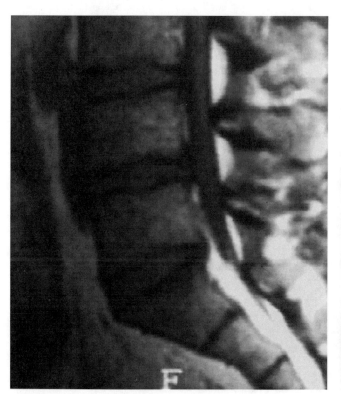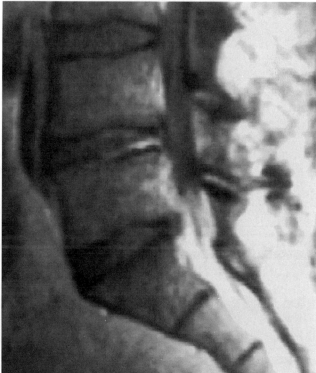

FIGURE 3-2 ■ T1-weighted image before *(left)* and after *(right)* the administration of intravenous contrast medium. In T1-weighted images, note the high signal intensity from epidural fat, the low signal intensity from cerebrospinal fluid, and the intermediate signal intensity of the intervertebral discs and medullary bone. Cortical bone has a very low signal intensity. After contrast medium, enhancement is noted in the intervertebral disc, indicating the presence of a radial tear.

effectively demonstrate herniations of the intervertebral disc that distort the epidural fat and facet joint
degeneration that causes bony sclerosis and foramenal
narrowing. T2-weighted images, acquired with a long
TR and a long TE, display high signal intensity from
cerebrospinal fluid and from intramedullary lesions,
intermediate signal intensity from the spinal cord, and
low signal intensity from bone and fat (Figure 3-3).
With a longer TR and TE, the images take longer to
acquire and have lower SNR. T2-weighted images are
especially useful for demonstrating intramedullary
lesions, such as demyelination, edema, and tumor
infiltration, because of the high signal intensity of
these processes. Because of the high signal intensity of
cerebrospinal fluid (CSF), these images are useful for
detecting narrowed subarachnoid spaces resulting

from degenerative changes or neoplastic processes.
T2-weighted images demonstrate high signal intensity
from normal intervertebral discs and diminished signal intensity from degenerating discs, which have less
glycosaminoglycans and water. They also detect the
HIZ in the annulus fibrosus, which may not be evident
in T1-weighted images. A fast spin echo (FSE) technique is used now to acquire T2-weighted images
because it shortens the acquisition time compared to
the conventional spin echo (SE). FSE T2-weighted
images may have less edge sharpness and less signal
intensity from the intervertebral disc. They also produce a higher signal intensity from fat compared to
conventional SE. A technique to reduce the signal
intensity of fat (fat saturation) may be used in conjunction with FSE.

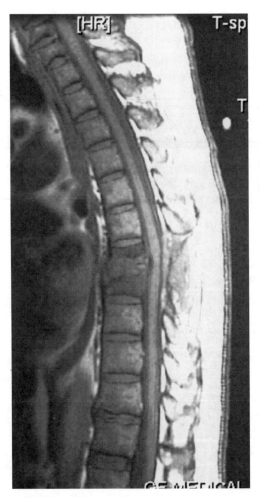
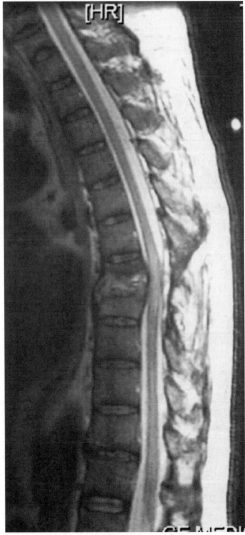

FIGURE 3-3 ■ T1 *(left)* and T2 *(right)* weighted images in a patient with discitis. In
the T2-weighted images, note the high signal intensity from the cerebrospinal fluid, from
the edematous region in the spinal cord, and from the intervertebral discs. Bone marrow
has a low signal intensity.

Contrast Media

Paramagnetic contrast media are used in MRI to increase the signal intensity in T1-weighted images of some structures. Tissues that have a blood supply, a fenestrated capillary endothelium, and an extravascular space demonstrate an increase in signal intensity in T1-weighted images acquired after the administration of intravenous paramagnetic contrast media. Within the central nervous system, normally protected by tight capillary junctions in the endothelium, enhancement does not occur. With a breakdown of the blood/brain barrier, contrast enhancement may be detected in the brain or spinal cord. Contrast enhancement characterizes most tissues outside of the central nervous system. Therefore, muscle, fat, meninges, marrow, and epidural veins demonstrate contrast enhancement to some degree. The intervertebral disc, lacking a blood supply, enhances little immediately after the injection of the contrast medium. Because contrast media diffuse into the intervertebral disc after intravenous administration, enhancement can be detected in the normal disc if larger amounts of contrast media are administered, and longer delays are used between contrast media administration and acquisition of the image.[15]

Radial tears in the intervertebral disc may demonstrate contrast enhancement. Two weeks after a radial tear is created experimentally in the annulus fibrosus, blood vessels and granulation tissue penetrate the tear.[22] Histological examination of degenerated intervertebral discs showing contrast enhancement and subsequently removed from patients, shows the presence of granulation tissue within the disc.[34] Anatomical sections through degenerating intervertebral discs may demonstrate granulation tissue within the disc (Figure 3-4). Granulation tissue demonstrates more rapid and more marked contrast enhancement than the normal disc.

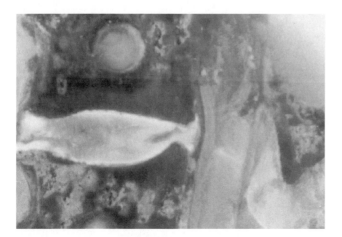

FIGURE 3-4 ■ Anatomical section in sagittal plane through a lumbar intervertebral disc, illustrating granulation tissue in degenerating intervertebral disc.

The contrast enhancement in postcontrast radial tears is detected in a much larger percentage of patients by contrast enhancement than by T2-weighted images.[29]

One of the indications for contrast media is to differentiate recurrent herniated disc and epidural scar. Following surgery, the sources of recurrent or residual leg pain commonly identified by MRI are herniated disc and scar tissue. Other causes of back pain in the postoperative patient are spinal instability, nonunion of a bony fusion, spinal stenosis, discitis, arachnoiditis and psychosocial disorders. MRI distinguishes scar from disc with an accuracy of 90%; CT makes that distinction with less accuracy. In the immediate postoperative period, detection of a recurrent herniated disc is complicated by the presence (in about 70% of cases) of a hematoma or an epidural mass of poorly organized connective tissue resembling a herniated disc in MRIs.[6]

MRIs, after administration of a contrast medium, intravenously demonstrate contrast enhancement in nerve roots that have been damaged or traumatized. When contrast enhancement is identified in a patient with a herniated disc, the enhanced nerve usually correlates with the nerve suspected clinically to be involved.[17] However, prominent radicular veins may simulate nerve root enhancement in some cases. Following laminectomy, nonspecific nerve root enhancement is often seen. The clinical significance of nerve root enhancement is uncertain at this point in time.

Paramagnetic contrast media for intravascular use in MRI include the ionic medium gadopentetate (Magnevist) and the nonionic media gadoteridol (ProHance) and gadodiamide (Omniscan). For most applications, the ionic and the nonionic media are comparable. The ionic and nonionic media produce different results in spine imaging. The ionic medium, because of the charge on the molecule, diffuses slowly into cartilage in the normal intervertebral disc or in herniated disc fragments. In the detection of recurrent herniated disc, therefore, the ionic medium may produce greater contrast between the disc fragment and the adjacent scar. The nonionic medium diffuses more readily into disc cartilage, reducing contrast between recurrent disc fragment and scar. The nonionic media, given in suitable amounts and at a suitable time before the images are acquired, produce detectable enhancement in normal intervertebral discs.[23, 35]

New Imaging Sequences

Inversion recovery techniques, compared to spin echo techniques, provide spine images with reduced signal intensity from fat. Fluid attenuated inversion recovery images (FLAIR), which are used to improve the conspicuousness of intracerebral lesions, may be used in spine imaging. FLAIR uses an inversion pulse to eliminate the signal intensity of cerebrospinal fluid without decreasing the signal intensity of the spinal cord. FLAIR increases the conspicuousness of lesions in the brain near CSF spaces. The technique appears less sensitive to demyelinating lesions when applied to spine imaging than when applied to cerebral imaging. FLAIR sequences, if optimized, have superior contrast at the CSF-cord interface and better conspicuity of lesions of the spinal cord and bone marrow compared to SE sequences for imaging the spine. Short tau inversion recovery (STIR) has been applied to spine imaging without the loss of sensitivity associated with the FLAIR sequence. Compared to SE, FLAIR has more limited anatomical coverage. Three-dimensional magnetization prepared rapid acquisition gradient echo (MP-RAGE) produces the suppression of CSF signal with greater anatomical coverage. Inversion recovery techniques, such as fast stir echo inversion recovery (FSEIR), or Faststir, may be more sensitive to bone marrow disorders than conventional T2-weighted imaging. GR (gradient recalled) images can be used to detect some vascular lesions in the spine. GR, which is affected by ferromagnetic substances in tissue (magnetic susceptibility), has greater sensitivity than spin echo sequence to hemosiderin, ferritin, or deoxyhemoglobin. In suspected cavernous hemangiomas, hematomas, or other lesions containing blood products, GR should be used. It improves the sensitivity of MRI to these lesions. Diffusion-weighted imaging, used most frequently for the diagnosis of stroke, may be useful in spine imaging. It has been reported to be effective in distinguishing pathological fractures from benign compression fractures.[4] In the former, diffusion is restricted so that the signal in the diffusion-weighted images shows a high signal process; in the latter, diffusion is not restricted, so that diffusion-weighted images do not show a high signal intensity. The effects of pulsation in the CSF and susceptibility effects complicate measuring diffusion in the spinal cord. To date, results have not been consistent.

INTERVERTEBRAL DISC

Anatomy

The normal intervertebral disc is a highly complex structure of specialized living connective tissue. The disc is composed of fibrocartilage, hyaline cartilage, and dense collagen tissue. It has anatomical relationships to the anterior longitudinal, posterior longitudinal, and transforamenal ligaments. The composition of the intervertebral disc changes with age.

Disregarding the anterior longitudinal ligament and the osseous and cartilaginous end-plates, the remaining tissue in the intervertebral disc can be divided into the following three parts for the purpose of description: outer annulus fibrosus, inner annulus

fibrosus, and nucleus pulposus. The outer annulus fibrosus has thick lamellae of dense connective tissue. The dense fibers in the outer annulus originate and insert in the bone contained within the adjacent ring apophysis. Each layer has fibers that run parallel at about 60° with respect to the end-plate. Fibers in adjacent layers run in different directions, although they make the same angle with respect to the end-plate. The major chemical constituent of the outer annulus is collagen, and the predominant cell type is the fibroblast. Histologically the outer annulus resembles a tendon such as the Achilles tendon. It contains 10% to 15% type VI collagen, which probably contributes to the stiffness of the intervertebral disc. In T2-weighted MRIs, it has a low signal intensity, like tendons.

The inner annulus contains lamellae that are composed of both collagen and glycosaminoglycans. Like the lamellae in the outer annulus, those in the inner annulus run obliquely. They insert and originate not in bone but in the hyaline cartilage that forms the cartilaginous end-plate. The predominant cell type is the chondrocyte.

The nucleus pulposus is fibrocartilage like the inner annulus but with a less organized fibrous structure. It also contains glycosaminoglycans, collagen, and chondrocytes, like the inner annulus fibrosus. The inner annulus fibrosus and the nucleus pulposus have high signal intensity in T2-weighted images, reflecting the glycosaminoglycans content.

The anterior and posterior longitudinal ligaments blend with the outer margin of the intervertebral disc. The anterior longitudinal ligament, which contains predominantly collagen and contacts the anterior and lateral surfaces of the disc, cannot be distinguished from the outer annulus fibrosus in MRIs. The posterior longitudinal ligament where it attaches to the posterior intervertebral disc margin cannot be distinguished from the posterior disc margin in MRIs. Where the ligament passes posterior to the epidural venous plexus behind the vertebral body, it may be distinguished in MRI.

Another morphological feature of the intervertebral disc that may be distinguished in MRIs is the intranuclear cleft. This term designates a region in the equator of the intervertebral disc characterized not by a cleft but by increased density of collagen, elastic, and reticulin fibers. The lower signal intensity of the cleft represents the lower concentration of glycosaminoglycans because of the higher fiber content.

The gelatinous structure of the inner annulus fibrosus and the nucleus pulposus confers flexibility to the spine. The glycosaminoglycans in the disc, which has a high concentration of chondroitin and keratin sulfates that have fixed negative charges, reversibly bind water in the disc and give it its gelatinous quality. The water in the disc is in equilibrium with the water in the extracellular space outside the disc. As pressure on the intervertebral disc increases, water escapes from the disc; as pressure diminishes, water returns. The discs change measurably in water content during the day, causing a change of an inch or more in height diurnally and a measurable change in signal intensity. As the disc degenerates, the glycosaminoglycans content diminishes, giving it a lower affinity for water and displacing the equilibrium between water concentration and pressure.

The intervertebral disc has several thousand cells (chondrocytes or fibroblasts) in each cubic millimeter. These cells produce precursors of collagen and glycosaminoglycans that are released into the disc matrix. The production of these precursors is necessary to replace the collagen and glycosaminoglycans in the disc that is degraded by collagenases and proteinases in the disc. The glycosaminoglycans and collagen in the disc turn over approximately every 180 days.

The cells in the intervertebral disc receive their nutrition via diffusion because the intervertebral disc has no perfusion from arteries or capillaries. Oxygen, glucose, sulfates, and other nutrients diffuse into the disc through the vertebral end-plates, and carbon dioxide and other waste products diffuse out. Diffusion into the intervertebral disc can be detected as an increase in signal intensity in the disc in MRIs after the intravenous administration of a paramagnetic contrast medium. Reduction in the diffusion into the intervertebral disc may contribute to disc degeneration by interrupting the normal synthetic processes in the cell population in the disc.

The structure of the intervertebral disc facilitates rotation between vertebrae. Several degrees of flexion, extension, or lateral bending are possible at levels with normal intervertebral discs. Axial rotation between adjacent vertebrae is restricted by the axial orientation of collagen fibers in the annulus fibrosus. At lumbar levels with normal discs, the axial rotation that occurs with the application of an axial physiological rotation torque is usually limited to 1°. Rotation of the vertebrae change the dimensions of the central spinal canal and neural foramen but not to a critical degree.[12]

Age-related Changes in the Intervertebral Disc

In the neonate, the disc appears as a gray translucent structure between the partially ossified vertebral bodies. In the periphery of the disc, an outer annulus with conspicuous lamellae and low signal intensity in MRIs is evident. In the center of the disc are some streaks, which represent syncytial cells, remnants of the primitive notochord. Adjacent to the disc, the unossified cartilage of the intervertebral disc has a similar color in anatomical sections and similar signal intensity in MRIs. The vertebral cartilage contains large blood vessels.

From birth to adolescence, the intervertebral disc rapidly changes in height, diameter, and structure as the skeleton matures. The lamellae in the outer annulus fibrosus become better defined by the second decade of life. The collagen content of the inner annulus and the nucleus pulposus increases rapidly in the first two decades of life, with an increase in the stiffness of the disc. The adolescent disc contains more nonaggregated glycosaminoglycans than the neonatal disc. Ossification of the vertebral body concludes in this time period. All blood vessels in the cartilage around the disc disappear. The change in the disc is also associated with changes in the nucleus pulposus. Notochordal cells in the center of the disc disappear.

After the second decade of life, change continues in the intervertebral disc at a slower rate. In all regions of the disc, the concentration of viable cells declines, especially in the central region. The proportion of aggregating proteoglycans and the size of the aggregants in the disc diminish. In the nucleus pulposus and inner annulus fibrosus, collagen and noncollagen proteins increase in concentration. As a result of these chemical and histological changes, the adult intervertebral disc becomes firm, white, and opaque, and its signal intensity in T2-weighted images diminishes slightly.

With aging, fissures and cracks develop in the annulus fibrosus. In the majority of intervertebral discs in people over the age of 50, transverse and concentric tears are present in the annulus fibrosus. Transverse tears are disruptions of the peripheral annular fibers near their attachment to the ring apophysis. They are found in discs that have no bulging of the annulus fibrosus, no loss of height or signal intensity, and no other signs of degeneration. They are, therefore, often characterized as age-related changes. The transverse tears that contain mucoid material may appear in T2-weighted MRIs as regions of increased signal intensity in the annulus fibrosus. If the transverse tears contain gas, they may appear as regions of low density on radiographs or of low signal intensity on MRIs. They may also demonstrate contrast enhancement. Concentric tears are small, crescent-shaped gaps between lamellae of the annulus fibrosus. They may occur in discs without other signs of degeneration. They seldom have sufficient mucoid material to permit their detection on MRI. They do not demonstrate contrast enhancement.

Some investigators classify the fissures in the annulus fibrosus and the increasing firmness of the nucleus pulposus as degenerative changes, and others classify them as age-related changes. These morphological changes are associated with changes in the biomechanical function of the disc. The stiffness of the intervertebral disc is diminished in the presence of transverse or concentric tears of the annulus fibrosus disc.[13] These changes are not associated with a biomechanical failure of the intervertebral disc.

Degenerative Changes

Degenerated discs, like discs with age-related changes, are characterized by decreased cell nutrition, decreased numbers of viable cells, loss of aggregating proteoglycans, modification of matrix proteins, diminished degredative enzyme activity, diminished water and glycosaminoglycans content, and increased collagen content. Therefore, degeneration has been characterized as accelerated aging of the disc. Alternatively, it has been characterized as a distinct process superimposed on normal aging. Discs with reduced height, reduced signal intensity, or bulging of the annulus have one feature that is not found in aging discs that have normal height and signal intensity; that is, a radial tear of the annulus fibrosus.[38,39] The radial tear represents a fatigue failure of the disc, possibly produced by a repetitive loading or axial torsion applied to the disc. Its role in the degenerative process is not well established. Disc degeneration may contribute to back pain through multiple mechanisms, including the loss of mechanical stability of the spine, the release of mediators that may sensitize nerve endings, the development of granulation tissue in the intervertebral disc, and the compression of spinal nerves in the spinal canal or neural foramen.

Radial Tear

Radial tears are clefts or fissures that extend radially from the central nucleus pulposus to the periphery of the intervertebral disc, significantly disrupting the integrity of the annulus fibrosus. The radial tear may affect the anterior disc only or the posterior disc only, or it may extend across the full equator of the disc with disruption of both the anterior and the posterior lamellae of the annulus fibrosus. Unlike concentric and transverse tears, the radial tear has been found by precise anatomical studies in almost all discs with other features of degeneration, but rarely in normal adult discs with normal height, normal end-plates, and normal signal intensity. Radial tears are most prevalent at the L4-L5 and L5-S1 disc levels.

The radial tear has multiple appearances in MRIs. In T2-weighted MRIs, the radial tear appears as a linear region of high signal intensity (the so-called "high intensity zone" or HIZ) within the low signal intensity region representing the peripheral annulus fibrosus. This high intensity represents mucoid material within the tear. In T1-weighted images obtained after contrast enhancement administration, a curvilinear region of contrast enhancement may be found that corresponds to the radial tear. The enhancement represents granulation tissue that invades the disrupted disc from the perivertebral tissues. It contains both blood vessels, which lack a tight capillary junction, and nerve end-

ings, which may include nociceptors. Therefore, granulation tissue may explain pain in some cases of suspected disc herniation.[21] Because cartilage heals by so-called "second intention," granulation tissue in the radial tear represents a natural healing process. In our experience, contrast enhancement in the disc, suggesting granulation tissue, is present in a minority of degenerating discs.

In patients with a radial tear of the annulus fibrosus, the pain may be indistinguishable from that produced by a herniated disc.[10] The radial tear of the annulus fibrosus may produce pain by one or more of several mechanisms. The presence of nociceptors within the disc is one possibility. The leakage of substances from the degenerating disc into the epidural space is another mechanism. Glycosaminoglycans, lactic acid, and immunogenic substances have been implicated as potential causes of pain after their escape from a degenerating intervertebral disc. Another possibility is the loss of stiffness and the increased motions of the spine at the level of a disc with a radial tear.

Tears in the annulus fibrosus are associated with diminished stiffness of the intervertebral disc. Radial, transverse, or concentric tears increase the motions or rotations that occur when a physiological force or torque is applied to the motion segment. The effect of the tears is greater on the resistance to an axial rotational torque than to a flexion, extension, or lateral bending torque (Figure 3-5). Radial tears are associated with a greater loss of stiffness than a transverse or concentric tear.[13] In such segments, physiological forces or loads, which in the presence of a normal disc produce only minimal anatomical changes, may cause critical narrowing of a neural foramen or of the central spinal canal. In the presence of a radial tear, spinal nerve roots may be intermittently compressed by changes in posture, by flexion/extension movements, or by rotational movements. Critical changes in the anatomical relationships within the neural foramina adjacent to a radial tear have been observed secondary to physiological forces that would not significantly affect a normal disc level.[12] The foramen narrowing resulting from a radial tear, however, is unlikely to be visualized in routine clinical imaging in which the patient is placed supine in a position of comfort with minimal loading of the spine.

MRI demonstration of a radial tear is an excellent predictor of a disc that will prove to be painful at discography. Intradiscal injection of a contrast medium or saline exactly reproduces the patient's pain in 77% of the discs with annular disruption and in 3% of normal intervertebral discs.[37] In another comparison of MRI and discography, discs with MRI evidence of a radial tear had "concordant pain" at discography, while 65 of 67 discs that appeared normal lacked con-

FIGURE 3-5 ■ Rotation of lumbar vertebrae subjected to a 5.7 nm axial rotational torque. Note that segments containing a disc with a radial tear rotate from 1.6 to over 4°, whereas segments with a normal disc rotate on average in a range of 0.4 to 2.3° (from 20).

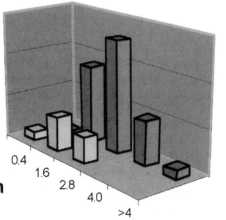

axial rotation
(degrees)

□ Normal disks
■ Radial tears

cordant pain.[2] The "normal" discs that had concordant pain were, in fact, abnormal discs mistakenly called normal because their appearance was "more nearly normal" in comparison to other more severely degenerated discs. In a third study, a radial tear, or "high intensity zone" in MRI, was found only in cases of grade 3 or grade 4 discograms.[3] The high intensity zone on MRI was 54% sensitive for a grade 4 discogram and 89% specific. The MRI finding was 82% sensitive and 89% specific for "concordant" pain production during discography. The positive predictive value of the high intensity zone for evidence of radial tear at discography was 86%. In other studies, the sensitivity of the MRI finding for predicting pain production at discography has ranged from 81% to 99%.[8,11,14,18,20, 24, 30, 32] The excellent correlation of a radial tear demonstrated by MRI and concordant pain demonstrated by discography has suggested that MRI accurately detects the painful level in selected patients (Figure 3-6).[14]

Herniation

The pathogenesis of pain from a herniated nucleus pulposus cannot be explained simply in terms of compression or displacement of a spinal nerve or nerve root. Pressure on a normal spinal nerve does not cause pain. Smyth's classic study in patients operated on for herniated discs showed that traction on a normal spinal nerve causes little symptomatology, whereas traction on a spinal nerve that had recently undergone decompression caused exquisite pain.[33] The study suggests that spinal nerves chronically traumatized by a herniated disc fragment behave differently from normal nerves when compressed. Chronic or intermittent compression of a spinal nerve or of roots leads to demyelination.[9] Demyelination changes the electrogenic properties of the axons so that graded pressure produces repetitive firing of the nerve. Graded pressure of demyelinated nerves results in repetitive depo-

larization of pain fibers that does not occur in normal nerves. In a demyelinated nerve root, weak mechanical stimuli, hypoxia, chemical mediators, inflammation, and sympathetic efferent activity may elicit nerve impulses ("ectopic hyperexcitability").

With a combination of T2- and T1-weighted MRIs in axial and sagittal projections, disc herniations can be demonstrated effectively. The fat in the epidural space deformed by the herniation is demonstrated best in the T1-weighted images. The relationship of the disc herniation to the spinal nerves in the neural foramen and in the dural sac can be evaluated. False negatives are exceptionally rare. Schwannomas, synovial cysts, and epidural hematomas produce most of the false positives. T2-weighted images demonstrate decreased signal intensity in intervertebral discs in most but not all cases. The herniated disc fragment may have different signal intensity than the parent disc. The radial tear in the annulus fibrosus, which is necessary for the herniation of the disc fragment, is not consistently demonstrated.

Disc Space Collapse

Collapse of the intervertebral disc is a late stage of disc degeneration, occurring long after the development of a radial tear in the annulus fibrosus. Loss of disc height likely represents a chronic depletion of glycosaminoglycans in the disc. The process may include loss of disc substance through the annulus fibrosus and through degradative enzymes, without compensatory synthesis of new collagen and glycosaminoglycans. The collapsed disc has typically low signal intensity, representing the loss of glycosaminoglycans and water. In those cases with high signal intensity in the collapsed disc space, a fissure has formed with mucoid material. Biomechanically, the collapse of the disc space changes the biomechanical properties of the segment. As disc height diminishes, the stiffness of the motion segment increases. Forces or torques applied to

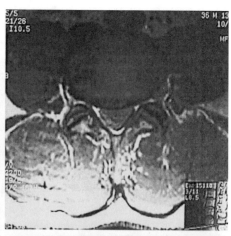

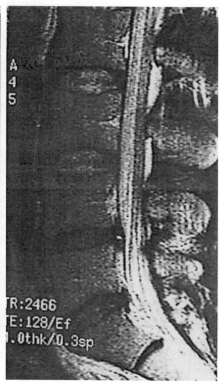

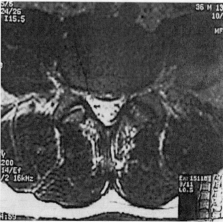

FIGURE 3-6 ■ **A,** T2-weighted sagittal MR image (left) illustrating a disc with decreased signal intensity. No high intensity zone is evident. In the late echo image (right), a small high intensity zone is evident. The axial images disclose no disc herniation; **B,** The discogram revealed concordant pain at L4-L5 and no pain at the other levels tested. The patient had an interbody fusion and relief of pain.

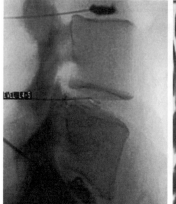

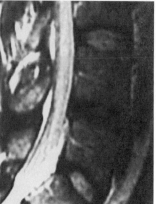

B

spinal levels with a collapsed disc produce less translation and rotation than the same forces applied to spinal levels with taller discs that have radial tears.[13] Spinal nerves in the neural foramen are less likely to be compressed as a result of physiological loading of the spine when a collapsed disc is present than when a taller disc is present.

With the collapse of the intervertebral disc, the ligamentum flavum shortens and thickens because of the elastic fibers within it. The thickening is often termed, inappropriately, *hypertrophy* of the ligamentum flavum. The thickened ligament may contain fissures or foci of calcification. The thickened ligament decreases the size of the central spinal canal and of the neural foramen. Spinal nerves in the neural foramen or the dural sac within the central spinal canal may be affected by the thickening of the ligamentum flavum. Ligamentum flavum thickening is a major factor in the development of spinal stenosis.

End-plate Changes

Adjacent to degenerating intervertebral discs, signal intensity within the bone marrow and end-plate may be abnormal. Three patterns have been identified. One pattern (Modic type I) is characterized by increased signal intensity in T2-weighted images and, if contrast medium is administered, by abnormal contrast enhancement Anatomically, this imaging pattern corresponds to increased vascularity in the vertebral end-plate and adjacent vertebral body. It corresponds to an increase in vascular tissue in the vertebral marrow adjacent to a degenerating disc, likely representing an early stage of disc degeneration. Some investigators suggest that it may be a sign of instability in the motion segment.[36] Another change (Modic type II) is characterized by increased signal intensity on T1-weighted images. It likely represents a conversion of red marrow to yellow marrow near the degenerating intervertebral disc. The clinical significance is not known. A third type of change is characterized by low signal intensity on T1- or T2-weighted images and corresponds to an increase in trabecular bone adjacent to the end-plate. On plain radiographs, sclerosis of the end-plate may be identified. It represents bony eburnation, a late stage of disc degeneration.

Discitis

MRI effectively demonstrates the changes in the vertebral end-plate and in the intervertebral disc resulting from discitis. The hallmarks of discitis are the destruction of the vertebral end-plate, increased signal intensity in the intervertebral disc and adjacent vertebral bodies, a soft tissue mass of granulation tissue surrounding the intervertebral disc, and contrast enhancement in the disc and adjacent inflammatory changes. Usually discitis is easily differentiated from disc degeneration, which lacks contrast enhancement in the disc and adjacent vertebral bodies, frank destruction of the end-plate, and a large soft tissue mass. Since imaging findings lag behind the pain and the elevated sedimentation rate of discitis, early cases may not have definitive findings.

SPINAL FACET JOINTS

Degenerative and inflammatory diseases of the facet joints may produce back pain. Either MRI or CT effectively demonstrates pathological changes in the facet joint, including articular cartilage destruction, subarticular erosion, sclerosis, hypertrophy, synovial cyst, and ankylosis.

Anatomy

The facet joint is the articulation between the superior and inferior articular processes at each spinal intervertebral level between C2 and S1. The anatomy of the facet joints varies from level to level. The flat or gently

curving articular surfaces of the facet joint can be approximated as a plane, which varies in inclination from one level to another. In the cervical region, the plane is oblique to the vertical or the axial plane. In the lumbar region, the plane is vertical and varying from nearly parallel to a sagittal plane (at L1) to nearly perpendicular to the sagittal plane (at L4 and L5).

The normal facet joint has a uniform layer of dense cortical bone and two thin layers of cartilage. Posteriorly, the facet joint has a tough, thick fibrous capsule, which covers the joint space and portions of the adjacent articular processes. Anteriorly, the facet joint has no capsule and no border except the ligamentum flavum. Within the periphery of the facet joint, a thin synovial lining is found. The synovium may extend a variable distance under the ligamentum flavum. In the first decade or two of life, the facet joints each contain a meniscus. The meniscus forms a bushing in the facet joint, as in the knee, that facilitates motion and weight bearing. In most adults over age 40, the meniscus has disappeared. Therefore, the meniscus itself is an unlikely cause of pain in adults.

Degeneration

Degeneration of the facet joint is characterized by loss of cartilage from the articular surface. Initially the degeneration has superficial crevasses described as *crabmeat degeneration*. With additional destruction of cartilage, the articular bone is exposed. At this stage, subarticular erosions, bony sclerosis, and hypertrophy occur in the articular processes. MRI and, to a greater extent, CT demonstrate the osseous and cartilaginous changes in the joint.

Intraspinal synovial cysts represent a combination of degeneration in the facet joint and cavitation in the ligamentum flavum. The cyst appears in images as an epidural soft tissue process adjacent to a degenerating facet joint, usually at L4-L5, and less commonly at other lumbar levels, thoracic levels, or cervical levels. The capsule of the cyst may be calcified. The contents of the cyst may be clear fluid, proteinaceous fluid, gas, or blood. The capsule enhances markedly after administration of an intravenous contrast medium. The enhancing capsule may mimic a meningioma or schwannoma.

Ankylosing Spondylitis

Ankylosing spondylitis causes characteristic imaging findings in the lumbar facet joints. The hallmark in imaging studies is the fusion of the facet joints without sclerosis. In addition, the intervertebral disc may appear denser than adjacent vertebrae in CT. The bamboo spine may be recognized in scout views or in sagittal images. Another feature of patients with ankylosing spondylitis and the cauda equina syndrome is inflammatory arachnoiditis, which causes diverticula of the dural sac and erosion of the adjacent laminae or vertebral bodies. The arachnoiditis, rather than an intradural mass, usually explains the neurological deficit in these cases.

Degenerative Spondylolisthesis

Degenerative spondylolisthesis, degeneration of the facet joints associated with a greater than 5 mm anterolisthesis of L4 or L5, is a common cause of back and leg pain, especially in women over the age of 65 years. Degenerative spondylolisthesis is found in 9.1% of women with back pain after the age of 65, compared to 5.8% of men. In women with back pain over age 75 years, it is diagnosed in 29%.[1] Back and leg pain are the primary symptoms in 80% of these patients, pseudo-claudication in 62%, and neurological deficit in 50%. Serial studies suggest that spondylolisthesis progresses at a rate of 2 mm per year. Risk factors for degenerative spondylolisthesis are age, gender, diabetes, and sacralization of L5.

In patients with suspected degenerative spondylolisthesis, MRI demonstrates the changes and aids in the selection of patients for fusions and decompressions. Sagittal MRIs demonstrate the slippage of one vertebra, usually L4, with respect to the adjacent one. Axial images demonstrate the sclerosis of the facet joints, hypertrophy, and, usually, the presence of fluid within the joint space. The dimensions of the sub-arachnoid space and the spinal canal must be evaluated both in the sagittal and the axial images. Because of the prevalence of asymptomatic spinal stenosis (7% of a series of normal volunteers [all ages] and 21% of normal volunteers over 60 years of age), criteria must be used that distinguish incidental narrowing of the spinal canal from critical narrowing.[5] No criteria are perfect for this distinction, perhaps because the degree of narrowing differs when the patient is supine for the MRI and when the patient is upright and active. Nonetheless, loss of the high signal intensity of CSF from within the dural sac on the axial T2-weighted images is considered evidence of sufficient narrowing to produce symptoms.

DYNAMIC IMAGING OF THE SPINE

Clinical instability has been defined as the failure of the spine to maintain normal patterns of deformation and to resist painful deformity under physiological loading.[27] The criteria for selecting patients for spinal fusion may be heavily weighted to the clinical findings because functional radiographs have little value except in the overtly unstable spine.[28] Physical examination by an "experienced observer" may be sufficient

to detect instability.[28] However, spinal fusion, according to some surgeons, should be reserved for patients with supporting functional imaging evidence of instability. A functional imaging study that accurately distinguishes stable and unstable segments would be helpful in selecting patients for fusion.

The primary imaging modality for diagnosing instability is flexion/extension radiography, despite its poor accuracy rate. False positives and false negatives are found with all methods for calculating instability from flexion/extension radiographs.[31]

Disc degeneration has a greater effect on the resistance of the disc to axial rotational torques than to flexion, extension, or lateral bending torques.[13, 25] Normal intervertebral discs resist axial rotation because of the radial orientation of collagen fibers in the annulus fibrosus. Although not effectively measured with radiographs, axial rotations can be measured with CT or MRI .[19] Axial rotatory motions of segments with normal and abnormal discs differ more significantly than the extension and flexion motions do. Functional imaging with applied axial rotatory torques may be useful in future studies to determine the effects of disc degeneration on the motions of spinal segments (see Figure 3-5).

REFERENCES

1. Andersson GB: What are the age-related changes in the spine? **Baillieres Clin Rheumatol** 12:161-173, 1998.
2. Anti-Poika I, Soini J, Talroth K, et al: Clinical relevance of discography combined with CT scanning: a study of 100 patients. **J Bone Joint Surg** 72B:480-83, 1990.
3. Aprill C, Bogduk N: High-intensity zone: a diagnostic sign of painful lumbar disc on magnetic resonance imaging. **Br J Radiol** 65:361-69, 1992.
4. Baur A, Stabler A, Bruning R, et al: Diffusion-weighted MR imaging of bone marrow: differentiation of benign versus pathologic compression fractures. **Images Radiology** 207(2):349-56, 1998.
5. Boden SD, Davis DO, Dina TS, et al. Abnormal magnetic-resonance scans of the lumbar spine in asymptomatic subjects: a prospective investigation. **J Bone Joint Surg** 72A:403-8, 1990.
6. Boden SD, Davis DO, Dina TS, et al: Contrast-enhanced MR imaging performed after successful lumbar disk surgery: prospective study. **Radiology** 182(1):59-64, 1992.
7. Buirski G: Magnetic resonance signal patterns of lumbar discs in patients with low back pain. A prospective study with discographic correlation. **Spine** 17(10):1199-204, 1992.
8. Collins DH, McElligott TF: Sulphate (35SO4) uptake by the chondrocytes in relation to histological changes in osteoarthritic human articular cartilage. **Ann Rheum Dis** 19:318-30, 1960.

9. Devor M: Neuropathic pain and injured nerve: peripheral mechanisms. **Br Med Bull** 47(3):619-30, 1991.

10. Fernstrom U: A discographic study of ruptured intervertebral discs. **Acta Chir Scandinav** 258(Supp):11-106, 1960.

11. Gibson MJ, Buckley J, Mawhinney R, et al: Magnetic resonance imaging and discography in the diagnosis of disc degeneration. **J Bone Joint Surg** 68B:369-73, 1986.

12. Hasegawa T, An HS, Haughton VM, et al: Lumbar foraminal stenosis: critical heights of the intervertebral discs and foramina. A cryomicrotome study in cadavera. **J Bone Joint Surg Am** 77(1):32-38, 1995.

13. Haughton VM, Schmidt TA, Keele K, et al: Flexibility of lumbar spinal motion segments correlated to type of tears in the annulus fibrosus. **J Neurosurg** 92(1 Supp):81-6, 2000.

14. Horton WC, Daftari TK: Which disc as visualized by magnetic resonance imaging is actually a source of pain? A correlation between magnetic resonance imaging and discography. **Spine** 6(Supp):S164-71, 1992.

15. Ibrahim MA, Jesmanowicz A, Hyde J, et al: Contrast enhancement of normal intervertebral disks: time and dose dependence. **Am J Neuroradiol** 15: 419-24, 1994.

16. Jensen MC, Brant-Zawadzki MN, Obuchowski N, et al: Magnetic resonance imaging of the lumbar spine in people without back pain. **N Engl J Med** 331(2):69-73, 1994.

17. Jinkins JR, Roeder MB: MRI of benign lumbosacral nerve root enhancement. **Semin Ultrasound CT MR** 14(6): 446-54, 1993.

18. Kornberg M: Discography and magnetic resonance imaging in the diagnosis of lumbar disc disruption. **Spine** 14:1368-71, 1989.

19. Lim TH, Eck JC, An HS, et al: Three-dimensional spinal motion analysis method. **Spine** 22:1996-2000, 1997.

20. Linson MA, Crowe CH: Comparison of magnetic resonance imaging and lumbar discography in the diagnosis of disc degeneration. **Clin Orthop** 250:160-63, 1990.

21. Modic MT, Ross JS, Obuchowski NA, et al: Contrast-enhanced MR imaging in acute lumbar radiculopathy: a pilot study of the natural history. **Radiology** 195(2):429-35, 1995.

22. Nguyen CM, Ho KC, Yu SW, et al: An experimental model to study contrast enhancement in MR imaging of the intervertebral disk. **Am J Neuroradiol** 10(4):811-14, 1989.

23. Nguyen CM, Ho KC, An H, et al: Ionic versus nonionic paramagnetic contrast media in differentiating between scar and herniated disk. **Am J Neuroradiol** 17(3):501-5, 1996.

24. Nordlander, Salen S, Unander-Scharin L: Discography in low back pain and sciatica. **Acta Orthop Scandinav** 28:90-102, 1958.

25. Nowicki BH, Haughton VM, Schmidt TA, et al: Occult lumbar lateral spinal stenosis in neural foramina subjected to physiologic loading. **Am J Neuroradiol** (9): 1605-14, 1996.

26. Osti OL, Fraser RD, Vernon-Roberts B: Annular tears and degeneration of the intervertebral disc - preliminary results of an experimental study. **Spine** 15:762-67, 1990.

27. Panjabi MM, Thibodeau LL, Crisco JJ III et al: What constitutes spinal instability? **Clin Neurosurg** 34:313-39, 1988.

28. Pope MH, Panjabi M: Biomechanical definitions of spinal instability. **Spine** 10:255-56, 1985.

29. Ross JS, Modic MT, Masaryk TJ: Tears of the anulus fibrosus: assessment with Gd-DTPA-enhanced MR imaging. **Am J Roentgenol** 154(1):159-62, 1990.

30. Schneiderman GB, Flannigan S, Kingston S, et al: Magnetic resonance imaging in the diagnosis of disc degeneration: correlation with discography. **Spine** 12:276-81, 1987.

31. Shaffer WO, Spratt KF, Weinstein J, et al: The consistency and accuracy of roentgenograms for measuring sagittal translation in the lumbar vertebral motion segment. An experimental model. **Spine** 15:741-50, 1990.

32. Simmons JW, Emery SF, McMillin JN, et al. Awake discography: a comparison study with magnetic resonance imaging. **Spine** 16 (Supp) S216-21, 1991.

33. Smyth MJ, Wright V: Sciatica and the intervertebral disc. **Bone Joint Surg** 40:(BR)1401–18, 1958, 1991.

34. Stabler A, Weiss M, Scheidler J, et al: Degenerative disk vascularization on MRI: correlation with clinical and histopathologic findings. **Skeletal Radiol** 25(2):119-26, 1996.

35. Sze G, Bravo S, Baierl P, et al: Developing spinal column: gadolinium-enhanced MR imaging. **Radiology** 180(2): 497-502, 1991.

36. Toyone T, Takahashi K, Kitahara H, et al: Vertebral bone marrow changes in degenerative lumbar disc disease. **J Bone Joint Surg** 765: 757-64, 1995.

37. Vanharanta H, Sachs BL, Spivey MA, et al: The relationship of pain provocation to lumbar disc deterioration as seen by CT/discography. **Spine** 12:295-98, 1987.

38. Yu S, Haughton VM, Sether LA, et al: Anulus fibrosus in bulging intervertebral discs. **Radiology** 169:761-63, 1988.

39. Yu S, Sether LA, Wagner M, et al: Tears of the anulus fibrosus: correlation between MRI and pathologic findings in cadavers. **Am J Roentgenol** 9:367-70, 1988.

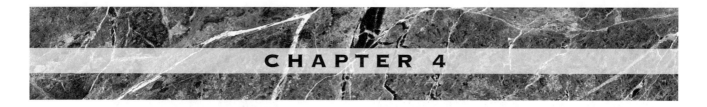

CHAPTER 4

Radiographic Evaluation of the Patient with Low Back Pain: The Role of Discography

ROBERT F. HEARY, M.D.

CESLOVAS VAICYS, M.D.

INTRODUCTION

No diagnostic procedure in the field of neurosurgery has generated greater controversy than discography. In order to gain an appreciation for the role of discography in the treatment of low back pain patients, there is a need to acquire a thorough understanding of the discography procedure itself. Proponents of discography require the following two basic premises to be upheld: (1) degenerative disc disease may be successfully treated, and (2) discography is a useful diagnostic procedure. Opponents of discography are those who believe either that degenerative disc disease is a nonsurgical entity and/or that discography is unable to accurately define this diagnosis.

This chapter provides an overview of the concept of degenerative disc disease and the discography procedure. In addition, the history of discography is reviewed, which includes references to numerous landmark studies both favoring and opposing this procedure. These varying views have led to the controversy surrounding the discography procedure. The indications for discography are reviewed in detail, and the specific technique of discography is described. The results of discography are analyzed both with respect to the imaging studies generated as well as the use of pain provocation as an interpretive factor. Comparisons between discography and other imaging studies used to evaluate disc abnormalities, such as computed tomography (CT) scans, plain film radiographs, and magnetic resonance (MR) imaging studies, are discussed. The reported complications of discography are reviewed. Finally, an attempt is made to present the reader with conclusions that will lead to a rational plan regarding the use of discography in the radiographic evaluation of the patient with low back pain.

DEGENERATIVE DISC DISEASE

Degenerative disc disease, as a diagnostic entity, is in itself a controversial topic. Various synonyms have been used to describe degenerative disc disease, such as internal disc disruption, mechanical low back pain, black disc disease, and axial back pain. The overriding premise in the concept of degenerative disc disease is that a lumbar intervertebral disc may degenerate and become the source of back pain. In this condition, the intervertebral disc loses hydration and subsequently degenerates. This degeneration is felt to be associated with low back pain. In addition, pain in the buttocks, thighs, and legs may be present; however, the classic description of degenerative disc disease provides that the back pain will be more severe than the extremity symptoms.

A herniated lumbar intervertebral disc is a distinctly different entity than a degenerative disc. In the case of a herniated lumbar disc, disc material is present outside the normal confines of the annulus fibrosis and typically will occur in a location where a lumbar nerve root will be irritated by the disc material. Not uncommonly, a herniated disc may be present simultaneously with a degenerative disc, at either the same level, or at adjacent levels, of the lumbar spine.

In pure degenerative disc disease of the lumbar spine, the patient will present with a history of low back pain as the primary complaint. Degenerative disc disease patients will frequently complain of difficulty with sitting intolerance. Frequently, the patient will describe the inability to sit still for even 20 minutes, and they are unable to perform many activities of normal daily living. Difficulties include an inability to sit in a classroom, in a conference, or in a movie theatre. In addition, patients with degenerative disc disease will often state that they are unable to ride in cars or buses for prolonged periods of time. The pain of degenerative disc disease is often worsened with changes in body position. These patients will typically use external structures to attempt to gain support for their low backs. This may include leaning on tables, utilizing lumbar braces or corsets, or lying down in a recumbent position in order to achieve relief. The neurological exams of patients with classic degenerative disc disease are usually normal. Motor power, sensory examination, and deep tendon reflexes are typically normal. In addition, no nerve root tension signs are present.

When the clinical history and physical examination is consistent with degenerative disc disease of the lumbar spine, radiographic imaging studies are frequently obtained. Depending upon the degree of degeneration, plain film radiographs may be completely normal, or abnormalities may be demonstrated. The abnormalities may include a loss of disc space height in more degenerated cases. In addition, lateral lumbar spine radiographs, with flexion and extension views, may demonstrate evidence of dynamic instability at the level of the degenerated disc. Evidence of bony degenerative changes may also be present at the level of the facet joints, which are best visualized on oblique view x-rays of the lumbosacral spine. CT scan examinations, with or without intravenous contrast, will rarely provide additional information regarding degenerative disc disease than that which can be obtained from a high quality lumbosacral spine plain radiograph series.

MR imaging is now widely used in the evaluation of patients with low back pain. Advantages of MR imaging include the lack of ionizing radiation, the noninvasiveness of the procedure, and the ability to accurately assess soft tissue structures, such as the intervertebral disc. In degenerative disc disease of the lumbar spine, MR imaging may provide variable results. The classic appearance of degenerative disc disease will be the loss of hydration of the intervertebral disc, which is best visualized on T2-weighted images in which the degenerative disc achieves a black appearance (Figure 4-1). A normal or nondegenerated disc typically will appear white on T2-weighted images. Significant controversy has occurred when MR imaging does not demonstrate any evidence of abnormal signal intensity in the intervertebral discs. In these instances, some authors will recommend performance of a discogram to attempt to define a degenerative disc.[65] These studies are reviewed later in this chapter. Myelography is frequently used to diagnose a herniated lumbar disc; however, myelograms do not allow for an assessment of the internal architecture of the disc, which is the primary abnormality in degener-

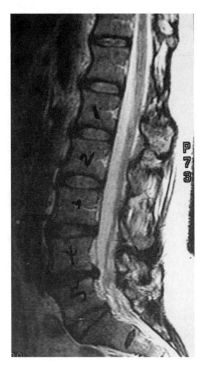

FIGURE 4-1 ■ Sagittal MR image (T2-weighted). Black disc at L4-L5 level with modest posterior protrusion; remaining discs appear normal.

ative disc disease. As such, myelograms are of little use in the diagnosis of degenerative disc disease.

When the clinical history, physical examination, and radiographic imaging studies are suggestive of lumbar degenerative disc disease, discography may be considered as a further diagnostic tool in order to determine the diagnosis.

THE HISTORY OF DISCOGRAPHY

In 1948, Lindblom published the first paper on the use of diagnostic disc puncture in the evaluation of patients with suspected lumbar disc pathology. The term *discography* was applied to this technique.[26] Over the next 20 years, discography became increasingly popular, particularly among orthopaedic spine surgeons.

Significant technological advances in the field of radiology have occurred over the past 50 years to improve the accuracy of needle placement in the lumbar intervertebral disc. Earlier discograms were performed and confirmed, with plain radiographs being used to confirm placement of the needle tip within the disc. Advances in fluoroscopy allowed for real time confirmation of accurate needle placement. Biplane fluoroscopy has become a standard in the performance of modern discograms (Figure 4-2). CT scans became available in the 1970s and these have been used by

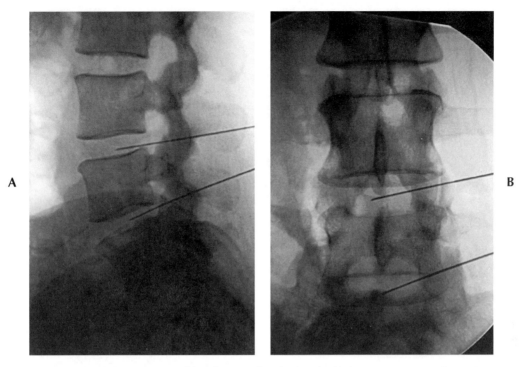

FIGURE 4-2 ■ **A,** Lateral lumbosacral radiograph demonstrates properly positioned small-bore discography needles (22 gauge) at the L4-L5 and the L5-S1 levels (needle tip should be in the middle third of the vertebral body on this projection); **B,** Anteroposterior (AP) lumbosacral radiograph demonstrates properly positioned discography needles at the L4-L5 and the L5-S1 levels (needle tip should be between the pedicles on this projection).

many authors to image the intervertebral disc following the performance of a discogram.

Holt, in 1968, performed a study of lumbar discography in 30 asymptomatic volunteers from a prison population. He determined that 36% of the disc injections demonstrated an abnormal radiographic appearance and 26% of the injections were associated with pain. This led Holt to question the benefit of lumbar discography, as the false-positive rate appeared excessively high.[20] Potential biases were present in this study. Prisoners were used as subjects, and it is unclear how thoroughly screened these subjects were for the presence of pre-existing lumbar spine conditions. In addition, Hypaque (diatrizoate) was the contrast medium used. This contrast agent came in direct contact with nerve roots, and pain may have been generated directly as a result of this highly irritant dye that leaked out of the abnormal discs.

In 1970, Crock defined internal disc disruption. In his article, Crock defined four types of abnormality of the lumbar intervertebral disc, and his definition of internal disc disruption is currently synonymous with the definition used for degenerative disc disease today.[12]

In 1987, Sachs and associates[44] published the "Dallas discogram description." These authors classified degenerative disc disease and annular disruption as separate phenomena. They also categorized clinical information, volumes of contrast dye used, and assorted additional miscellaneous information. Important contributions made by the Dallas discogram description include quantifying the volume of contrast dye injected in an intervertebral disc. The maximum volume able to be injected was recorded. The theory was that an incompetent, deteriorated disc will accept more dye, whereas a normal disc will be able to accept a lesser volume of contrast dye. In addition, clinical information related to the generation of pain during injection of the dye was recorded. Specifically, a comparison was made between the pain elicited by injection of the dye with the patient's original presenting complaint of pain. Pain at the time of injection was rated as either none, dissimilar to the usual pain, similar to the usual pain, or an exact reproduction of the original pain. This definition of an exact reproduction of the patient's original pain during injection of dye has become popularly referred to in the present time as *concordant* pain (Figure 4-3). This study was published at a

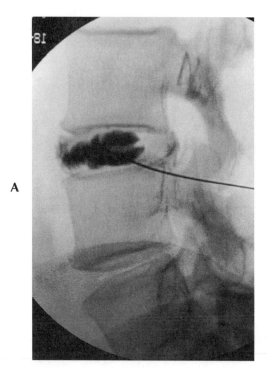
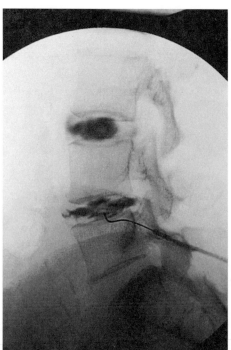

FIGURE 4-3 ■ **A,** Fluoroscopic lateral view of L3-L4 discogram. This "control" level shows normal pooling of contrast dye with some anterior filling and no posterior filling; **B,** Same patient as **A:** fluoroscopic lateral view after L4-L5 discogram, which demonstrates a markedly degenerated disc. (This L4-L5 level was accompanied by a positive "concordant" pain response.)

time prior to the widespread use of magnetic resonance imaging. Sachs and associates recommended discography when revision spine surgery was considered or when the clinical information from the patient did not agree with either the myelographic or CT scan information.[44]

In 1988, Simmons and associates wrote a detailed analysis of the study performed by Holt in 1968. In this critical analysis of Holt's study, Simmons and associates noted that the procedure of discography performed in the 1980s had evolved significantly from a technological sense. They cited the advantages of the use of fluoroscopy, different contrast dyes including contrast dyes of lower osmolarity and nonionic forms, and the use of CT scan imaging following the discography. In addition, Simmons and associates were critical of the number of nondiagnostic studies obtained by Holt. Simmons and associates concluded that discography procedures performed in the 1980s were markedly different than, and superior to, the procedure as performed in the 1960s. As a result, these authors suggested that the negative impression of discography propagated by the article by Holt, in 1968, was not valid.[51]

Nachemson, in a 1989 editorial, condemned the use of discography. He described the use of "clinical judg-

ment" in the performance of discography as "at best a disguise for ignorance, at worse, an excuse for quackery." This editorial by a well-respected member of the orthopaedic spine community continued to spark significant controversy over whether discography was a legitimate procedure for determining a painful degenerative disc in the lumbar spine that may benefit from surgical intervention.[35] During the first 40 years discographies were performed, the inconsistent results led to much debate regarding this procedure. Although many of the early studies were methodologically flawed, as well as oftentimes technically inadequate, a wealth of literature both supporting and refuting the procedure had been published.

THE INDICATIONS FOR DISCOGRAPHY

Discography is an invasive diagnostic procedure. *Provocative discography* refers to the assessment of the pain response associated with the injection of dye during a discography procedure. Discography or, more appropriately, provocative discography, is indicated to determine whether noninvasive radiographic imaging studies and appropriate history and clinical examination findings have correctly identified a painful degenerative disc. In clinical practice, provocative discography is performed as part of the diagnostic work-up in a patient who may be a candidate for a more invasive surgical procedure.

Prior to performing discography, patients with suspected painful degenerative disc disease should undergo prolonged conservative work-ups. The minimal timeframe for conservative management has been variously reported to be between two to six months.[4,31,42,43] In the conservative treatment regimen, patients are encouraged to attempt to maintain an ideal body weight. For obese patients, this may involve referral to a medical specialist to assist in a weight loss program that may be safely performed. Physical therapy, which attempts to strengthen both back and abdominal musculature, is another standard form of conservative therapy.[62] A trial of medical therapy, usually involving the use of nonsteroidal anti-inflammatory drugs, is also indicated.[31,42] More recently, Cox-2 inhibitors have also been used to attempt to improve medical management.

As a general rule, nonnarcotic medications are preferable for the medical management of patients with suspected painful degenerative disc disease. Well-documented problems with narcotic medications include the development of tolerance and addiction, which may limit the value of these medications in chronic low back pain patients. Additional conservative measures that have been attempted include the use of epidural steroid injections, as well as trials of bracing.[31] In addition, an assortment of less invasive conservative measures including chiropractic treatment, acupuncture, and biofeedback have been attempted in conservative treatment regimens. An additional useful conservative treatment regimen is the performance of a formal evaluation of the psychological condition of the low back pain patient.[41] Psychological profiles are able to help in determining patients with somatization disorders and patients who may demonstrate secondary gain following Workers' Compensation cases and/or litigation. Among the various conservative treatment measures advocated, physical therapy remains the most commonly used technique.

Low back pain may be the result of degenerative disc disease. However, low back pain may also result from disease of the facet joints, the sacroiliac joints, spinal stenosis, lumbar disc herniation, and segmental instability.[3] Clinical and radiological evaluations are used to attempt to differentiate among these other sources of low back pain and degenerative disc disease. In patients who are able to undergo MR imaging, this procedure has become the radiological test of choice to evaluate the lumbar disc for signs of degeneration. A patient who has a clinical history and a physical examination suggestive of degenerative disc disease and who has failed conservative treatment regimens should be a candidate for a magnetic resonance imagery (MRI) study.

An assortment of indications for provocative discography has been described. The most common indication for discography is a painful degenerative lumbar disc.[2,6,11,18,47,50,52] Numerous investigators have used discography as a diagnostic study to determine whether the patient would benefit from a spinal fusion procedure.[2,11,31,47,61] More recently, discography has been advocated for patients considering evaluation and treatment via lesser invasive methods, such as intradiscal electrothermy.[43] Some authors have used discography to evaluate whether a disc within a fused segment is a pain generator.[2,18] Other authors have stated that prior failed spinal surgery can be a serious confounding factor, and as such, discography is not valuable in these patients.[14] An additional frequent indication for discography is the evaluation of a disc adjacent to a prior spinal fusion.[2,18]

A common indication for discography includes the patient with multiple black discs on T2-weighted MR imaging where an attempt is made to determine which of the black discs is a pain generator.[18,21,47] The most controversial indication for discography is the patient with no abnormalities demonstrated on MRI where discography is performed to attempt to determine a painful MRI negative degenerative disc.[6,18,65]

In 1990, Boden and associates investigated asymptomatic patients and found that one third of these patients with no history of low back pain had abnormal MRIs of the lumbar spine.[5] This landmark study convinced the majority of spine surgeons that an abnormal MR image, in and of itself, is not adequate for determining the presence of a painful degenerative lumbar disc. Likewise, Buirski and Silberstein have stated that MRI may only be used to assess nuclear anatomy and not to assess symptomatology of a lumbar disc.[8] Despite these data, Horton and Daftari have stated that if a single level abnormality on MRI has a high probability for provoking pain, discography may be avoided.[21]

Despite conflicting reports in the literature, the optimal indications for provocative discography include the patient with a clinical history and physical examination consistent with degenerative disc disease who also has an abnormal MRI, with a black disc demonstrated on T2-weighted imaging. These patients would also have had an appropriate unsuccessful course of conservative therapy, as well as other causes of low back pain ruled out. Furthermore, a psychological profile that does not suggest significant secondary gain issues should be performed.

THE TECHNIQUE OF DISCOGRAPHY

Discography is an invasive diagnostic procedure that requires a moderate degree of technical skill. There is a substantial learning curve to mastering this technique.

The procedure requires an adequate understanding of the bony and soft tissue anatomy of the lumbar spine. In addition, knowledge of anesthetic and sedative techniques is useful to obtain the optimal information from the discography procedure. The discographer may be the spine surgeon or another healthcare professional skilled in the technique. Positioning for the procedure may be either in a prone position or a lateral position.[3,29,31,47,52] Meticulous sterile technique is mandatory to prevent infectious complications.[3,29,31] In order to limit exaggerated pain responses from an irritated lumbar spinal nerve, most discographers approach from the asymptomatic or less symptomatic side.[3,31,47]

Adequate use of local anesthesia on the nondiscal structures is essential.[29,31,52] It is important not to anesthetize the annulus proper; however, the skin and extra spinal soft tissues should be well anesthetized. In addition, sedation may be used.[29,52] Recently developed, very short-acting sedative medication, such as propofol, allow for the patient to be well sedated during the positioning of the needles. Upon discontinuation of the intravenous propofol solution, the patient will completely reverse from the sedation within a few minutes. This allows for the patient to be completely awake and alert in order to accurately monitor the pain provocation response.

The entry site on the skin typically lies between 8 to 10 cm lateral to the midline.[29,31] Either a single or a double needle technique may be used. Of clinical importance, the needle, which perforates the annulus, should be of a small gauge. This will typically involve use of a needle no larger than 22 gauge to penetrate the annulus.[2,31,47,52] McCutcheon and Thompson describe the situation in which contrast extravasation occurred in a retrograde fashion through a needle tract from a 20 gauge needle, which can lead to a false positive interpretation of the plain film images.[30] In addition, the needle tip should attempt to reach the anatomical midline in both a sagittal and coronal plane.[3,29,31,47] Current discography technique typically uses biplane fluoroscopy to confirm appropriate location of the tip of the needle.[3,18,47] Numerous authors have stressed the importance of accurate needle placement in obtaining the maximal degree of diagnostic information.[3,7,23,56]

Once the needle is correctly positioned and the patient is fully awake and alert with no lingering effects from short-acting sedation, contrast dye is injected into the disc. During the injection of dye, a pain response is monitored from the patient.[3,18,31,47,52] In particular, the presence or absence of pain, whether it be similar or dissimilar to the usual pain, and the presence of an exact reproduction of the pain, termed *concordant pain,* is reported.[13] Factors that may be responsible for an inaccurate pain response by the patient include poor needle placement, an overreaction to the painful stimulus by the patient, an exaggerated pain

response resulting from an extradural extravasation of dye, and pain resulting from the needle placement rather than the injection of dye.[7] An inaccurate needle placement into the annulus fibrosis may be painful and might produce atypical pain. This may result in a false positive discography study. Injections into the annulus fibrosis may be recognized by acceptance of a very small volume of contrast with a firm end point during injection.[3] In addition, improper needle placement may lead to nerve root sheath injection, subarachnoid injection, or irreversible damage to the disc.

In addition to recording the presence of pain, recent studies have documented recording the presence of resistance to injection, the volume of dye, and the pressure transduced.[3,13,18,28,31,47,52,54] Adams and associates found that fissured and ruptured discs were more common in older spines. They determined that older discs accepted a greater volume of injected fluid and required a lower injection pressure.[1] Derby and associates performed precise manometric measurements of the pressure during discography. They developed specific diagnostic categories for pressure measurements, including chemical, mechanical, indeterminant, and normal pressures. These parameters were defined as:[13]

- *Chemical*—less than 15 pounds per square inch pressure upon injection
- *Mechanical*—between 15 to 50 pounds per square inch
- *Indeterminant*—pressure between 51 to 90 pounds per square inch
- *Normal*—pressures of greater than 90 pounds per square inch without pain.

Following the injection of the dye, plain film radiographs or fluoroscopic images are taken to document the radiographic appearance of the disc.[3,47] Some investigators also perform a postdiscography CT scan (Figure 4-4).[3,52] Disc morphology can be rated as either normal, presence of annular tears or fissures, presence of end-plate defects, and presence or absence of leakage of contrast dye.[47]

Milette and Melanson determined that technical failures were present in 2.7% of discograms. Reasons for technical failures included impossible disc puncture, impossible contrast injection, and impossible opacification of the disc.[33] An excessively narrow intervertebral disc space may be responsible for a technical failure. In addition, the L5-S1 disc space requires greater technical expertise and may be difficult to image, particularly with less experienced discographers. Schellhas and Pollei have emphasized the need to perform a diagnostic disc injection at a "control" disc.[47] A controlled disc injection is obtained when the radiographic images are within normal limits and there is no provocation of pain with the injection. The

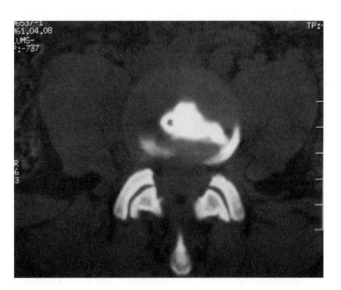

FIGURE 4-4 ■ Axial CT scan following discogram demonstrates a left-sided annular tear with pooling of dye in multiple layers of the annulus fibrosis.

presence of a "controlled" disc injection increases the specificity of a positive discography result at another level.

THE RESULTS OF DISCOGRAPHY

Discography results are typically classified into those related to radiographic imaging studies and those related to the provocation of pain. Both of these areas provide useful diagnostic information that may be used in further treatment planning.

Yasuma and associates performed an anatomical study of discography. In this study, they determined that discograms may present a false negative result when a protrusion or prolapsed disc involved the annulus fibrosis but did not involve the nucleus pulposus. Likewise, extensive annulus fibrosis degeneration may be present in a patient who has a normal discogram, which would result in a false negative study.[63] Other authors have also highlighted the importance of the annulus fibrosis with respect to pain generation.[11,16,34] In a cadaveric study of discography, Gunzburg and associates found that tears in the posterior annulus were more common than discographic tears in the anterior annulus.[16]

Similarly, Colhoun and associates found that provocation of back pain symptoms was most common when tears were present in the posterior annulus fibrosis. Degenerative disc and internal disc disruption were less frequently associated with the provocation of pain.[11] Moneta and associates analyzed 833 discograms in 306 patients and determined that the outer annulus fibrosis was the origin of pain reproduction during discography.[34]

Degenerative disc changes are more common in the lower lumbar segments than in the upper lumbar segments.[53] Milette and associates found that a loss of disc height or abnormal signal intensity on MRI was significantly associated with disc disruptions, which extended into or beyond the outer annulus on discography, and a higher incidence of similar or exact pain reproduction was present in these cases.[32]

Numerous investigators have found no difference between sexes in the provocation of pain during discography.[28,34] Some studies have demonstrated no difference in pain provocation based on the patient's age during discography.[34] Other studies have demonstrated different patterns of pain with respect to the patient's age, with younger patients demonstrating more pain.[28] There is no difference in the average number of painful discs between smokers and nonsmokers.[31]

PROVOCATIVE DISCOGRAPHY

In Sachs and associates sentinel article in 1987 on Dallas discogram description, they defined the correlation between the production of pain and the injection of dye during discographic procedures. These investigators classified pain into the following four categories: no pain, pain dissimilar to the usual pain, pain similar to the usual pain, and pain that is an exact reproduction of the usual pain. The final category of exact reproduction of usual pain has been termed *concordant pain*.[44] This grading system has been widely accepted and is the standard used in most series of discography.[18,28,50,59]

Some inconsistency exists in the reporting of pain provoked by discography procedures. There is general agreement that concordant pain is a positive response; however, studies differ as to whether similar or dissimilar pain evoked by discography is considered a positive discographic pain response. Most studies describing the results of discography cite a positive pain provocation response in approximately 70% of patients undergoing lumbar discograms.[7,19,30,34] In addition to commenting on positive pain generating discograms, most investigators also require the presence of a "controlled" disc injection. A controlled disc injection is a lumbar intervertebral disc that has dye injected that does not produce a pain response. In cases in which all discs injected invoke a pain response, meaning that no controlled disc injection is obtained, the discographic procedure should be considered nondiagnostic.

Numerous factors affect whether a positive pain response will occur following discography. When significant degenerative changes are present in a disc, the incidence of a positive pain response increases (Figure 4-5).[2,46,60] Likewise, the presence of significant annular disruptions is also associated with an increased positive pain response.[46,60] The

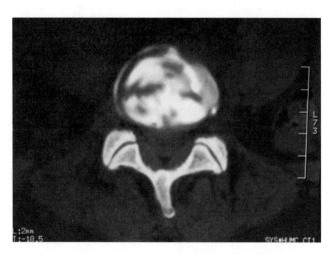

FIGURE 4-5 ■ Axial CT scan following discogram demonstrates diffuse degenerative changes throughout the entire disc.

presence of facet tropism, or asymmetry, has not been found to be associated with an increased pain response.[57] Abnormal disc protrusions, which occur either centrally, paracentrally, or in an intraforaminal location, are more likely to invoke a pain response than extraforaminal disc protrusions.[28] Furthermore, pain is more likely to be found in discograms performed at the lowest two motion segments (L4-L5 and L5-S1) than in discograms performed at more rostral levels.[28,31] Patients with chronic somatization states or chronic pain syndromes, particularly those with active compensation claims, are more likely to report painful discographic injections than are patients without chronic pain.[9] Intervertebral discs with sequestered fragments or extraligamentous extrusions are more likely to invoke the pain response than disc herniations that are subligamentous or merely disc protrusions.[28] Heggeness and associates performed discograms on patients following discectomy procedures. They found that a pain response was more likely to occur in previously operated discs than in the unoperated discs.[19] Aprill and Bogduk reported a fivefold increase in the reproduction of pain in discs that were radiographically pathological compared to discs that had a normal discographic appearance.[2]

Pain drawings have been used in some discographic studies to permit the patient to demonstrate where pain occurs following discographic injections. Pain drawings, which demonstrate pain in the lower extremities, are more likely to be associated with painful injections than are discographic procedures that do not produce leg pain.[36,37] Ohnmeiss and associates have attempted to localize the involved painful disc based on pain drawings performed following discographic procedures. They have found that when

pain radiates into the leg anteriorly, the most commonly affected level is the L3-L4 disc. When pain is in the posterior thigh or leg without pain in the anterior drawing, positive discograms were more likely to occur in the L4-L5 or L5-S1 disc. Pain drawings, which showed pain limited to the low back and buttocks, were more often associated with the absence of disc pathology.[37] Ohnmeiss and associates have used pain drawings to help identify patients who may demonstrate an exaggerated response to discography. Using these pain drawings, the overall accuracy of differentiating patients with false positive pain was 78%.[38]

IMAGING STUDIES

Discography typically consists of two separate phases. The imaging phase includes images obtained at the time of discography, which may be plain film radiographs but are more frequently fluoroscopic images, as well as CT scans, which are frequently obtained following the discography procedures. In addition, the second phase of the discographic procedure includes the provocation of pain. As previously discussed, patients with appropriate history and physical examination findings consistent with degenerative disc disease will frequently undergo MRIs. If the MRI confirms the diagnosis of degenerative disc disease, and a failure of conservative treatment has occurred, then consideration of provocative discography may be entertained.

Plain film radiographs are frequently obtained in the evaluation of low back pain secondary to degenerative disc disease. In addition, dynamic imaging studies include flexion/extension lateral views of the lumbar spine looking for evidence of instability. Quinnell and Stockdale performed a study comparing flexion/extension lateral lumbar spine radiographs with discography. Interestingly, all single-level, discographically abnormal studies were correctly diagnosed by flexion/extension radiographs. Furthermore, the presence of a single-level abnormality on flexion/extension views did not exclude the presence of another discographically abnormal level.[40] Some investigators have performed flexion/extension views following the contrast infusion during discography.[45,49] Although the findings have not been consistently reported, discograms with normal morphology demonstrate pooling of dye in a more anterior position within the disc during extension. The clinical significance of this finding is not clear.[49]

Many investigators have reported the use of CT scanning following discography to augment the diagnostic information provided.[3,25,27,30,44,55,60] The abnormal images described may be consistent with either disc degeneration or disc herniations. Discograms are particularly useful in diagnosing lateral disc herniations that may not be visible with myelography.[25,27,30,44] In addition, axial and sagittal reconstructive images may facilitate the precise localization of a herniated disc as either central, paracentral, lateral, or far lateral.[3] The CT scans obtained following discography may be useful in determining evidence of degeneration as well as in identifying annular tears. Investigators more interested in the pain provocation response may not obtain CT scans following discography. In these instances, the images obtained by fluoroscopy will usually suffice.

Myelography is an invasive study which can accurately diagnose herniated lumbar intervertebral discs. Myelograms do not provide information about the internal architecture of the intervertebral discs. Whereas both myelography and discography may be useful in diagnosing herniated lumbar intervertebral discs, in practice, myelography is usually indicated when disc herniation is the working diagnosis, and discography is used when degenerative disc disease is being sought.

Significant controversy exists regarding whether MRI or provocative discography is a more accurate test to diagnose degenerative disc disease. There are numerous published reports of patients with abnormal discograms who had normal MRI studies. Similarly, there are numerous studies that document abnormal MRIs in patients who have normal discograms.

MR imaging is a noninvasive study. As such, many surgeons prefer to use this study as a screening tool prior to the more invasive discography procedure. Boden and associates documented abnormal MRI studies in one third of clinically asymptomatic patients.[5] This study has led many investigators to consider MRI to be excessively sensitive in the diagnosis of painful degenerative disc disease. The earliest sign of a degenerated or dehydrated disc on MRI is a black signal intensity on T2-weighted images of the intervertebral disc. Whereas MRI may be overly sensitive, numerous investigators have found that if a disc appears more degenerated on MRI, it is more likely to be associated with pain.[8,22]

In 1992, Aprill and Bogduk introduced the concept of the high-intensity zone (HIZ). They define an HIZ as a focus of high signal intensity on T2-weighted imaging within the posterior annulus of a degenerative disc. These authors felt that the HIZ represented inflammation in the annulus secondary to trapped nuclear material. Furthermore, they postulated that the high intensity zone is predictive of a painful degenerative disc responsible for low back pain.[2] Subsequently, other investigators have also found the presence of an HIZ on MR imaging to be a reliable marker of a painful outer annulus disruption.[45,48] Advocates of discography have previously claimed that discograms are superior for determining annular pathology.[22,39,65] At the present time, it is unclear whether discography or a high intensity zone on MRI is more sensitive for accurately diagnosing a painful

annular disruption. Ricketson and associates stated that an HIZ probably represents neovascularity or granulation tissue within the posterior annulus, which is induced by inflammation. Whereas these authors stated that an HIZ was never seen in a morphologically normal disc, they cautioned that the presence of an HIZ on MR imaging is not necessarily associated with a positive concordant pain response.[42]

Additional advances in MR imaging include the use of the bony vibration test. Vanharanta and associates found that pain provoked by the vibration test can improve the specificity of MRI in the diagnosis of symptomatic lumbar disc herniations.[58] Likewise, Yrjama and associates stated that the combination of an MRI with a positive bony vibration test gives more information on the origin of back pain than MRI alone.[64]

COMPLICATIONS OF DISCOGRAPHY

Although discography is an invasive procedure, the complication rate of discography in experienced hands is quite low. The most frequently reported complication is bacterial discitis.[17,18,29,33] Aseptic discitis may also occur.[7] Fraser and associates reported a discitis rate of 2.7% when a large bore needle was used. This rate decreased to 0.7% when stiletted needles and a two needle technique were used.[15] Guyer and Ohnmeiss, in 1995, published the position statement from the North American Spine Society Diagnostic and Therapeutic Committee. In this report, they summarized the overall incidence of discitis to be 0.15%.[18] Although rare, bacterial discitis is a serious complication that requires prolonged antibiotic treatment.[17,39]

Other than discitis, complications related to discography are extremely rare. Isolated reports have described the complications of retroperitoneal hemorrhage, urticaria, spinal epidural abscess, and dural violation.[3,24,29] Although an assortment of complications is possible following an invasive procedure in the spine, the overall complication rate in experienced hands remains extremely low with discography. Although not truly a complication, the technical difficulty of an inability to access the L5-S1 interspace has been frequently noted in most large series. Common suggestions to avoid complications include the use of biplane fluoroscopy to confirm needle placement, the use of a two needle technique, the use of nonionic contrast dye, use of antibiotic in the dye solution, and avoidance of discography procedures in patients with known bleeding diatheses. Overall, the complication rate for provocative discography is acceptable.

SUMMARY

Provocative discography remains a controversial diagnostic study. The majority of medical literature on this subject has been reported by investigators who believe in the efficacy and use of this diagnostic tool. Detractors of provocative discography have questioned the value of this procedure. Nachemson, in 1989, condemned the use of discography.[35] More recently, Carragee and associates, in 2000, have published reports questioning the validity of this study.[9,10]

We advocate the use of "blinded" provocative discography in selected situations. The appropriate discography patient should have a clinical history and physical examination consistent with the diagnosis of degenerative disc disease. Specifically, useful historical information includes the presence of predominantly low back pain as well as the presence of sitting intolerance. The physical examination should not demonstrate nerve root tension signs. Appropriate candidates for discography should have experienced a prolonged attempt at aggressive conservative therapy that failed. At a minimum, the conservative treatment regimen should include a course of physical therapy and an optimization of ideal body weight, if possible. Additional conservative measures have been previously outlined. In those patients with suggestive evidence of degenerative disc disease, an MRI of the lumbar spine, which demonstrates a black disc on T2-weighted images, is suggestive of a painful degenerative disc. Recent advances with MR imaging, including the presence of high intensity zones and the use of vibration tests, have attempted to correlate positive MRI findings with low back pain. At the present time, the specificity and sensitivity of MR imaging for the diagnosis of a painful degenerative lumbar disc disease is inadequate. As such, we would not recommend a spinal fusion procedure based solely on the presence of a suggestive clinical history and physical exam and a positive MR imaging study.

In a patient who has failed a conservative treatment regimen with an appropriate history and physical examination, a normal psychological profile, and a positive MR imaging study, a "blinded" provocative discogram is indicated. The *blinded* study refers to performance of the lumbar discogram by a discographer who is unaware of the results of the previously obtained MR imaging study. Routinely, this study will evaluate the L3-L4, L4-L5, and L5-S1 disc spaces. A positive blinded provocative discogram will have both a positive concordant pain response and abnormal imaging at the level that matches the findings of the abnormal MRI. By having the discographer "blinded," a potential bias in the interpretation of the diagnostic result is removed. The theory is that blinding the discographer will increase the specificity of the study. A blinded provocative discogram should only be used for patients who are candidates for further invasive treatment, such as a spinal fusion procedure or, possibly, the recently described procedure of intradiscal electrothermy (IDET).

If the information obtained from the history, physical examination, psychological profile, and MR imaging study, in a patient who has failed conservative therapy, correlates precisely with the results of a blinded provocative discogram, then the likelihood that a degenerative lumbar intervertebral disc is a pain generator that will respond positively to further treatment is increased. As such, in appropriately selected patients, provocative discography is a useful adjunctive diagnostic tool.

REFERENCES

1. Adams MA, Dolan P, Hutton WC: The stages of disc degeneration as revealed by discograms. **J Bone Joint Surg** 68B:36-41, 1986.
2. Aprill C, Bogduk N: High-intensity zone: a diagnostic sign of painful lumbar disc on magnetic resonance imaging. **Br J Radiol** 65:361-69, 1992.
3. Bernard TN Jr: Lumbar discography followed by computed tomography—refining the diagnosis of low-back pain. **Spine** 15:690-707, 1990.
4. Birney TJ, White JJ Jr, Berens D et al: Comparison of MRI and discography in the diagnosis of lumbar degenerative disc disease. **J Spinal Disord** 5:417-23, 1992.
5. Boden SD, Davis DO, Dina TS et al: Abnormal magnetic-resonance scans of the lumbar spine in asymptomatic subjects: a prospective investigation. **J Bone Joint Surg** 72A:403-8, 1990.
6. Brightbill TC, Pile N, Eichelberger RP et al: Normal magnetic resonance imaging and abnormal discography in lumbar disc disruption. **Spine** 19:1075-7, 1994.
7. Brodsky AE, Binder WF: Lumbar discography—its value in diagnosis and treatment of lumbar disc lesions. **Spine** 4:110-20, 1979.
8. Buirski G, Silberstein M: The symptomatic lumbar disc in patients with low-back pain—magnetic resonance imaging appearances in both a symptomatic and control population. **Spine** 18:1808-11, 1993.
9. Carragee EJ, Tanner CM, Khurana S et al: The rates of false-positive lumbar discography in selected patients without low back symptoms. **Spine** 25:1373-81, 2000.
10. Carragee EJ, Tanner CM, Yang B et al: False-positive findings on lumbar discography—reliability of subjective concordance assessment during provocative disc injection. **Spine** 24:2542-7, 1999.
11. Colhoun E, McCall IW, Williams L et al: Provocation discography as a guide to planning operations on the spine. **J Bone Joint Surg** 70B:267-71, 1988.
12. Crock HV: A reappraisal of intervertebral disc lesions. **Med J Australia** 1:983-9, 1970.
13. Derby R, Howard MW, Grant JM et al: The ability of pressure-controlled discography to predict surgical and nonsurgical outcomes. **Spine** 24:364-72, 1999.
14. Fairbank JCT, Deans W: Letter to the editor. **Spine** 15:839-40, 1990.
15. Fraser RD, Osti OL, Vernon-Roberts B: Discitis after discography. **J Bone Joint Surg** 69B:26-35, 1987.

16. Gunzburg R, Parkinson R, Moore R et al: A cadaveric study comparing discography, magnetic resonance imaging, histology, and mechanical behavior of the human lumbar disc. **Spine** 17:417-23, 1992.

17. Guyer RD, Collier R, Stith WJ et al: Discitis after discography. **Spine** 13:1352-4, 1988.

18. Guyer RD, Ohnmeiss DD: Contemporary concepts in spine care—lumbar discography. Position Statement from the North American Spine Society Diagnostic and Therapeutic Committee. **Spine** 20:2048-59, 1995.

19. Heggeness MH, Walters WC III, Gray PM Jr: Discography of lumbar discs after surgical treatment for disc herniation. **Spine** 22:1606-9, 1997.

20. Holt EP Jr: The question of lumbar discography. **J Bone Joint Surg** 58A:720-26, 1968.

21. Horton WC, Daftari TK: Which disc as visualized by magnetic resonance imaging is actually a source of pain—a correlation between magnetic resonance imaging and discography. **Spine** 17 (Suppl 6):S164-71, 1992.

22. Ito M, Incorvaia KM, Yu SF et al: Predictive signs of discogenic lumbar pain on magnetic resonance imaging with discography correlation. **Spine** 23:1252-60, 1998.

23. Ito S, Muro T, Urasaki T et al: Re-evaluation of discograms not classified into usual classifications. **J Spinal Disord** 12:151-56, 1999.

24. Junilla J, Niinimaki T, Tervonen O: Epidural abscess after lumbar discography. **Spine** 22:2191-3, 1997.

25. Kornberg M: Computed tomography of the lumbar spine following discography. **Spine** 12:823-25, 1987.

26. Lindblom K: Diagnostic puncture of intervertebral discs in sciatica. **Acta Orthop Scand** 17:231-39, 1948.

27. Linsom MA, Crowe CH: Comparison of magnetic resonance imaging and lumbar discography in the diagnosis of disc degeneration. **Clin Orthop** 250:160-63, 1990.

28. Maezawa S, Muro T: Pain provocation at lumbar discography as analyzed by computed tomography/discography. **Spine** 17:1309-15, 1992.

29. McCulloch JA, Waddell G: Lateral lumbar discography. **B J Radiol** 51:498-502, 1978.

30. McCutcheon ME, Thompson WC: CT scanning of lumbar discography—a useful diagnostic adjunct. **Spine** 11:257-59, 1986.

31. McFadden JW: The stress lumbar discogram. **Spine** 13:931-33, 1988.

32. Milette PC, Fontaine S, Lepanto L et al: Differentiating lumbar disc protrusions, disc bulges, and discs with normal contour but abnormal signal intensity—magnetic resonance imaging with discographic correlations. **Spine** 24:44-53, 1999.

33. Milette PC, Melanson D: A reappraisal of lumbar discography. **J Can Assoc Radiologists** 33:176-82, 1982.

34. Moneta GB, Videman T, Kaivanto K et al: Reported pain during lumbar discography as a function of anular ruptures and disc degeneration—a re-analysis of 833 discograms. **Spine** 19:1968-74, 1994.

35. Nachemson A: Editorial comment: lumbar discography—where are we today? **Spine** 14:555-57, 1989.

36. Ohnmeiss DD, Vanharanta H, Ekholm J: Degree of disc disruption and lower extremity pain. **Spine** 22:1600-5, 1997.

37. Ohnmeiss DD, Vanharanta H, Ekholm J: Relation between pain location and disc pathology: a study of pain drawings and CT/discography. **Clin J Pain** 15:210-17, 1999.

38. Ohnmeiss DD, Vanharanta H, Guyer RD: The association between pain drawings and computed tomographic/discographic pain responses. **Spine** 20:729-33, 1995.

39. Osti OL, Fraser RD: MRI and discography of annular tears and intervertebral disc degeneration—a prospective clinical comparison. **J Bone Joint Surg** 74B:431-35, 1992.

40. Quinnell RC, Stockdale HR: Flexion and extension radiography of the lumbar spine: a comparison with lumbar discography. **Clin Radiol** 34:405-11, 1983.

41. Rankine JJ, Gill KP, Hutchinson CE et al: The clinical significance of the high-intensity zone on lumbar spine magnetic resonance imaging. **Spine** 24:1913-20, 1999.

42. Ricketson R, Simmons JW, Hauser BO: The prolapsed intervertebral disc—the high-intensity zone with discography correlation. **Spine** 21:2758-62, 1996.

43. Saal JA, Saal JS: Intradiscal electrothermal treatment for chronic discogenic low back pain: a prospective outcome study with minimum 1-year follow-up. **Spine** 25:2622-27, 2000.

44. Sachs BL, Vanharanta H, Spivey MA et al: Dallas discogram description—a new classification of CT/discography in low-back disorders. **Spine** 12:287-94, 1987.

45. Saifuddin A, Braithwaite I, White J et al: The value of lumbar spine magnetic resonance imaging in the demonstration of annular tears. **Spine** 23:453-57, 1998.

46. Schechter NA, France MP, Lee CK: Painful internal disc derangements of the lumbosacral spine: discographic diagnosis and treatment by posterior lumbar interbody fusion. **Orthopaedics** 14:447-51, 1991.

47. Schellhas KP, Pollei SR: The role of discography in the evaluation of patients with spinal deformity. **Orthop Clin North Am** 25:265-73, 1994.

48. Schellhas KP, Pollei SR, Gundry CR et al: Lumbar disc high-intensity zone—correlation of magnetic resonance imaging and discography. **Spine** 21:79-86, 1996.

49. Schnebel BE, Simmons JW, Chowning J et al: A digitizing technique for the study of movement of intradiscal dye in response to flexion and extension of the lumbar spine. **Spine** 13:309-12, 1988.

50. Schwarzer AC, Aprill CN, Derby R et al: The prevalence and clinical features of internal disc disruption in patients with chronic low back pain. **Spine** 20:1878-83, 1995.

51. Simmons JW, Aprill CN, Dwyer AP et al: A reassessment of Holt's data on: "The questions of lumbar discography." **Clin Orthop** 237:120-24, 1988.

52. Simmons JW, Emery SF, McMillin JN et al: Awake discography—a comparison study with magnetic resonance imaging. **Spine** 16 (Suppl 6):S216-21, 1991.

53. Soini J, Antti-Poika I, Tallroth K et al: Disc degeneration and angular movement of the lumbar spine: comparative study using plain and flexion-extension radiography and discography. **J Spinal Disord** 4:183-87, 1991.

54. Southern EP, Fye MA, Panjabi MM et al: Disc degeneration—a human cadaveric study correlating magnetic resonance imaging and quantitative discomanometry. **Spine** 25:2171-5, 2000.

55. Tervonen O, Lahde S, Rydberg J: Lumbar disc degeneration—correlation between CT and CT/discography. **Acta Radiologica** 31:551-54, 1990.

56. Urasaki T, Muro T, Ito S et al: Consistency of lumbar discograms of the same disc obtained twice at a 2-week interval: influence of needle tip position. **J Orthop Sci** 3:243-51, 1998.
57. Vanharanta H, Floyd T, Ohnmeiss DD et al: The relationship of facet tropism to degenerative disc disease. **Spine** 18:1000-5, 1993.
58. Vanharanta H, Ohnmeiss DD, Aprill CN: Vibration pain provocation can improve the specificity of MRI in the diagnosis of symptomatic lumbar disc rupture. **Clin J Pain** 14:239-47, 1998.
59. Vanharanta H, Sachs BL, Ohnmeiss DD et al: Pain provocation and disc deterioration by age—a CT/discography study in a low-back pain population. **Spine** 14:420-23, 1989.
60. Vanharanta H, Sachs BL, Spivey MA et al: The relationship of pain provocation to lumbar disc deterioration as seen by CT/discography. **Spine** 12:295-98, 1987.
61. Weinstein J, Claverie W, Gibson S: The pain of discography. **Spine** 13:1344-8, 1988.
62. Wilson DH, MacCarty WC: Discography: its role in the diagnosis of lumbar disc protrusion. **J Neurosurg** 31:520-23, 1969.
63. Yasuma T, Ohno R, Yamauchi Y: False-negative lumbar discograms. **J Bone Joint Surg** 70A:1279-90, 1988.
64. Yrjama M, Tervonen O, Kurunlahti M et al: Bony vibration stimulation test combined with magnetic resonance imaging—can discography be replaced? **Spine** 22:808-13, 1997.
65. Zucherman J, Derby R, Hsu K et al: Normal magnetic resonance imaging with abnormal discography. **Spine** 13:1355-9, 1988.

CHAPTER 5

Geometrical Considerations for the Surgical Management of Low Back Pain

JORGE J. LASTRA, M.D.

BYRON H. WILLIS, M.D.

EDWARD C. BENZEL, M.D., F.A.C.S.

INTRODUCTION

Low back pain is a complex, multifaceted entity that represents one of the most common reasons for patients to seek the consultation of a physician.[10] Most low back pain is self-limited, with 90% to 95% of affected individuals returning to normal, pain-free activities within three months of onset.[2,12] The remaining patients are classified as having chronic low back pain. They represent a significant challenge to the physician. Confounding an accurate diagnosis is the high percentage of asymptomatic patients with radiographic evidence of degenerative disc disease in the age group in which low back pain complaints are greatest.[26]

The spine surgeon must approach the problem of low back pain in a logical, stepwise manner. This entails a thorough knowledge of the relevant structural and neural spinal anatomy. The geometrical anatomy of the spine can provide a basis for an analytical and structured approach to addressing normal and dysfunctional spinal motion. The spine surgeon can use biomechanical principles to identify the best techniques to eliminate or reduce any dysfunctional spinal motion postulated to be the source of spine pain.

ANATOMY OF SPINAL NOCICEPTIVE INNERVATION

The innervation of the lumbar spinal motion segment and associated soft tissue structures has been extensively studied. The sinuvertebral nerve is implicated in the innervation of ventral pain sensitive structures.[6] The nerve is formed by the fusion of an autonomic branch from a gray ramus communicans and a spinal nerve branch just distal to the dorsal root ganglion.[37] The nerve splits into multiple branches and innervates the periosteum of the vertebral body, the posterior longitudinal ligament, the dorsal aspect of the annulus fibrosus, the ventral aspect of the dura mater, and associated blood vessels.[6,13,14,18,31] This innervation runs one segment rostral and two segments caudal, resulting in considerable overlap of spinal segments.[6,18] The dorsal surface of the dura mater is sparsely innervated. The inner annulus and nucleus of the disc is not innervated. Branches of the ventral ramus of the spinal nerves, autonomic branches from the gray rami communicans, and branches from the sympathetic trunk innervate the ventral and lateral outer annulus and anterior longitudinal ligament. Branches off the dorsal ramus of the spinal nerve innervate the facet joints.[21,27] Innervation of the ligamentum flavum and interspinous ligaments is controversial.

CLASSIFICATION OF SPINE PAIN

Clinical manifestations of spine pain can be delineated based on the primary pathological process. They include spine pain without neural compression, spine pain with neural compression, spine pain referred from extraspinous tissues, and spine pain secondary to paraspinal muscle spasm. Multiple underlying etiologies exist and have considerable overlap as they relate to each clinical syndrome and to each anatomical abnormality.

Spine Pain without Neural Compression

This type of pain can be isolated to a specific region of the spine (localized) or can radiate in general patterns that have no localizing value (referred). Localized spine pain is typically deep, boring, and aching in nature, exacerbated by spine loading (activity), and alleviated by unloading (rest).

Pain referred from the spine is typically deep, ill-defined, and poorly localized in nature. It radiates to the buttock, thigh, and occasionally the calf, typically without any involvement of the foot. There is no objective weakness, atrophy, or sensory loss; however, occasional attenuation of deep tendon reflexes may be seen.

Spine Pain with Neural Compression

Low back pain with radiculopathy and/or myelopathy suggests an underlying element of neural compression either peripherally, with involvement of nerve roots, or centrally, with compression of the spinal cord. This type of pain can be subclassified into radicular and funicular pain. *Radicular pain* is caused by irritation of a nerve root with the pain distribution encompassing a subset of the dermatomal area subserved by that root. *Dermatomal radicular pain* is defined as sharp, stabbing, and shooting pain that is superimposed on a chronic aching pain. The distribution is typically well defined and localizes the involved nerve root with a high degree of accuracy. The pain is typically aggravated by activities that increase the stretch or compression on the root, such as coughing, sneezing, straining, extension, lateral bending, or straight leg raising. Myotomal radicular pain is characterized as deep, aching, diffuse, and dull in nature. It is associated with nerve root compression and typically involves the myotome of the associated ventral nerve root.

Funicular pain arises from compression or irritation of the spinothalamic tracts or posterior columns of the spinal cord, causing sharp jabbing sensations on a background of burning, diffuse, poorly localized pain. It can be provoked by cutaneous stimulation or movement of the spine. The pain distribution can cover both the trunk and any combination of extremities, depending on the location of the spinal cord compression.

Neurogenic claudication is another neural compression syndrome. The pain of neurogenic claudication is typically in the lower back with ill-defined and poorly localized pain radiating down the lower extremities, often accompanied by paresthesias. The pain may also come on slowly with prolonged extension of the lumbar spine. The relief of pain is prolonged and associated with reduction of lumber extension and/or reduction of activity (e.g., ambulation).

Referred Spine Pain

Pain that originates in tissues anatomically distant from the spine may be referred to the low back. This type of pain is often dull, aching, and poorly localized, although this may vary based on the underlying pathological process. The spine is usually not tender to palpation, and a full range of motion is typical on physical examination. Visceral pain can be referred to the back through common neural pathways or may cause inflammation or pressure on structures adjacent to the spine.

Visceral pain afferent fibers travel through both the parasympathetic and sympathetic divisions of the autonomic nervous system. In the parasympathetic system, the pain afferents travel via the vagus nerve and pelvic splanchnic nerves. In the sympathetic nervous system, the afferent pain fibers enter the sympathetic chain and subsequently travel to the corresponding spinal nerve root via the white rami communicans. The common pathways of these pain afferents and the associated spinal nerve roots give rise to referred pain.

Pain Secondary to Paraspinal Muscle Spasm

This type of pain is typically of acute onset with a history of injury or excessive activity, resulting in a painful, tender muscle. This type of pain can be well localized, aching, or cramping in character. There is often evidence of muscle spasm on physical examination. Muscle spasm is a common response to muscle injury, nerve irritation, or tissue inflammation. Paraspinal muscle spasm often represents a reflexive defense to guard against continued mechanical irritation of inflamed or otherwise damaged tissues.

Another type of spinal pain, the myofascial pain syndrome, can be either local or referred in nature.[32,33] The involved muscle group typically generates local pain or pain that is referred to a specific area. The region of pain may be tender to palpation and there may be subjective weakness of the underlying muscle groups. Myofascial pain syndromes are associated with hyperirritable foci known as trigger points that, when stimulated, reproduce the patient's pain.

Mechanical Low Back Pain

Mechanical low back pain is a subtype of spine pain without neural compression. This entity has a distinct clinical syndrome and has distinct associated radiographic abnormalities as described below.

Clinical Syndrome

The clinical syndrome of mechanical low back pain associated with an abnormal spinal motion segment consists of the following:

1. Deep agonizing pain not associated with paraspinous muscle spasm, neural deficit, or neural compression syndromes.

2. The association of the pain with activity or with stresses placed on the allegedly painful motion segment.

3. The diminution or elimination of the pain upon minimization or elimination of stresses on the allegedly painful motion segment.[3]

Radiographic Abnormalities

Plain radiographic evidence of abnormal spinal motion can be either direct or indirect. Indirect evidence of abnormal spinal motion at the allegedly painful motion segment includes the following:

1. Decreased disc space height.
2. Sclerosed and irregular end-plates.
3. Osteophyte formation.
4. Loss of lumbar lordosis.
5. Vacuum disc.
6. Fixed subluxation.[3]

Direct evidence of abnormal spinal motion is excessive motion visible on flexion/extension films. The degree to which these findings are present can help to determine if significant instability is present. White and Panjabi use 4mm of translation and 10° of angulation to define spinal instability on dynamic films.[39] The utility of these findings is limited without corroborating clinical and historical data from the patient. It is well known that a high percentage of the population over the age of 60 has radiographic evidence of spondylosis, with only a small fraction being symptomatic.[5,38] Magnetic resonance imaging (MRI) is used extensively in the evaluation of patients with back and leg pain. Loss of T2 signal in the intervertebral disc, annular tears, end-plate signal changes, and marrow signal changes immediately adjacent to the end-plates all contribute to a diagnosis of degenerative disc disease and suggest abnormal spinal motion at the involved segments.[41]

Discography is a diagnostic modality that attempts to identify the pain generating spinal segment by reproducing the patient's pain. This is accomplished by increasing the intradiscal pressure in the studied disc. Many studies have investigated the usefulness of this procedure, and the results indicate that discography may be beneficial for patients with definite abnormalities on MRI scans but not in the context of a normal MRI.[20,30]

BIOMECHANICAL CONSIDERATIONS IN THE DEVELOPMENT OF MECHANICAL LOW BACK PAIN

The spine is designed to provide a certain degree of preprogrammed intrinsic motion via the coupling of multiple motion segments. Each motion segment is comprised of two vertebrae, their intervertebral discs, associated facets, and paraspinal soft tissue. A spinal motion segment can be characterized by a stress/strain curve for each degree of freedom of movement. The human spine functions within the linear (elastic) portion of the stress/strain curves for normal loading situations. Each load applied to a given spinal motion segment can be broken down into component vectors related to axial loading, rotational loading, bending moments, and shear stresses. Loads applied to the normal spine typically lie on the linear portion of the stress/strain curve. Excessive loads move onto the nonlinear portion of the curve where permanent mechanical deformation may occur. Extreme loads may lead to frank structural failure. The ability of each spinal motion segment to withstand certain loads without permanent deformation depends on the modulus of elasticity of the given segment in the given loading plane. As loads increase, or as the modulus of elasticity of the spinal motion segment changes, the segment will be "operating" closer to the limit of the linear range of its stress/strain curve, causing repetitive microtrauma. Thus, degeneration of a spinal motion segment can be accelerated by either increasing the applied load or by altering the geometry of the segment to effectively magnify the load "seen" by the motion segment.

An individual predisposition to degeneration of the spine can be modeled as an alteration of the modulus of elasticity of the spinal segment. The anatomical correlate of this predisposition may be poor collagen production, which would result in weak ligaments, annular fibers, and joint tissues. Through excessive loading of the spine and forcing the spinal motion segment to function at the limits of the linear portion of the stress/strain curve, tissue damage may result. The resulting tissue damage can lead to new or increased abnormal spinal motion. This abnormal motion causes certain anatomical changes in the motion segment that can be seen using modern imaging strategies and that are well documented. The anatomical abnormalities can lead to neural compression. Dysfunctional spinal motion is the postulated underlying mechanism for mechanical low back pain through stimulation of spinal nociceptors.

MANAGEMENT OF MECHANICAL LOW BACK PAIN

The diagnosis of *mechanical low back pain* is made based on a characteristic history and appropriate objective findings upon physical examination and imaging studies. These findings should corroborate the historical and subjective findings that lead to the diagnosis of mechanical low back pain. Once the diagnosis has been made, the next step is to engage the patient as an active participant in his or her care. This includes an assessment of the patient's motivation to participate in both nonoperative and postoperative treatment strategies. A poor clinical outcome will be more likely in poorly motivated patients, independent of the type of treatment. A comprehensive plan should be agreed upon by both the patient and the primary caregiver of the spine. The goals of the initial plan should include patient education, improvement in mental and physical condition, lowering of surgical risk by modifying behavior, and reduction or elimination of low back pain by nonoperative treatment modalities.

NONSURGICAL MANAGEMENT OF LOW BACK PAIN

Components of a comprehensive nonoperative plan include the following:

1. An aerobic exercise program for sedentary patients.
2. A stretching exercise program.
3. A strengthening exercise program.
4. A weight loss program for overweight patients.
5. A tobacco cessation program.
6. A drug withdrawal program for patients addicted to pain medications or alcohol.
7. A psychiatric treatment program for depressed patients.
8. An educational program.

Aerobic Exercises

Aerobic exercises improve a patient's physical condition and sense of well being. Some examples include walking, swimming, cycling, and running. Several exercises should be selected, depending on patient characteristics, pain pattern, and patient preference.

Stretching Exercises

Pain can cause stiffness of the lumbar spine because of voluntary or involuntary guarding to minimize the pain associated with dysfunctional spinal motion. Abnormal spinal movement can lead to an alteration of normal sagittal balance, resulting in a compensatory stressing of paraspinous, gluteal, and lower extremity muscles.

Flexibility can be improved with stretching exercises. Simple exercises include flexion bending (Figure 5-1). This can be monitored and objectively assessed by measuring the distance between the fingers and the floor at each visit. Similarly, extension exercises may be performed (Figure 5-1). These exercises improve patient flexibility and well being in a goal-oriented manner.

Strengthening Exercises

The abdominal and paraspinal muscle groups assist with normal spinal motion, provide support, and min-

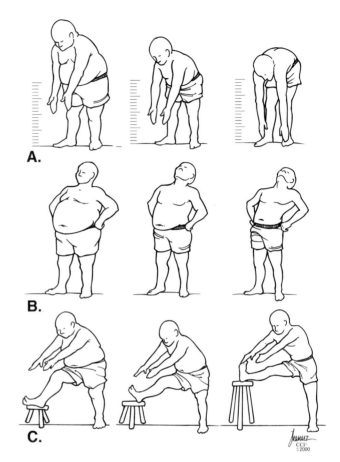

FIGURE 5-1 ■ Stretching exercises. A, Toe touching. Note the method of measuring and monitoring progress; **B,** Back extension; and **C,** "Foot on stool" exercise. This augments both flexion and rotation flexibility. (From Benzel EC: **Biomechanics of Spine Stabilization: Principles and Clinical Practice.** New York: McGraw-Hill, Inc. 1995, with permission.)

imize abnormal movement of the spine. The strengthening of these muscles can assist with spinal stability while at the same time reducing abnormal movement that can incite pain.

Strengthening exercises for the paraspinal muscles include prone leg lifts, airplane, or rocking chair exercises (Figure 5-2). Strengthening exercises for the abdominal muscles include supine leg lifts and sit-ups (Figure 5-2).

Weight Loss Program

Obesity increases the axial load applied to the spine and the predisposition for abnormal segmental movement and degeneration. As a result of more weight ventral to the spine, a compensatory hyperlordosis of the lumbar spine can result in accelerated degeneration of the facet joints. A weight loss program in which the patient monitors caloric intake, with regular

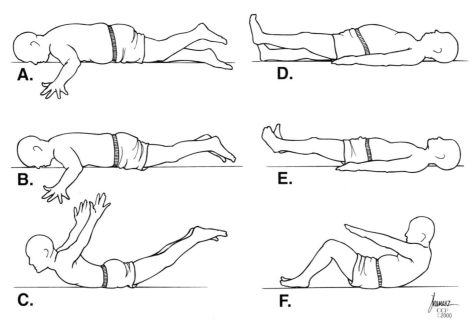

FIGURE 5-2 ■ **Strengthening exercises.** Paraspinous and other dorsal low back muscles can be strengthened by prone leglifts, beginning with one leg at a time (**A**) and progressing to both legs (**B**) and, finally, to the head, chest, and both legs (the "airplane" or "rocking chair" maneuver) (**C**). Abdominal muscles can be strengthened by leg lifts, beginning with one leg at a time (**D**) and progressing to both legs (**E**) and, finally, to sit-ups (**F**). (From Benzel EC: **Biomechanics of Spine Stabilization: Principles and Clinical Practice**. New York: McGraw-Hill, Inc. 1995, with permission.)

weight monitoring and quantification of improvement, is ideal.

Tobacco Cessation Program

Tobacco use is related to back pain.[11] Smoking cessation can help reduce back pain and can improve exercise tolerance. Smoking cessation can also help improve fusion rate in the event that surgery is eventually required.

Drug Withdrawal Program

The patient with alcohol dependency needs pre-operative detoxification to minimize alcohol withdrawal and to decrease perioperative and surgical risk. The patient who is dependent on pain medication because of chronic pain will benefit from the pre-operative reduction in narcotic medications.

Psychiatric Treatment

Many patients develop depression because of low back pain and can harbor back pain as a manifestation of depression. The identification of such patients and the initiation of appropriate treatment are exceedingly important to the efficacy of any treatment plan.

Patient Education

Patient education should be comprehensive and should include details about many of the above topics. A thorough knowledge of what causes the patient's pain and what can relieve the pain will help the patient be a more involved and active participant in his or her care.

SURGICAL MANAGEMENT

The correlation between fusion rate and the relief of mechanical low back pain is varied in the literature and is dependent on the fusion technique employed. One report by Stauffer and Coventry reported 89% good results with an 80% radiographic fusion rate using dorsolateral fusion[34]. Findlayson, in a similar series of 20 patients, had only six patients reporting a good outcome.[16] Wood and associates, in 1995, reported a 70% to 85% success rate of fusions using transpedicular instrumentation.[40] Overall, the pseudoarthrosis rates of instrumented versus noninstrumented fusions

(0% vs. 33%) and clinical improvement (77%–95% vs. 59%–70%) suggest that dorsolateral fusion for degenerative disc disease should include fixation.[15,19,20,24,35,42]

It is evident from the above studies that clinical relief of back pain is not perfectly correlated with fusion rate. This suggests that either dysfunctional spinal motion is not the sole cause of mechanical low back pain or that better selection criteria should be defined.

The patient who is motivated, but who has not improved with an aggressive nonoperative management program, should be considered for surgery. The patient should understand the surgical procedure, the benefits, the risks, and the rehabilitation process. The surgeon must be certain that the patient's expectations of the surgery are appropriate and reasonable.

GEOMETRICAL CONSIDERATIONS

The spinal fusion strategy should be based on geometrical and biomechanical factors. These factors include the following:

1. Applied forces at the disc interspace.
2. Subsidence.
3. Restoration of disc height.
4. Angular deformation and sagittal balance.
5. Graft bed preparation.
6. Strut position.
7. Strut integrity.
8. Strut geometry.
9. Ligamentous disruption.
10. Load sharing versus load bearing.[4]

Applied Forces at the Disc Interspace

Spinal segmental motion involves bidirectional motion along (translation) or about (rotation) the three axes of the Cartesian coordinate system (Figure 5-3)[29,39] The magnitude of each applied force vector is dependent on the underlying orientation of the spinal elements. This alignment will determine if shear stresses, axial loading, or rotational forces predominate at a given motion segment. For example, at the L5-S1 disc interspace, the end-plates are not aligned perpendicular to vertically applied axial loads, leading to increased shear stresses at that particular disc interspace (Figure 5-4).[4] The larger shear force component of applied loads at this level should be taken into account during construct planning. Translation is theoretically more prone to occur postoperatively with fusion at L5-S1. Interbody struts, including cages, are typically ineffective in preventing this translational movement. In this case, the placement of dorsal fixation should be considered. Although cages are designed to function as interference screws and to

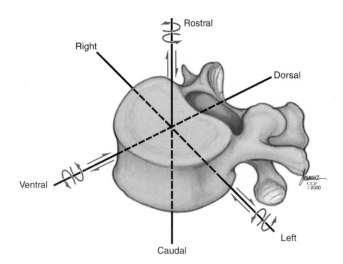

FIGURE 5-3 ■ **The Cartesian coordinate system centered on the vertebral body.** Motion occurs in a bidirectional manner along (*straight arrows*) and about (*curved arrows*) each axis.

limit translational motion (Figure 5-5), they are usually ineffective in this regard.

Subsidence

Postoperative decrease in disc space height following anterior interbody fusion is seen with some frequency. This postoperative axial deformation, or *subsidence*,

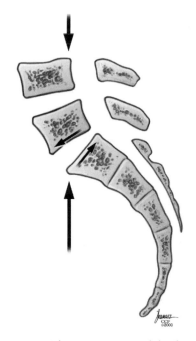

FIGURE 5-4 ■ The orientation of the lumbosacral disc interspace causes a portion of applied axial forces (*vertical arrows*) to be converted to shear forces (*diagonal arrows*).

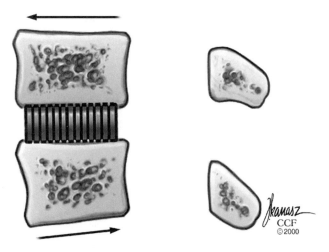

FIGURE 5-5 ■ TIFCs provide minimal resistance to shear forces (*arrows*).

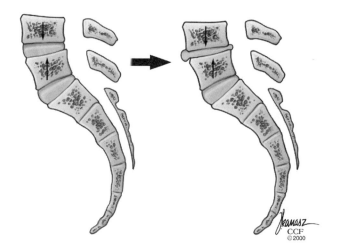

FIGURE 5-6 ■ The lumbar spine loses intervertebral disc height with time because of repetitive axial loading (*vertical arrows*).

can be secondary to several factors. Some of the common causes of subsidence are the following:

1. Pistoning of an interbody strut into the vertebral body because of fracture of the end-plate or excessive removal of the end-plate during graft bed preparation.
2. A mismatch of the modulus of elasticity between the strut and the vertebral body, resulting in either graft or end-plate fracture.
3. Inadequate area of contact between the strut and the vertebral body, resulting in excessive pressures at the end-plates.
4. Poor geometrical interface between the strut and the graft bed.
5. Graft absorption secondary to stress shielding.
6. Graft dislodgment.

Restoration of Disc Height

After a fusion procedure, the spine will have a predisposition to subside until fusion is achieved. A solid fusion does not subside. One of the goals of threaded interbody fusion cage (TIFC) placement is to restore the intervertebral disc height, which in turn expands the neural foramina, decompressing neural structures.[8,36]

The distracted intervertebral space has significant axial and nonaxial loads placed upon it and will seek the state of lowest potential energy or highest entropy. *Entropy* is a measure of the degree of disorder of a system.[1] The second law of thermodynamics states that systems will change spontaneously from states of lower probability to states of higher probability.[1] The restoration and distraction of the interspace with a strut (TIFC) decreases the entropy. The axial and nonaxial loads placed on the intervertebral space result in a strong tendency toward disc inter-

space collapse and subsidence (Figure 5-6). A strategy that permits a state of high entropy (disc collapse), but that encourages fusion, as well as spinal alignment (sagittal balance) and neural decompression, may be more prudent.[4]

Angular Deformation and Sagittal Balance

The restoration and maintenance of sagittal balance is an important concept when designing a spinal fusion construct. Progressive kyphosis can occur postoperatively and can be exacerbated by the subsidence of an interbody strut.[22] The loss of lumbar lordosis creates a moment arm that encourages further kyphotic deformation by moving the instantaneous axis of rotation (IAR) ventrally. This deformation will increase the moment arm of applied forces, resulting in larger moments for given axial loading forces. In other words, "deformity begets deformity."

The placement of a cylindrical strut into a disc interspace can alter the trapezoidal relationship of the end-plates by making them parallel (Figure 5-7). This is

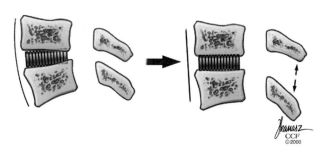

FIGURE 5-7 ■ Loss of lordosis at a single motion segment results after placement of a cylindrical implant into a trapezoidal shaped disc space. Distraction of the dorsal elements can occur (*vertical arrows*).

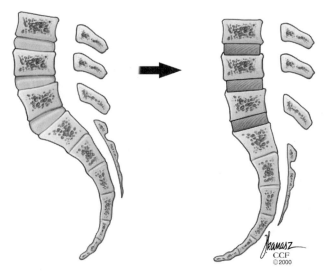

FIGURE 5-8 ■ Loss of lordosis of the lumbar spine caused by multiple level TIFC placement.

more dramatic with multiple level interbody cylindrical implants (Figure 5-8). A loss of lordosis and a disturbance of sagittal balance can result. This may become a source of persistent back pain.[4]

Graft Bed Preparation

Meticulous preparation of the strut and the graft bed is imperative for the success of a lumbar fusion. Insufficient debridement of the end-plates with inadequate exposure of the cancellous bone may result in pseudoarthrosis. Excessive end-plate debridement may result in end-plate fracture with a resultant loss of load-bearing capacity. The construct will then be predisposed to subsidence with the possible progression to kyphotic deformity.

Interbody struts by themselves provide little translational resistance (Figure 5-9A). Translational resistance may be increased with deep mortises in the vertebral bodies that encompass the strut (Figure 5-9B).

However, this technique damages the end-plates, reducing axial load-bearing capacity. A thorough knowledge of the anticipated applied load vectors can help determine whether axial or shear forces will predominate at a given spinal level, and the graft bed can be prepared appropriately.

Strut Position

The IAR is a dynamic axis that describes the point about which a motion segment rotates. With spinal flexion, the IAR tends to move ventrally, and with spinal extension, the IAR tends to move dorsally (Figure 5-10). With the addition of spinal instrumentation or a spinal fusion, the IAR tends to move toward the spinal implant (Figure 5-10). Axial loads applied ventral to the IAR will generate a flexion bending moment about the IAR. Axial loads applied dorsal to the IAR will generate an extension bending moment about the IAR. A strut placed in line with the pre-existing IARs (e.g., mid-vertebral bodies) has superior axial load-bearing capacity but provides little resistance to angular deformation from applied bending moments. A strut placed at a distance from the IAR resists applied bending moments (Figure 5-11).[3] For example, a dorsal onlay fusion has poor axial load-bearing capacity but resists bending moments and angular deformation by acting as a tension band fixator (Figure 5-12). The ability of a dorsal onlay fusion to resist applied bending moments is enhanced by increasing the distance from the fusion mass to the IAR, thereby increasing the moment arm of the construct (this assumes an intact middle column).

Strut Integrity

Strut integrity is essential to minimize collapse, reabsorption, and fracture of the interbody construct.[4] The

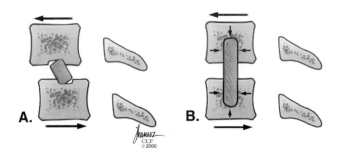

FIGURE 5-9 ■ **A**, Shallow mortices do not effectively resist significant translational forces (*horizontal arrows*); **B**, Deep mortices resist translational forces (*small horizontal arrows*) but have reduced axial load-bearing capacity (*vertical arrows*).

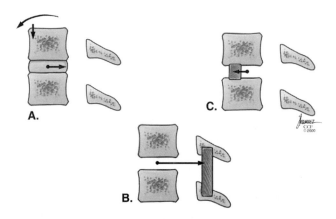

FIGURE 5-10 ■ **A**, The IAR (*dot*) shifts dorsally when an axial load is applied ventral to the IAR, creating a bending moment (*curved arrow*); **B** and **C**, A solid fusion causes the IAR to move toward the fusion mass.

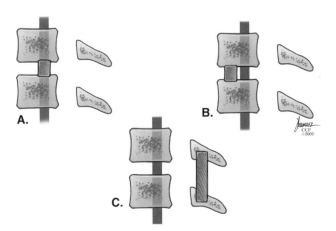

FIGURE 5-11 ■ **A**, Bone graft placement close to the IAR (*thick black line*) improves axial load-bearing capacity; **B**, A graft placed ventral to the IAR improves resistance to flexion where a graft placed dorsal to the IAR improves resistance to extension; **C**, Angular motion resistance is improved the further the fusion mass from the IAR, as in the dorsal onlay fusion.

strut and graft bed should each have a comparable modulus of elasticity. The *modulus of elasticity* characterizes the mechanical nature of a material and is defined as the amount of deformation a solid body will undergo in response to a force applied (the stress/strain ratio). The higher the modulus of elasticity, the stiffer the material. If the modulus of elasticity of a strut is greater than that of a graft bed, there is propensity for pistoning of the strut through the end-plate into the vertebral body, dislodgment, and subsidence (Figures 5-13*A,B*). A small area of contact between an interbody strut and graft bed can exacerbate pistoning (Fig-

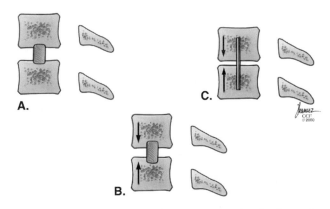

FIGURE 5-13 ■ **A** and **B**, A strut with a high modulus of elasticity will piston through a soft end-plate and vertebral body; **C**, Pistoning is encouraged if a strut has a small area of contact with the end-plate.

ure 5-13*C*). If the modulus of elasticity of the strut is less than the graft bed, there is propensity for strut collapse, fracture, and reabsorption.

Strut Geometry

The capacity to resist axial loads and to minimize micromotion via an interbody fusion is proportional to the surface area of contact between the bone graft and the graft bed.[4] The fusion rate increases as the surface area of contact increases. A larger surface area of contact between the graft and graft bed provides increased resistance to axial loads and reduces micromotion once fusion has occurred.

The contour of the strut should mimic the contour of the graft bed (Figure 5-14) and should mimic the

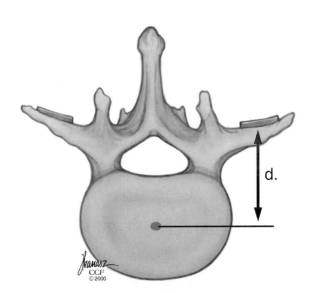

FIGURE 5-12 ■ A lateral intertransverse fusion positioned a distance "d" from the IAR.

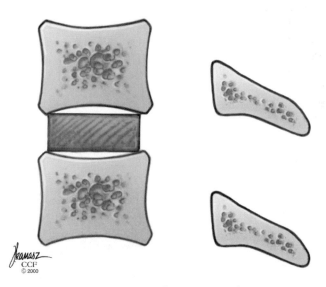

FIGURE 5-14 ■ Nonuniform contact between an intervertebral strut and elliptical shaped vertebral end-plates.

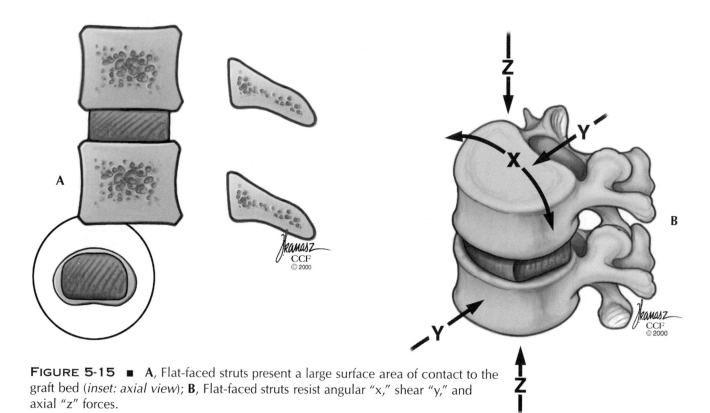

FIGURE 5-15 ■ **A**, Flat-faced struts present a large surface area of contact to the graft bed (*inset: axial view*); **B**, Flat-faced struts resist angular "x," shear "y," and axial "z" forces.

wedge-shaped lumbar intervertebral space. The strut should provide a maximum surface area of contact between the bone graft and the graft bed. A large surface area of contact between a strut (e.g., TIFC) and the graft bed does not imply a large surface area of contact between the bone graft and the graft bed. Metal may provide the majority of the contact.

Struts (e.g., TIFCs) are grouped into two categories based on the manner in which they interface with the graft bed, flat- or round-faced. Flat-faced struts can be square, rectangular, round, or oval. They present a relatively large area of contact to the graft bed (Figure 5-15A). They function in resisting compressive, angular, and translational deformation (Figure 5-15B).[4]

Round-faced struts, mostly characterized by the TIFC, present a round surface to the graft bed. Single cages that present a round surface to the graft bed function poorly in resisting angular deformation (Figure 5-16A) but adequately as paired cages (Figure 5-16B).[4] There is a relatively small surface area of bone graft contact with the graft bed (Figure 5-17A), particularly if not placed properly (Figure 5-17B).[4]

The placement of a cylindrical strut (e.g., TIFC) into an elliptical wedge-shaped lumbar interspace results in a nonuniform area of contact between the cage and the graft bed (Figure 5-18). Coronal cross-sectional views (planes A, B, and C in Figure 5-18) demonstrate the nonuniform nature of the contact between the implant and the end-plate. Minimal contact exists in plane A. This may provide a load-bearing capacity resistance in flexion but allows for micromotion across the inter-

space. No bone-to-bone contact exists at this location, diminishing the fusion rate. Optimal contact exists between the implant and the end-plate in plane B. The width to contact of the implant with the end-plate is still very narrow. The implant in plane B has a greater capacity to bear axial loads than the implant in plane C. The implant in plane C sits deep in the end-plate and invades the vertebral cancellous bone, resulting in a greater propensity to piston in this region.

Ligamentous Disruption

Dorsal interbody strut insertion requires the disruption of the dorsal ligaments and bony elements, including the facet joints in order to insert a large enough strut to achieve the desired interspace distraction (Figure 5-19).[8,17,36] Disruption of the facet joints results in significant loss of stiffness with regard to flexion and rotation and may cause predisposition to postoperative deformity. The increased interspace height is desired, with the assumption that this technique will place the ligamentous tissues in tension and increase the overall stiffness of the interspace because of reduced mobility across the segment.

Load Sharing versus Load Bearing

Load sharing occurs when a strut shares a portion of the overall construct's applied load with another implant or the spine itself. *Load bearing* occurs when the strut bears the entire load applied to the construct.[4]

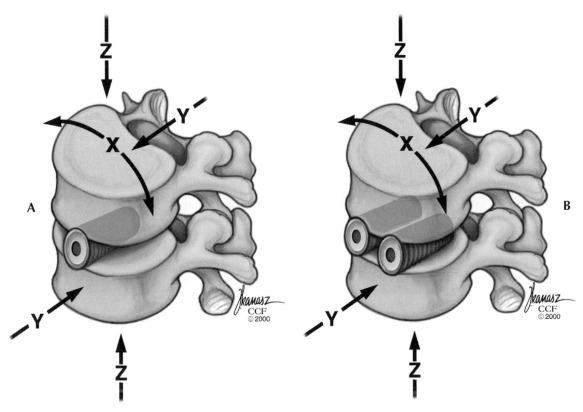

FIGURE 5-16 ■ **A**, A single round-faced cage functions poorly in resisting angular "x," shear "y," and axial "z" forces; **B**, Paired cages have improved load-bearing capacity in all planes.

An interbody strut without the assistance of dorsal instrumentation bears the majority of applied axial loads. Rigid dorsal instrumentation shares applied loads if used in combination with an interbody strut.

The proportion of axial load transferred through the interbody strut depends on intraoperative preloading of the dorsal instrumentation. If the dorsal construct is preloaded under compression, the graft is loaded and

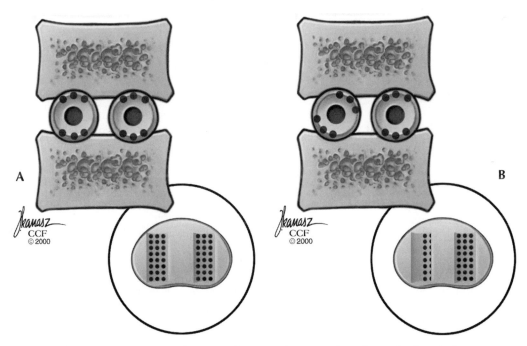

FIGURE 5-17 ■ **A**, Area of contact between bone graft and vertebral end-plate through holes (*dots*) in the TIFCs; **B**, Reduced area of contact if placed improperly (*insets: axial views*).

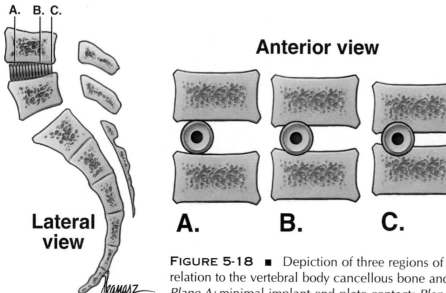

FIGURE 5-18 ■ Depiction of three regions of contact of a cylindrical implant in relation to the vertebral body cancellous bone and end-plate (planes A, B, and C). *Plane A:* minimal implant-end-plate contact; *Plane B:* optimal contact; *Plane C:* excessive penetration into cancellous bone.

the dorsal instrumentation is unloaded when the patient is upright. This creates an ideal setting for bone fusion while reducing the load on the dorsal implant. When the dorsal instrumentation is placed without preloading, the interbody strut and dorsal instrumentation share applied axial loads. When the construct is preloaded in distraction, the dorsal implant bears both the preloaded forces and the applied axial loads, effectively shielding the interbody strut from axial loading and bone-fusing forces.

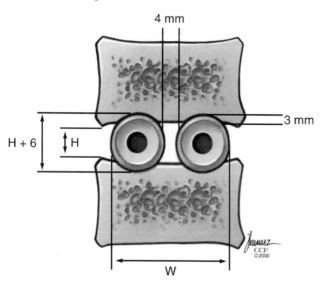

FIGURE 5-19 ■ In order for TIFCs to achieve the desired disc interspace distraction, excessive resection of the dorsal elements is required. The width ("W") necessary to achieve this interspace distraction is $2(H + 6mm) + 4mm = 2H + 16mm$. "H" is the desired interspace distraction height. A penetration of 3mm of the implant in the end-plate and a distance of 4mm between the implants is assumed.

A minimal threshold for interbody motion must be maintained for a successful fusion. Too little motion may result in shielding the bone graft from bone healing enhancing forces by the implant. Excessive motion may result in pseudoarthrosis, construct failure, and persistence of low back pain.[4]

SURGICAL PROCEDURES FOR MECHANICAL BACK PAIN

Mechanical back pain may be managed by segmental fusion after appropriate nonoperative management has failed. Multiple techniques for segmental spinal fusion exist.

Dorsolateral Intertransverse Fusion

Dorsolateral intertransverse fusion is an onlay type of fusion consisting of placing bone graft between the transverse processes bilaterally. The fusion mass abuts the lateral aspects of the involved facet joints. The advantages of this procedure include ease of exposure, simultaneous direct neural decompression, and less need for extensive intervertebral disc removal. The disadvantages of this procedure include significant soft tissue dissection to expose the transverse processes and limited axial load-bearing capabilities of the fusion mass. The biomechanical disadvantages of this type of fusion become greater the further the fusion mass from the IAR (see Figure 5-11). This can lead to either excessive intervertebral motion with persistent low back pain or frank pseudoarthrosis.

Posterior Lumbar Interbody Fusion

Posterior lumbar interbody fusion (PLIF) was popularized by Cloward in the fifties.[9] The procedure is technically demanding and requires meticulous end-plate and graft preparation to obtain an optimal area of contact between the intervertebral bone graft and the vertebral end-plates. The popularity of this procedure was enhanced by the introduction of interbody cages. A PLIF procedure performed with or without a TIFC should be performed with the same fundamental clinical, surgical, and biomechanical strategies in mind.

PLIF has the advantage, as any dorsal approach does, of facilitating a dorsal decompression of the dural sac and nerve roots. With this procedure, the fusion is closer to the IAR than with the lateral inter-transverse fusion. This provides a greater ability to resist axial load. The graft is exposed to greater compressive loads, with an enhanced biomechanical advantage regarding fusion.[39] There is greater axial load-bearing capacity and less micromotion in the disc interspace compared to the dorsolateral intertransverse fusion.

The traditional PLIF technique is associated with several factors that can lead to construct failure. These include epidural bleeding, inadequate graft shaping, graft retropulsion, insufficient donor bone volume, and graft fracture.[7]

Anterior Lumbar Interbody Fusion

Anterior lumbar interbody fusion (ALIF) has recently increased in popularity. This has, in part, been related to the increased use of minimally invasive surgical techniques. The interest in minimally invasive surgery is related to perceived decreases in surgical morbidity, hospitalization, cost, and rehabilitation time.

One of the major advantages of ALIF is exposure of the disc space, resulting in a relatively safe placement of a wide bone graft with substantial area of contact with the vertebral end-plates. The ventral approach provides for easier placement of a trapezoidal bone graft to better match the contour of the intervertebral space and to reduce iatrogenic loss of lumbar lordosis. ALIF also can eliminate the necessity of dorsal neural decompression in selected cases, possibly reducing the surgical risks associated with re-exploration procedures.

The disadvantages of ALIF include venous and arterial thrombosis, venous and arterial laceration, hemorrhage, retrograde ejaculation, and impotence.[23] ALIF is often combined with dorsal spinal instrumentation, further increasing the risks of surgery.[25,28]

CONCLUSIONS[4]

1. The cross-sectional area of contact between the strut and the graft bed (in particular end-plates) is directly proportional to the construct's capacity to resist axial loads and to minimize micromotion. This distributes the axial forces over a greater area and avoids stress risers (regions of high stress).

2. Placement of the strut close to the IAR (mid-dorsal vertebral body region) minimizes the application of excessive bending moments.
3. Meticulous graft bed preparation and the preservation of the end-plate decrease the possibility of pistoning. This increases the fusion rate and the axial load resistance capacity.
4. Strut type must be carefully selected. The integrity of the strut and graft beds should be comparable regarding the modulus of elasticity (hardness). If a TIFC is used in poor vertebral bone, subsidence is inevitable. Pistoning, end-plate fractures, cage extrusion and graft nonunion may result.
5. Wedge-shaped intervertebral disc geometry and the trapezoidal design of the strut to closely match the interspace graft beds may minimize micromotion, loss of stability, and fusion failure. This design and the proper sizing of the strut increase the surface area of contact and maintain (restore) lumbar lordosis.
6. Bone is formed where bone healing enhancing stresses (e.g., compression) are present, and it is absorbed where these stresses are absent (Wolff's law). Thus, an adequate understanding of the following concepts is imperative for the planning of a fusion: (a) load bearing, (b) load sharing, and (c) stress shielding.
7. The tendency of the lumbar spine to change from a state of less entropy (healthy disc interspace, less disorder) to a state of higher entropy (collapsed disc interspace, more disorder) with time should be carefully considered. Perhaps a strategy that permits higher entropy but that encourages fusion and spinal alignment and provides neural element decompression is more prudent than the philosophy of the restoration of disc interspace height.

REFERENCES

1. Albers B, et al: **Molecular Biology of the Cell**, 3rd edition. New York: Garland Publishing, Inc. 1994.
2. Andersson G, Svenson H, Oden A: The intensity of work recovery in low back pain. **Spine** 8:880, 1983.
3. Benzel EC. **Biomechanics of Spine Stabilization: Principles and Clinical Practice**. New York: McGraw-Hill, Inc., 1995.
4. Benzel EC, Lastra JJ, Kalfas I, et al: The biomechanics of interbody fusion and the shortcomings of lumbar fusion with cages and interbody bone dowels. Submitted to **Clin Neurosurg**.
5. Boden SD, Davis DO, Dina TS, et al: Abnormal magnetic resonance scans of the lumbar spine in asymptomatic subjects. A prospective investigation. **J Bone Joint Surg Am** 72:403-8, 1990.
6. Bogduk N: The innervation of the lumbar spine. **Spine** 8:286-93, 1983.

7. Brantigan JW: Pseudoarthrosis rate after allograft posterior lumbar interbody fusion with pedicle screw fixation. **Spine** 19(11):1271-1278, 1994.

8. Chen D, Fay LA, Lok J, et al: Increasing neuroforaminal volume by interbody fusion in the reduction of foraminal stenosis. **Spine** 20(1):74-79, 1995.

9. Cloward R: The treatment of ruptured lumbar intervertebral discs by vertebral body fusion. **J Neurosurg** 10:154, 1953.

10. Cypress BK: Characteristics of physician visits for back symptoms: a national perspective. **Am J Public Health** 73:389-95, 1983.

11. Deyo RA, Bass JE: Life style and low back pain: the influence of smoking and obesity. **Spine** 14:501-6, 1989.

12. Deyo RA, Diehl AK, Rosenthal M: How many days of bed rest for acute low back pain? A randomized clinical trial. **N Engl J Med** 315:1064-70, 1986.

13. Edgar MA, Ghadially JA: Innervation of the lumbar spine. **Clin Orthop Rel Res** 115:35-41, 1976.

14. Edgar MA, Nundy S: Innervation of the spinal dura mater. **J Neurol Neurosurg Psychiatry** 29:530-34, 1966.

15. Ferguson R, Tencer A, Woodard P, et al: Biomechanical comparisons of spinal fracture models and the stabilizing effects of posterior instrumentations. **Spine** 13:453-60, 1988.

16. Findlayson D, Birche M, Morris E, et al: Is there a place for fusion in simple backache? **J Bone Joint Surg Br** 67:151, 1985.

17. Goh JCH, Yu CS, Thambyah A, et al: Influence of PLIF cage size on lumbar spine stability. North American Spine Society Proceedings 12th Annual Meeting. New Orleans: October 22-25, 1997, 267-68.

18. Groen G, Baljet B, Drukker J: The nerves and nerve plexuses of the human vertebral column. **Am J Anat** 188:282-96, 1990.

19. Grubb SA, Lipocomb HJ: Results of lumbosacral fusion for degenerative disc disease with and without instrumentation: two to five year follow-up. **Spine** 17:349-55, 1992.

20. Heggeness MH, Doherty BJ: Discography causes end plate deflection. **Spine** 18:1050-3, 1993.

21. Jackson HC, Winkelman RK, Bickel WH: Nerve endings in the human lumbar spinal column and related structures. **J Bone Joint Surg** 48A:1272-81, 1966.

22. Kitchel SH: Improvement in sagittal plane alignment following anterior lumbar interbody fusion with threaded titanium cages. North American Spine Society Proceedings 12th Annual Meeting. New Orleans: October 22-25, 1997 108-9.

23. Kuslich Sd, Ahern JW: Analysis of complications in large personal series of lumbar interbody fusions using the BAK instrumentation. North American Spine Society Proceedings 12th Annual Meeting. New Orleans: October 22-25, 1997, 104-5.

24. Lorenz M, Zindrick M, Schwaegler F, et al: A comparison of single level fusions with and without hardware. **Spine** 16(Suppl. 8):455-58, 1991.

25. Mathews HH, Evans MT, Molligan HJ, et al: Laparoscopic discectomy with anterior interbody fusion. **Spine** 20(16):1797-1802, 1995.

26. Miller J, Schmatz C, Schultz A: Lumbar disc degeneration correlation with age, sex, and spine level in 600 autopsy specimens. **Spine** 13:173-78, 1988.

27. Parke WW: Applied anatomy of the spine, in Rothman RH, Simeone FA, (eds.): **The Spine**. Philadelphia: W.B. Saunders, 1982.

28. Penta M, Sandhu A, Fraser RD: Magnetic resonance imaging assessment of disc degeneration 10 years after anterior lumbar interbody fusion. **Spine** 20:743-47, 1995.

29. Ray CD: Spinal interbody fusions: a review, featuring new generation techniques. **Neurosurgery Quarterly** 7(2):135-56, 1997.

30. Schneiderman G, Flannigan B, Kingston S, et al: Magnetic resonance imaging in the diagnosis of disc degeneration. Correlation with discography. **Spine** 12:276-81, 1987.

31. Sherman MS: The nerves of bone. **J Bone Joint Surg** 45A:522-28, 1963.

32. Simons DG, Travell JG: Myofascial origins of low back pain. **Postgrad Med** 73:66-108, 1983.

33. Simons DG, Travell JG: Myofascial pain syndromes, in Wall PD, Melzak R, (eds.): **Textbook of Pain**. Edinburgh: Churchill Livingstone, 1984.

34. Stauffer RN, Coventry MB: Posterolateral lumbar spine fusion-analysis of Mayo Clinic Series. **J Bone Joint Surg Am** 54:1195-1204, 1972.

35. Truumees E, Sidhu K, Fischgrund JS: Indications for fusion in lumbar disc disease. **Sem Spine Surg** 11(2):147-62, 1999.

36. Vamvanij V, Fay LA, Hai Y, et al: Changes in spinal canal dimensions using interbody distraction for spondylolisthesis. North American Spine Society Proceedings 12th Annual Meeting. New Orleans: October 22-25, 1997, 25-26.

37. Wiberg G: Back pain in relation to the nerve supply of the intervertebral disc. **Acta Orthop** 19:211-21, 1947.

38. Wiesel SW, Tsourmas N, Feffer HL, et al: A study of computer-assisted tomography 1. The incidence of positive CAT scans in an asymptomatic group of patients. **Spine** 9:549-51, 1984.

39. White AA, Panjabi MM: **Clinical Biomechanics of the Spine**, 2nd edition. Philadelphia: J.B. Lippincott Company, 1990.

40. Wood GW, Boyd RJ, Carothers TA, et al: The effect of pedicle screw/plate fixation on lumbar/lumbosacral autogenous bone graft fusions in patients with degenerative disc disease. **Spine** 20:819-30, 1995.

41. Yu S, Haughton VM, Sether LA, et al: Criteria for classifying normal and degenerated lumbar intervertebral discs. **Radiology** 170:523-26, 1989.

42. Zdeblick TA: The treatment of degenerative lumbar disorders. A critical review of the literature. **Spine** 20:126S-37S, 1995.

CHAPTER 6

The Facet Syndrome

◼

GORDON TANG, M.D.

REGIS W. HAID, JR., M.D.

GERALD RODTS, M.D.

INTRODUCTION

Estimates for the lifetime incidence of low back pain (LBP) ranges from 60% to 80%, whereas point prevalence has been reported to be from 20% to 30%. Low back pain limits activity more than any other cause in people less than 45 years of age. Between the ages of 45 and 65, only cardiac and arthritic conditions create as much disability. Low back pain accounts for more than a tenth of all new patient visits to physicians and results in 3% of all patient discharges in the United States. The socio-economic costs have been estimated at two billion dollars each year, with medication costs alone estimated at $192 million in 1990.[9] Despite ergonomic improvements, all industrialized countries have witnessed a steady increase in LBP problems, and approximately 500,000 Workers' Compensation and personal injury cases dealing with LBP are recorded each year.

Despite its prevalence, the etiology of low back pain is infrequently defined. The pain is poorly classified, and routine diagnostic tests often illustrate no specific findings. Attempts to pinpoint the diagnosis are rendered unnecessary because 90% of patients undergo substantial improvement independent of the course of treatment. Although recurrences may be common, only 5% to 10% of recurrences progress to chronicity. In one of the most comprehensive studies to date, the National Low Back Pain study followed 2,374 patients referred for neurosurgical or orthopedic evaluation. Of this group, final diagnoses included disk protrusion or herniation in 37%, spondylosis in 21%, stenosis in 14%, and spondylolisthesis in 7%. Twenty percent of patients ultimately underwent surgical intervention.[1]

The role of the facet joint in etiology of chronic low back pain has long been a controversial topic. In 1933,

Ghormley first drew attention to the facet joint as a source of low back pain.[10] His hypothesis was furthered by Putti's cadaveric study in 1927 demonstrating osteoarthritic changes of the facet joints.[27] Ghormley, in 1933, coined the term *facet syndrome*.[10] Suggesting that facet joints created back pain, Ghormley advocated fusion as a surgical remedy. The successful treatment of disc prolapse by Mixter and Barr drew attention away from the facet joint and toward the intervertebral disc as the primary source of back and leg pain.[22] The concept of the facet joint as a pain generator resurfaced in the 1960s with the recreation of low back pain by the injection of hypertonic saline into the facet joints by Hirsch.[13]

ANATOMY OF FACET JOINTS

The biomechanical role of the facet joint indirectly supports its potential role in low back pain. The lumbar facet joints demonstrate a progressive 30° to 60° angulation in the axial plane. The L1 facet joints slope at 35°, the L2 slope at 30°, the L3 slope at 34°, the L4 slope at 41°, the L5 slope at 53°, and the S1 slope at 58°.[29] The progressive coronal orientation and increased surface area of the lower facets are designed to accommodate greater loads. Biomechanically, the facet joints withstand a compressive load, principally with the back in extension. In flexion, the facet joints bear most of the shear forces. Disk space narrowing, as seen in degenerative disc disease, increases loading onto the facets (Figure 6-1).[5,18,33] Excessive loads may cause the inferior facet joint to pivot about the pars and stretch the capsule. The decreasing height and anterior-to-posterior dimension of the lower facets shield the force applied to the pedicles; the increasing cross-sectional area also

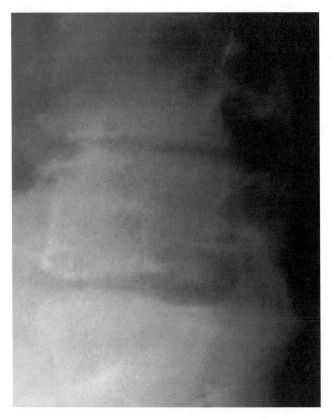

FIGURE 6-1 ■ Lateral lumbar spine radiograph depicts severe disk space collapse at L4-L5 resulting in greater shear forces at the facet joint.

participates in counteracting loading stress on the spine.

The presence of pain fibers in the facet joint also argues for the role of the facet as generators of low back pain. Small diameter, high threshold fibers are found in the facet joint capsules of humans. The nociceptive type IV receptor system is found in the fibrous joint capsule, representing a plexus of unmyelinized nerve fibers and types I and II corpuscular mechanoreceptors. Substance P, calcitonin gene-related peptide, vasoactive intestinal polypeptide, and the autonomic fiber markers neuropeptide Y and tyrosine hydroxylase have all been found in the synovial villi of the facet joints.[2,11] Physiologically, the following three classes of fibers and responses have been noted at the facet joint: phasic discharges consistent with velocity detectors, low-threshold group II and group III receptors located in the muscles and tendons inserting into the joint subserving propioception, and high-threshold, slowly adapting mechanoreceptors consistent with nocicpetive fibers.

The facet joints are innervated by medial branches of the lumbar dorsal rami and possibly receive innervation from the adjacent dorsal ramus, the dorsal root ganglion, and the next more caudal medial branch.[16]

At L1 through L4, the medial branches cross the transverse process at the medial superior edge and cross the root of the superior articular process. The medial branch then passes medially and is covered by the mammiloaccessory ligament, where it splits into proximal and distal zygapophysial branches. The proximal branch innervates the adjacent facet joint, and the distal branches innervate the next lower level. The medial branch may also innervate the interspinous ligaments and multifidus muscles. With medial branch stimulation, patients often report a deep pain similar to muscle spasm symptoms. The diverse cross innervations provide an anatomical basis for the variability in the clinical syndrome of facet pain and may help to explain the ineffectiveness of limited facet blocks.

CLINICAL FINDINGS

A multitude of causes for pain arising from the facet joints is given in the literature. These include compression of nerve roots by hypertrophic osteoarthritic changes at the facets (lateral stenosis) and tension of nerve roots by scar tissue. These well-known and well-characterized nerve root syndromes are not addressed here. The focus here is pain from the facet joint itself, either from an arthritic mechanism or as a component of lumbar hypermobility and instability that overstresses the facet joint.

The classic description of facet syndrome describes low back pain that is dull and nonlocalizing. The pain can be stabbing, burning, drilling, and deep. Pain increases during the day and disappears when lying down. Pain may radiate posterolaterally into the thigh or calf. Radiation into the feet suggests another diagnosis. No neurologic findings are expected, although motor weakness owing to pain may be encountered. In cases of hypertrophic facet arthritis, a clear-cut distinction between pure facet syndrome and spinal stenosis may be impossible to make. Some have suggested that pain provocation by coughing, sneezing, or Valsalva can occur more frequently with facet pain. Pain is often exacerbated by hyperextension, especially combined with rotation or lateral bending as well as tenderness over a joint. Bracing may be helpful in identifying patients with motion-induced pain but is nonspecific and does not define where the pain may come from.

Study of clinical predictors of subsequent response to facet block has yielded mixed results. Fairbank and associates found that acuteness of back pain, pain augmented by sitting and bending, and back pain occurring with straight leg raising are associated with responders.[8] Helbig and Lee identified paravertebral tenderness, symptoms elicited by extension-rotation movements, back pain in conjunction with groin or thigh pain, and pain extending below the knee as pre-

TABLE 6-1 ■ **Factors Associated with Poor Response to Lumbar Surgery**

Older age
Prior history of low-back pain
Normal gait
Maximum pain on extension following forward flexion in the standing position
Absence of leg pain, muscle spasm
Pain not worsened when rising from forward flexion
Pain well relieved by recumbency
Pain not worsened by extension-rotation
Lack pain aggravation by Valsalva

dictors of response to facet blocks.[12] Two well-designed studies by Jackson and Revel and associates came to similar conclusions.[14,28] Each suggested that older age, lack of aggravation of pain by Valsalva, and to some extent, pain relieved by recumbency all predicted relief from facet blocks (Table 6-1).

As facet arthropathy remains a diagnosis of exclusion, meticulous attention should be paid to other possible etiologies. Radicular pain, true weakness, sensory deficits, and reflex changes are all relative contraindications to the diagnosis of facet arthropathy unless they can be clearly attributed to another etiology that does not create the most troubling pain for the patient. Psychosocial influences should be excluded, as described by Waddell.[32]

RADIOGRAPHIC FINDINGS

In pathologic studies, 68% of patients over age 60 were found to have facet joint arthritis.[26] Asymptomatic patients will frequently have morphologically altered facet joints. Therefore, interpretation of radiographs should be done primarily for the purpose of exclusion and should never be relied upon to indicate LBP from a facet source. Given the need to ascertain exclusion of other diagnoses and the prevalence of prior lumbar surgery, a post myelographic computerized tomography (CT) myelogram is usually warranted to provide the best view of the bony anatomy and to accurately depict the degree of foraminal compromise. Sagittal and coronal reconstructions provide particular attention to signs suggestive of lumbar instability, such as pseudoarthrosis, osteophytic spurs, pars defects, and minimal spondylolisthesis (Figures 6-2, 6-3, 6-4). Whereas the finding of degenerative changes does not assure the diagnosis of facet syndrome, the lack of abnormalities essentially excludes the possibility of significant back pain arising from the facet joint. In patients with entirely normal studies, facet injections do not appear to be indicated. A bone scan will often illustrate inflammation at the facet joints. Little literature, however, exists to define the sensitivity and

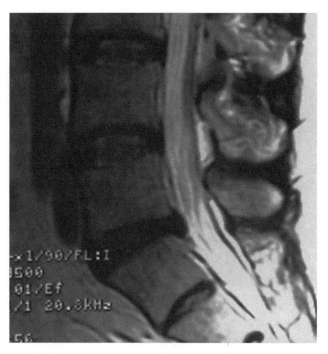

FIGURE 6-2 ■ Sagittal T2-weighted MRI illustrates "dark disc" disease, which may prompt a provocative discogram to ascertain discogenic pain from degenerative disc disease.

specificity of this test. Magnetic resonance imaging (MRI) with and without contrast can also be helpful in the diagnosis of persistent or recurrent pain in patients with prior surgery. Work-up should also include all studies typically prescribed for the identification of instability, including supine and standing flexion/extension radiographs.

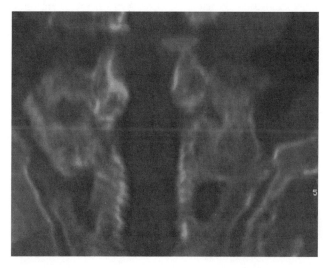

FIGURE 6-3 ■ Coronal reconstruction of a CT of the lumbar spine illustrates pseudoarthrosis in the fusion mass.

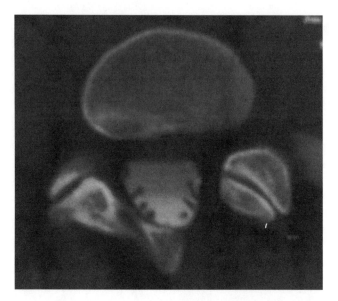

FIGURE 6-4 ■ Axial CT image illustrates facet hypertrophy in association with spina bifida. This patient had mechanical low back pain with instability on dynamic films that was remedied by posterior segmental fixation.

NONOPERATIVE MANAGEMENT

Physiotherapy

There has been extensive study of the nonoperative treatment of low back pain. However, as the diagnosis of the facet syndrome is often uncertain, there are no data to support any one form of conservative management over another when the facet joint is presumed to be the source of low back pain. In a recent review of randomized, controlled trials, van Tulder and associates identified 28 trials on intervention for acute back pain and 20 for chronic back pain.[30] Those authors found strong evidence of the effectiveness of nonsteroidal anti-inflammatories (NSAIDs) and muscle relaxants and the ineffectiveness of exercise for the treatment of acute low back pain. Regarding chronic back pain, strong evidence, especially of short-term improvement, was reported for exercise, back school, and manipulation. The primary goal of treatment of chronic back pain is the return to work or usual activities, with relief of pain being secondary. It is notable that a recent randomized clinical trial of three active therapies of chronic pain concluded that benefit was not derived from any physiologic adaptation, but rather from an alteration of the patients' perceptions of what constitutes disability.[21]

Therapeutic Facet Injections

Corticosteroid injections into the facet joints were first used in 1976 by Mooney and Robertson, who reported

significant long-term improvement in 52% of patients.[23] Other reports have noted success rates from 10% to 63%.[4,20,24] Two randomized controlled trials have addressed the therapeutic benefit of facet injections with corticosteroids. In a study by Lilius and associates, 109 patients were randomized to either intra-articular steroids mixed with an anesthetic, a peri-capsular injection, or saline.[17] Neither the method, the type of injectate, nor the duration of symptoms correlated to outcome. In Carette and associates, 190 patients with chronic low back pain without neurologic findings underwent injections of lidocaine into the L4-L5 and L5-S1 facet joints, either unilaterally or bilaterally.[3] Of these, 110 (58%) patients reported a reduction of 50% or more in their pain following the injections. Eleven patients (6%) had complete reduction of pain with the injections. All but two patients had return of pain after two weeks. Ninety-seven patients of this group were then randomized to either methylprednisolone or to placebo injections into the facet joint. One month following injection, the two groups did not differ in any outcome measure. Three months following injection, 36% of patients in the methylprednisolone group reported marked improvement as compared to 28% in the placebo arm. At six months, 46% of patients treated with methylprednisolone reported marked improvement as compared to 15% for the placebo group. These numbers were adjusted down to 31% in the methylprednisolone group and 17% for the placebo group when the numbers were re-analyzed in an attempt to factor out the contribution of concurrent interventions. The authors of this study concluded that corticosteroids were not beneficial.

Whereas data to support the use of therapeutic facet injections remain inconclusive, we have found such injections to be beneficial in select patients. On occasion, patients who are otherwise poor candidates for surgical procedures, patients who refuse surgical intervention, or patients whose surgical intervention failed will derive marked short-term relief from facet injections. Following repeated injections, in conjunction with physical therapy and NSAIDs, some patients may avoid surgery altogether. Facet injections may also be useful as a temporary measure while patients consider the various therapeutic options. In our experience, long-term pain relief is exceptional.

Radiofrequency Facet Denervation

Patients who experience dramatic benefit from facet blockade may be candidates for radiofrequency facet denervations. Although radiofrequency facet denervation has been practiced for more than two decades, there have been relatively few studies with clear patient selection criteria and standardized long-term outcomes. In one study with detailed analysis, North and associates reported on 82 patients selected for diagnostic medial branch posterior primary ramus blocks.[25] Forty-two patients reported at least 50% relief and received radiofrequency denervation. Of those, 45% reported at least 50% improvement in pain at a mean follow-up of 3.2 years. Of note, 13% of patients who received temporary blocks nonetheless had greater than 50% reduction of pain at follow-up, illustrating both a placebo effect as well as the self-limited nature facet pain in some patients. Recently, van Kleef and associates concluded a randomized prospective double-blind trial of facet denervation in 31 patients who responded to medial branch blocks.[31] One year following radiofrequency denervation, 7 of 15 patients in the radiofrequency arm reported a successful outcome as compared to 2 of 16 in the sham group. As in other studies, the results suggest a gradual return of pain over time. Patients who have failed prior surgery may be particularly suitable candidates.

SURGICAL MANAGEMENT

Diagnostic Facet Injections and Patient Selection

In addition to therapeutic injections, facet joints are also often injected in order to determine whether the patient is suitable for a surgical remedy to pain. The capacity of the facet joint has been recorded as 1.5 to 2 cm.[4] Therefore, in contrast to therapeutic injections, diagnostic injections should be limited to small volumes of anesthetic. Injection of excess volume allows the inferior recess of the capsule to rupture and the fluid to extrude laterally, diffusing into the branches of the ramus posterior and medially, throughout the ligamentum flavum, the epidural space, and intervertebral foramen. Some have supported injecting larger volumes, arguing that extravasation allows for anesthesia of periscapular tissues innervated by noncapsular branches of the posterior rami, which are denervated during the fusion operation. In this way, the anesthetic quality of the block may still be a useful predictor of outcome. In diagnostic blocks, a strictly intra-articular injection may be ensured by a concurrent arthogram.

A number of studies have examined the value of facet blocking in predicting outcome following lumbar arthrodesis. Unfortunately, no clear conclusions can be reached. Esses and Moro retrospectively reviewed 296 patients who underwent facet injections in a 10-year span.[7] Of those, 126 patients received follow-up, and 82 patients underwent subsequent surgery. Results of preoperative facet blockade were correlated with postoperative outcome. No statistical correlation could be found between blockade response and surgical outcome. The lack of specific patient data precludes more detailed analysis that could assess the study's potential limitations. In this study, surgery was not confined to the areas of the facet blocks, and the decision for surgery was not based on the patient's response to the facet block. The study has also been criticized for examining pain response only at 15 minutes following injection and for using uncontrolled blocks. It is also notable in this series that the only positive finding was the correlation of pre-operative employment status with postoperative employment status. Other typical predictors of surgical outcome, such as Workers' Compensation status, pending litigation, or number of levels fused, did not correlate with surgical outcome.

Jackson retrospectively examined the pre-operative response to facet blockade in 36 patients who had undergone surgical fusion.[15] As with Esses and associates, response to facet blockade was not the sole criterion to determine whether the patient was a surgical candidate, and fusion was not limited to the levels of facet blockade.[6] All 36 patients did well despite the fact that only 26 patients had improvement with blocking. The uniformly good outcome makes this study difficult to interpret. One could argue that all patients with a positive block did well, and only false negatives occurred. As fusion may treat a number of painful conditions, the high false-negative rate does not argue for or against facet blockade as a diagnostic test.

Lovely and Rastogi examined the predictive role of facet blocking for outcome following lumbar arthodesis in 91 patients who underwent 197 facet blocks.[19] Of those, 28 patients had significant relief from facet blocks, defined as greater than 70% relief for longer than six hours on three separate blocks. Including an additional two surgical patients, 23 patients had successful fusion. Of the 23 patients with solid fusion, 19 (82.6%) had greater than 90% relief of preoperative pain, and 3 (13%) had partial relief, with only one failure. Prolo scores improved from a pre-operative mean of 3.95 to a post-operative mean of 7.7. Of the seven patients with pseudoarthrosis, five of the seven had less than 50% relief, and two had partial (50%-90%) relief. Prolo scores improved from a mean of 3.6 to a mean of 5.3. Although in the course of the procedure the facet joint capsule was denervated, the pain was not remedied. This finding suggests that in most cases, a solid arthodesis must be obtained for a good outcome.

It is the opinion of the authors that facet injections are rarely indicated to select patients who would benefit from fusion procedures. History and physical examination, in conjunction with routine diagnostic tests such as MRI, CT, CT myelogram, and static and dynamic radiographs are sufficient in the overwhelming majority of patients. Facet blocks are useful in the occasional patient when the diagnosis is uncertain or when there is some question regarding the patient's suitability for a fusion procedure. Facet blocks may also be helpful to determine if a specific level is symptomatic in an attempt to limit the length of a fusion. Some of the value of facet injections, as with discograms, may also lie in their negative predictive value. Whereas there is uncertainty that patients with relief from a facet block may benefit from either decompression or fusion of that level, patients with no relief from a facet block may be assumed to have a lower likelihood of success.

Review of our series indicates 280 facet blocks from September 1992 to June 1998. Of these, 48 of the patients (17%) went on to undergo spinal procedures, including both lumbar and cervical fusions. In an average follow-up of 15 months after surgery, 80% of the patients had significant relief of their axial pain, remained free from narcotics, and had resumed regular activities. Of the 48 procedures, 41 were fusion procedures, including 11 cases of articular mass plates for cervical spine disease, nine lumbar interbody fusions, and seven facetectomies with foraminotomies without fusions. The remainder were posterior segmental fusions.

Surgical Approaches

Given the ill-defined nature of the facet syndrome, it is not surprising that there is no consensus on the surgical approach to patients who obtain relief following a facet block. The lack of a gold standard for the diagnosis of low back pain from facet disease precludes any meaningful study of surgical approaches. In theory, a simple facetectomy obliterates the joint and denervates the joint capsule, thereby affording complete relief. In practice, facet arthropathy is likely to be a component of a degenerative process that may involve multiple facet articulations and may accompany or be the consequence of concomitant degenerative disk disease. Radiographic findings such as disc space narrowing and Modic changes should alert one to the possibility of concomitant discogenic pain. In the setting of a positive discogram with negative controls, medial facetectomies combined with a posterior lumbar interbody fusion may be the surgery of choice for single level disease. Addressing the facet disease alone with a facetectomy and foraminotomy leaves accompanying discogenic pain from degenerative disease untreated and does not address accompanying lumbar instability. When there is little possibility of lateral stenosis, an anterior interbody fusion stabilizes and relieves stress from the facet joint while eliminating pain from degenerative disc disease. As multilevel interbody fusions harbor significantly worse outcomes, multilevel disease is best addressed with multiple facetectomies and posterior segmental fixation.

CONCLUSION

The diagnosis and treatment of facet syndrome remain controversial. Nonetheless, there is some agreement that the facet joint can be a significant source of low back pain, although most studies suggest the incidence is low. History and radiographic findings are nonspecific, and the diagnosis relies on clear-cut relief from facet blockade. However, the decision for fusion should not rest solely on response to facet blockade. Instead, response to a facet injection should be considered in association with all other factors. The treatment plan of facet arthropathy should take into account the overall degenerative process in the lumbar spine and thereby address both the pain generator as well as the underlying lumbar stability.

REFERENCES

1. Ackerman SJ, Steinberg EP, Bryan RN, et al: Patient characteristics associated with diagnostic imaging evaluation of persistent low back problems. **Spine** 22:1634-40, 1997.
2. Ahmed M, Bjurholm A, Kreicbergs A, et al: Sensory and autonomic innervation of the facet joint in the rat lumbar spine. **Spine** 18:2121-6, 1993.
3. Carette S, Marcoux S, Truchon R, et al: A controlled trial of corticosteroid injections into facet joints for chronic low back pain. **New Engl J Med** 325:1002-7, 1991.
4. Destouet JM, Gilula LA, Murphy WA, et al: Lumbar facet joint injection: indication, technique, clinical correlation and preliminary results. **Radiology** 145:321-25, 1982.
5. Dunlop RB, Adams MA, Hutton WC: Disc space narrowing and the lumbar facet joints. **J Bone Joint Surg Br** 66:706-10, 1984.
6. Esses SI, Botsford DJ, Kostuik JP: The role of external spinal skeletal fixation in the assessment of low-back disorders. **Spine** 14:594-601, 1989.
7. Esses SI, Moro JK: The value of facet joint blocks in patient selection for lumbar fusion. **Spine** 18:185-90, 1993.
8. Fairbank JC, Park WM, McCall IW, et al: Apophyseal injection of local anesthetic as a diagnostic aid in primary low back pain syndromes. **Spine** 6:598-605, 1981.
9. Frymoyer JW, Cats-Baril WL: An overview of the incidences and costs of low back pain. **Orthop Clin North Am** 22:263-71,1991.
10. Ghormley RK: Low back pain. With special reference to the articular facets, with presentation of an operative procedure. **JAMA** 101:1773-7, 1933.
11. Giles LGF, Taylor JR: Innervation of lumbar zygapophyseal joint synovial folds. **Acta Orthop Scand** 58:43-46, 1987.
12. Helbig T, Lee CK: The lumbar facet syndrome. **Spine** 13:61-64, 1988.
13. Hirsch D, Inglemark B, Miller M: The anatomical basis for low back pain. **Acta Orthop Scand** 33:1, 1963.

14. Jackson RP, Jacobs RR, Montesano PX: Facet joint injection in low back pain: A prospective statistical study. **Spine** 13:966-71, 1988.

15. Jackson RP: The facet syndrome: myth or reality? **Clin Orthop** 279:110-21, 1992.

16. Kaplan M, Dreyfuss P, Halbrook B, et al: The ability of lumbar medial branch blocks to anesthetize the zygapophysial joint: A physiologic challenge. **Spine** 23(17):1847-52, 1998.

17. Lilius G, Laasonen EM, Myllynen P, et al: Lumbar facet joint syndrome: a randomized clinical trial. **J Bone Joint Surg Br** 71:681-84, 1989.

18. Lorenz M, Patwardhan A, Vanderby R Jr: Load-bearing characteristics of lumbar facets in normal and surgical altered spinal segments. **Spine** 8:122, 1983.

19. Lovely TJ, Rastogi P: The value of provocative facet blocking as a predictor of success in lumbar spine fusion. **J Spinal Disord** 10:512-17, 1997.

20. Lynch MC, Taylor JF, et al: Facet joint injection for low back pain. A clinical study. **J Bone Joint Surg Br** 68:138-41, 1986.

21. Mannion AF, Muntener M, Taimela S, et al: A randomized clinical trial of three active therapies for chronic low back pain. **Spine** 23(23):2435-48, 1999.

22. Mixter WJ, Barr JS: Rupture of the intervertebral disc with involvement of the spinal canal. **N Engl J Med** 211:210-15, 1934.

23. Mooney V, Robertson J: The facet syndrome. **Clin Orthop** 115:149-56, 1976.

24. Moran R, O'Connell D, Walsh MG: The diagnostic value of facet joint injections. **Spine** 12:1407-10, 1986.

25. North RB, Han M, Zahurak M, et al: Radiofrequency lumbar face denervation: analysis of prognostic factors. **Pain** 57(1):77-83, 1994.

26. Parthria M, Sartoris D, Resnick D: Osteoarthritis of the facet joints: accuracy of oblique radiographic assessment. **Radiology** 164:227-30, 1987.

27. Putti V: New conceptions in the pathogenesis of sciatic pain. **Lancet** ii:53-60, 1927.

28. Revel M, Poiraudeau S, Auleley GR, et al: Capacity of the clinical picture to characterize low back pain relieved by facet joint anesthesia. Proposed criteria to identify patients with painful facet joints. **Spine** 23(18):1972-6; discussion 1977, Sep 15, 1998.

29. Schneck CD: The anatomy of lumbar spondylosis. **Clin Orth** 183:20-37, 1985.

30. van Tulder MW, Koes BW, Bouter LM: Conservative treatment of acute and chronic nonspecific low back pain. A systematic review of randomized controlled trials of the most common interventions. **Spine** 22:2128-56, 1997.

31. van Kleef M, Barendse GA, Kessels A, et al: Randomized trial of radiofrequency lumbar facet denervation for chronic low back pain. **Spine** 24(18):1937-42, 1999.

32. Waddell G: **The Back Pain Revolution**. London: Churchill Livingstone, 1998.

33. Yang KH, King AI: Mechanism of facet load transmission as a hypothesis for low back pain. **Spine** 9:557-65, 1984.

CHAPTER 7

Posterolateral Fusion in the Management of Low Back Pain

Peter H. Nguyen, M.D.

Gregory R. Trost, M.D.

INTRODUCTION

A major health dilemma in many industrialized countries, low back pain (LBP) remains one of the most common reasons for individuals to seek medical attention. It is estimated that 70% to 90% of adults will experience at least one episode of LBP, and 15% to 20% of all adult males will suffer from disabling back conditions.[9,37] The economic impact of back pain management, including the costs of surgical procedures and hospitalization, the costs of supportive therapies, and the costs of time lost from work and productivity, has been estimated to be in the tens of billions of dollars annually in the United States.

Spinal fusion has traditionally played a vital role in the stabilization and healing processes in the treatment of spinal conditions such as scoliotic deformities, infections, and traumatic spinal fractures. Its indication for degenerative spinal diseases (DSD), however, remains unclear and, often times, controversial. Although only a small fraction of patients with LBP undergo some form of lumbar surgical intervention, spinal fusion alone accounts for more than 70,000 operations each year in this country. Among all, posterolateral fusion (PLF), with or without instrumentation, alone or in combination, continues to be the technique most preferred by orthopedic and neurological spine surgeons.[13,18,66]

Technological advancements in diagnostic tools and instrumentation hardware and the development of new surgical techniques have enabled surgeons to address many spinal conditions that would have been formidable otherwise. Greater correction of deformity, early stabilization and mobilization, and desirable clinical improvements are some of the favorable outcomes reported.

HISTORICAL BACKGROUND

Early therapeutic indications for spinal fusion were primarily for the management of spinal instability secondary to infections, or pathological or scoliotic deformities, and not for the treatment of DSD. The first to perform posterior spinal fusion for the treatment of Pott's disease, Albee, in 1911, implanted an interspinous tibial graft to provide internal fixation and to promote spinal stabilization.[1] Cleveland and King similarly applied interspinous bone graft to enhance fusion and to improve structural stability.[65] Hibbs, in 1917, reported the role of spinal fusion in the prevention of progressive deformity of degenerative scoliosis.[23] Similar results have been reported throughout the literature, with different bone graft materials used for internal splint fixation. In early attempts to treat and eradicate spinal tuberculosis, Hodgson pioneered the anterior spinal approach.[25]

Although initially performed for spinal infections and scoliosis, spinal fusion has quickly expanded to treat developmental deformities and spinal trauma. In 1929, the intriguing concept of spinal fusion for the treatment of DSD became popularized when Hibbs and Swift reported favorable results in their fusion series performed for degenerative spine conditions.[24] Mixter and Barr, in 1934, and Howorth, in 1943, went on to advocate spinal fusion for the treatment of ruptured lumbar discs.[26,43] Watkins and Campbell, in 1953, in the midst of the fusion era, introduced a new surgical technique that was later known as the *posterolateral fusion technique*. It involved the fusion of facet joints, pars interarticularis, and bases of transverse processes.[59] Wiltse later modified the technique and included the lamina into the fusion bed.[62] Since its introduction, PLF has remained the most popular fusion procedure.

The use of instrumentation to augment bony fusion dates back to the end of the 19th century. Hadra, in 1891, described the first interspinous wiring technique, which used silver wire.[18,66] Lang, in 1902, achieved spinal stability using steel rods and a cellulose cylinder affixed to affected spinal segments.[33] Early instrumentation hardware, however, was limited to interspinous wiring and sublaminar wiring and was used mainly to treat symptomatic scoliosis.

Improvements in tools and techniques continued over the next several decades. For example, Luque introduced the use of multiple sublaminar wires and Cotrel and Dubousset used laminar hooks to achieve spinal stability. Ingenious introduction of the pedicle screw by Roy-Camille and Magerl marked a breakthrough in the field of complex spine surgery because the treatment of degenerative spinal diseases often involved extensive removal of the posterior bony elements. Roy-Camille popularized the semirigid screw and plate system, whereas Steffee championed the rigid pedicle screw and plate interface model.[54,55] Recent interest in interbody fusion has sparked the development of carbon-fiber interbody cages by Brantigan and of titanium metal alloy cages by Bagby and Kuslich.[5,30]

Recent innovations in the field of bone graft materials and advancements in our understanding of the biology of bone fusion have stimulated the field of spinal fusion research.[2,3,40] New surgical adjuncts, such as endoscopy, laparoscopy, and stereotactic image-guided techniques, have provided surgeons a wide spectrum of surgical opportunities.

INDICATIONS

No medical treatment has received as much public scrutiny as the management of LBP. Despite its long tradition and popularity, spinal fusion for DSD has remained controversial. To date, there remains a lack of consensus in the standards of care and indication criteria for surgical LBP management. Furthermore, the lack of a "gold" standard assessment for spinal fusion results has created difficulties in surgical outcome evaluation and in determining the therapeutic effectiveness of fusion procedures.[13,18,66]

Advances in instrumentation hardware, surgical techniques, and diagnostic imaging tools have provided a smooth transition in fusion indications from well-established conditions such as scoliosis, infections, and traumas to the more controversial entities of spinal instability and DSD. Commonly encountered DSD conditions are degenerative disc disease (DDD), spinal stenosis, isthmic and degenerative spondylolisthesis, degenerative scoliosis, and pseudoarthrosis/failed back syndrome. PLF has been widely performed to treat all of the previously mentioned DSD conditions.

With the exception of interbody fusion, posterolateral fusion has biomechanical advantages over other types of posterior fusion techniques.[13,18,32,51,59,66] The intertransverse arthrodesis is anatomically positioned closer to the center of rotational and bending forces and, therefore, helps to minimize the added stress placed upon the fusion sites by spinal segmental motion. The locally exposed muscle also provides a generous vascular supply to the fusion graft bed. Altogether, these factors serve to increase the overall graft fusion success. The modified Wiltse technique, with sacrospinalis muscle splitting, enables the surgeon to gain access to the fusion site and allows safe pedicle screw placement.[62]

Major disadvantages of the midline PLF approach are the long incision and the wide dissection needed in order to obtain adequate bony exposure of the involved transverse processes, the lamina, and the facet joints. This wide exposure can result in muscular ischemia and can decrease the blood supply to the fusion bed. Furthermore, despite the solid fusion seen in patients who have undergone PLF, a number of patients continue to have persistent lumbar pain, a condition sometimes termed *fusion disease*. Because the bone grafts are placed so they are lying free in the fusion bed, there is an increased risk for graft displacement. This can result in the migration of the fusion mass to a different level and can cause undesirable pseudoarthrosis.

Disc Herniation/Herniated Nucleus Pulposus (HNP)

There is no substantial evidence in the current literature to support the routine use of spinal arthrodesis in the treatment of HNP. Several independent, retrospective studies have demonstrated the effectiveness of simple decompressive discectomy in the treatment of herniated disc disease.[8,9,49] Clinical improvements, such as alleviation of pain and sensorimotor deficits, faster recovery, and early return to work, have been reported to be significantly higher in the surgically treated group in comparison to the medically treated group. Hakelius and associates have found that these clinical improvements, however, appeared to equalize after six months, and no statistical clinical difference was seen at seven-year follow-up.[66] Nashold and Hrubec reported that 50% of their patients treated for HNP continued to have debilitating back symptoms regardless of the type of treatments used, and additional surgery was warranted (14.7% in the surgical group vs. 13.9% in the nonsurgical group).[48] They concluded that there is no difference in long-term outcome between conservative medical therapy and direct decompressive surgery.

Early authors advocated routine spinal arthrodesis in addition to discectomy for the treatment of lumbar disc herniation. In 1934, Mixter and Barr and associates identified herniated nucleus pulposus as the etiology for back and radicular pain and treated patients surgically with satisfactory outcome.[43] They subsequently recommended concomitant spinal fusion because they believed that, following surgical removal of the disc, structural weakness existed at the intervertebral disc space, causing progressive disc space collapse and eventually resulting in structural instability. Howorth and associates, in 1943, similarly advocated spinal arthrodesis as an adjunctive method for the management of HNP.[18]

Retrospective series comparing discectomy with fusion to discectomy alone have failed to show any clinical improvement with decompression and fusion when compared to decompressive discectomy alone. Many authors have reported increased morbidity and significant complication rates with the added fusion.[29,35,66] Lehmann and associates, in a 20-year follow-up study, reported a 40% incidence of spinal instability and spinal stenosis in patients treated with simultaneous fusion for HNP.[35] Likewise, Knutsson and associates found 20% spinal instability after 13 years in patients who had undergone L4-S1 fusion surgery, with 5% of these patients clinically symptomatic.

The concept of using concomitant fusion with discectomy has fallen out of favor because of a lack of support in the literature. In conclusion, decompressive discectomy has been proven to be therapeutic for leg and back pain secondary to HNP. There is, however, no evidence that routine spinal arthrodesis with discectomy will improve surgical outcome in the management of lumbar disc herniation, with the exception of multiple recurrent disc herniations.

Spinal Stenosis/Spondylosis

Spinal spondylosis represents a spectrum of nonspecific, generalized spinal degenerative conditions in which marked central, lateral recess, and foraminal stenosis are frequently observed. Because of the physical and mechanical constraint resulting from the overall reduction in the diameter of the spinal canal, decompressive surgery is generally accepted as the definitive treatment of choice.[12,18,22,38,51,66]

Indications for fusion in lumbar stenosis are often based on initial clinical and/or radiographic evidence and less frequently on intra-operative findings that suggest the presence of spinal instability at the time of spinal canal decompression. Extensive spinal decompression, such as generous or complete intra-operative facetectomy with or without pars resection, can often lead to structural instability. Currently, there is inadequate literature addressing the criteria for simultaneous spinal fusion with decompressive surgery for the treatment of spinal stenosis. Nevertheless, decompressive laminectomy with concomitant spinal fusion has long been shown to improve back and radicular symptoms and to reduce the incidence of postoperative slippage and, thus, has resulted in improved clinical outcomes.[22,51,66]

The applicability of spinal fusion for spinal stenosis has solely been empirical and has been based on the experience from retrospective studies. The incidence of increasing lumbar spinal instability has been reported repeatedly in the literature, ranging anywhere from 10% to 60% following extensive decompression for lumbar stenosis.[38,53,61] The risk of developing postoperative instability has been strongly associated with the presence of concomitant degenerative spondylolisthesis. White and Wiltse and associates reported a 60% chance of developing increased postoperative slip in patients with lumbar stenosis and degenerative spondylolisthesis.[61] Two thirds of patients who had undergone decompression with partial facetectomy were found by Lombardi and associates to have increased postoperative slip, resulting in poorer clinical outcome.[38]

Routine fusion with decompression for patients with concomitant degenerative spondylolisthesis resulted in 64% to 100 % good or excellent results.[53] Feffer and associates treated 19 patients with lumbar stenosis and degenerative spondylolisthesis and found 100% good clinical outcome in patients who underwent fusion compared to 72% without fusion.[12] Bolesta and Bohlman and associates reported 100% good clinical outcome with decompression and fusion and only 50% good clinical outcome with decompression alone.[66] Therefore, simultaneous spinal arthrodesis with decompression for lumbar stenosis has been shown to improve radicular symptoms and back pain and to decrease postoperative spondylolisthesis.

Johnson and associates recognized the following potential risk factors for spinal instability development following decompression surgery:

1. Female gender.
2. Pre-operative unstable flexion/extension study.
3. Pre-existing degenerative spondylolisthesis.
4. Complete facetectomy.[32]

Reynold and Wiltse advocated fusion in patients younger than 60 years of age who have pre-existing degenerative spondylolisthesis, and in those who are younger than 50 years of age and have pre-existing isthmic spondylolisthesis.[51] Herkowitz and Kurtz reported 64% fusion rate with noninstrumented PLF, with reduced postoperative slip.[22] The addition of instrumentation, especially pedicle screw fixation, has helped to increase the rate of successful fusion and to improve clinical outcome in more recent years.

In general, patients with spinal stenosis typically respond well to decompressive surgery. However, in the situation in which extensive disruption of facet joints, pars, or both is identified intraoperatively, fusion with or without instrumentation should be considered. Furthermore, posterolateral fusion, with or without instrumentation, can improve clinical outcome in patients with spinal stenosis and concomitant degenerative spondylolisthesis.

Isthmic Spondylolisthesis

It is estimated that 5% to 8% of the general population may have bilateral pars interarticularis defects, but fewer than 50% of these individuals will eventually progress to any clinically relevant spondylolisthesis.[19,52,66] Early treatment for symptomatic spondylolysis and spondylolisthesis has relied heavily on nonsurgical modalities such as external bracing devices, physical therapy for truncal strengthening, and the use of nonsteroidal antiinflammatory drugs (NSAIDs). Steiner and Micheli and associates reported a 9% progression to symptomatic spondylolysis or low-grade slip that eventually required fusion.[56] Turner and Bianco found that 34% of their patients deteriorated with pain and debilitating musculoskeletal complaints to the point requiring surgical intervention.[58]

Surgical treatments for isthmic spondylolisthesis have been discussed extensively in the literature, including simple repair of pars defects, decompression alone (Gill procedure), complex in situ fusion, decompression with in situ fusion, and combined reduction/fixation with simultaneous fusion. Review of literature from retrospective fusion series has suggested that combined fusion with concomitant decompression is the preferred treatment for isthmic spondylolisthesis.[19,21,32,36,42,52] With the historical success of alleviation of symptoms, posterolateral fusion has been shown to be effective in the treatment of isthmic spondylolisthesis. The reported fusion rate for isthmic spondylolisthesis ranges from 27% to 100% for various fusion techniques and from 66% to 89% for PLF.[18,19,66] Overall, risk factors that may result in unsatisfactory outcomes include the following:

1. Male gender.
2. Middle age.
3. Smoking habit.
4. Pre-operative radicular symptoms.[19]

Harrington introduced instrumentation with PLF in 1967, using distraction rods, sublaminar hooks, and a transiliac sacral bar. Following his initial attempt to use pedicle screw instrumentation for spinal stability, Har-

rington reported that there is no advantage in reducing the listhesis.[20] Compared to earlier procedures, such as posterior intralaminar fusions performed for isthmic spondylolisthesis, many have found PLF with or without anterior fixation to be more successful than other posterior fusions and to provide better relief of symptoms.[21,52] To date, fusion with instrumentation has been well received by surgeons worldwide, and instrumentation with pedicle screw placement has been an integral part of the treatment of isthmic spondylolisthesis.

Lenke and associates reported a discouragingly low 50% solid fusion with noninstrumented in situ fusion but, surprisingly, greater than 80% good clinical outcome.[36] Reynold and Wiltse reported 90% of patients with high grade L5-S1 slips treated with in situ fusion to have resolved hamstring pain. Subsequently, 71% of patients remained free of symptoms.[51] With bilateral posterolateral fusion, Riley and associates were able to achieve 85% good or excellent outcome with symptomatic relief of back and leg pain.[52] Compared to historical controls, Jacobs and associates reported a 90% fusion rate using transfacet screw fixation methods.[31]

The incidence of postoperative slip for patients who had undergone PLF for isthmic spondylolisthesis has been reported to range from 11% to 72%. Possible causes include excessive bending stress or deformation of fusion mass, leading to subsequent pseudoarthrosis. Despite high fusion success rates reported in many series, it remains challenging for many to correctly diagnose solid fusion. Boxall and associates assessed 10 patients with isthmic spondylolisthesis who had bilateral PLF and diagnosed all patients to have solid fusion from using radiographic evidence.[4] However, following surgical exploration due to persistent symptoms, 70% of these patients were found to have pseudoarthrosis. Interestingly, McGuire and Amundson and associates, in their study of 27 patients, failed to see any statistically significant improvement in fusion rate with the addition of instrumentation.[42] They reported a 72% versus 78% fusion rate with noninstrumented versus rigid pedicle screw fixation and concluded that instrumentation did not enhance bony fusion rate, at least when fusion is determined radiographically.

Despite the controversy in fusion surgery, there is convincing evidence that PLF has been successful in fusion enhancement and in the improvement of clinical symptoms in the treatment of isthmic spondylolisthesis. The addition of pedicle screws or other instrumentations such as transfacet screw fixation has also been shown to be advantageous in fusion outcome.[31,50]

Discogenic Pain

Crock was the first to examine the mechanism of pain of discogenic origin. He went on to coin the term *internal disc derangement* to describe unremitting lumbar spinal pain that persisted more than four months, pain that is not responsive to conservative care, and that can be reproduced with discography.[7] In a sense, discogenic pain syndrome represents a continuum of pathologies that mainly involve the diseased intervertebral disc. They are also known as degenerative disc disease, internal disc derangement, annular tear, and dark disc disease. In many instances, these pain entities can be diagnosed either by magnetic resonance imaging (MRI) or by discography.[6,44,45,63]

The success in discogenic pain management depends heavily on the ability to eliminate the pain, which appears to originate from within the disc space. This may require complete disc ablation and elimination of disc motions. Thus, the goal of surgery is to completely immobilize all disc motions. Biomechanical studies have demonstrated that the most effective treatment for eliminating motion between two vertebral bodies is through the disc space. In fact, the mechanical strength in anterior lumbar interbody fusion (ALIF) has been found to be twice as strong compared to that of PLF.[34,64]

Early nonfusion treatments for pain of discogenic origin have included discectomy, percutaneous discectomy, and chymopapain injection. These treatment modalities, however, were found to be ineffective. Recent literature suggests that fusion may be the appropriate treatment for discogenic pain syndrome. Contemporary spinal fusions used have been PLF with or without instrumentation, posterior lumbar interbody fusion (PLIF), (ALIF), combined anterior and posterior fusion, and with the use of interbody cages made from metal alloys or prepared cadaveric bone grafts. Crock has long recommended the ALIF technique for this disease entity.[7]

Posterolateral fusion, the most time-honored fusion technique, has been found to be inadequate in eliminating pain of discogenic origin. Despite excellent fusion rate of higher than 80% reported in several fusion series, clinical correlation, which ranged from 57% to 67%, has been somewhat disappointing for PLF. The addition of pedicle screw fixation, according to Zucherman and associates, has resulted in 89% successful fusion rate but with only 60% clinical success.[68] Weatherley and associates documented five patients with continued low back pain despite satisfactory solid PLF who went on to have complete resolution of symptoms following subsequent ALIF.[60]

Colhoun found an 88% satisfactory result in his nonconsecutive series of patients who underwent fusion following positive discography.[6] Others have reported the clinical outcome and fusion success rate ranging from 73% to 89% for the anterior approach. In the case of combined anterior and posterior fusion, several clinical series have reported the overall clinical success rate to be as high as 60% to 80%.

Although fusion rates in many ALIF series have been in the range of 70% to 80%, there were associated complications reported, such as significant loss in disc height and a high incidence of nonunion. Dennis and associates found 100% of patients with ALIF to have evidence of disc space height loss postoperatively. Others reported nonunion rates and bone graft collapse and resorption rates as high as 34%.[67] Knox and Chapman looked at patients who underwent ALIF and found 35% had good clinical outcome with one-level fusion and none had good outcomes for two-level fusion. In their series, there is a very high rate of pseudoarthrosis.[28]

Zdeblick compared the fusion outcome of different surgical techniques in the management of DDD and reported 80% fusion rate with PLF, 91% with PLIF, and 100% with ALIF using interbody fusion cages in a prospective randomized study of patients with one-level degenerative disc disease at L5-S1.[67] Kuslich and associates had a 91% fusion rate and a 92% clinical success rate in their series using an interbody cage.[30]

In short, because the pain originates mainly within the disc space, PLF alone, with or without instrumentation, has not been successful in the treatment of DDD despite the high fusion rate. There is convincing evidence that ALIF with or without simultaneous posterior fusion is the preferred fusion procedure for this DSD entity.

Instrumentation versus Noninstrumentation

Noninstrumented PLF results in a solid arthodesis in 50% to 100% of patients treated for DSD. In the early '50s, Watkins and Campbell reported a 68% fusion rate.[59] Herkowitz and Kurtz similarly achieved a 64% fusion rate with noninstrumented in-situ PLF in the treatment of patients with isthmic spondylolisthesis. Lenke and associates reported a 50% fusion rate in a series of 56 patients with known isthmic spondylolisthesis who underwent bilateral PLF without decompression and instrumentation.[36]

In order to improve these less than optimal results, the use of instrumentation was added. McAfee and associates reported an increased fusion rate with the use of spinal instrumentation, first in animal models and later in a clinical series.[41] In a prospective series of 124 patients treated for different DSD conditions, Zdeblick and associates reported a 65% fusion rate without the use of instrumentation.[47,66] Using the semirigid pedicle screw and Luque II plate system, they found the fusion rate to increase to 77%, and to 95% when rigid instrumentation was used.[65] In a retrospective study of patients with isthmic spondylolisthesis, Deguchi and associates reported no statistical difference in single-level fusion rate whether or not instrumentation was used.[10] They did, however, observe better fusion results with two-level fusion with instrumentation

(79%) compared to noninstrumentation fusion (57%). McGuire and Amundson found no statistical significance resulting from the addition of instrumentation in 27 patients with isthmic spondylolisthesis. They reported a 72% fusion rate for noninstrumentation and a 78% fusion rate with rigid pedicle screw fixation.[42]

In a series of 68 patients who underwent spinal fusion, Lorenz and associates found a 58.6% pseudoarthrosis rate in the noninstrumented group and a 0% pseudoarthrosis rate in patients instrumented with pedicle crew fixation.[39] Clinical improvement was strongly correlated with fusion success; only 41.4% in the nonhardware group improved, whereas 76.9% in the instrumented group improved following fusion surgery. Kaneda and associates followed patients treated for unstable degenerative spondylolisthesis. These patients underwent medial facetectomies and PLF with distraction and compression rod instrumentation and had a 96.3% successful fusion rate.[27] All patients had complete resolution of pre-operative bladder and neurogenic claudication at the time of follow-up (mean follow-up of 30 months).

Although instrumentation use can improve fusion outcome, the addition of hardware has not been without added risks. Instrumentation use has been associated with increased complications, which are well documented in the literature. Furthermore, McAfee and associates report an increased risk for the development of osteopenia in patients who underwent fusion with instrumentation.[41] Osteopenia is frequently located within the fused segments spanned by the hardware devices.[46] This is known as *stress-reduction osteopenia*. Dalenburg and associates have found that this device-related osteopenia can be prevented or reduced if the longitudinal segment of the implant is allowed to loosen.[18]

In summary, the addition of instrumentation to PLF appears to result in higher rates of fusion. There may be a positive effect on patient outcome, as well. The use of such instrumentation is not without short- and long-term complications. The potential benefits of instrumentation use must be balanced against the potential complications in any given clinical scenario.

TECHNIQUE

Without bony fusion, instrumentation will eventually fail. Adequate quantity and quality of bone graft as well as meticulous preparation of the recipient bed will undoubtedly enhance the likelihood of a bony fusion. In addition, the use of instrumentation has been associated with an increase in the probability of a successful fusion. Instrumentation is not, however, required in all cases, as previously discussed.

The patient is placed in the prone position on the Jackson operating table (the type of table preferred by the authors). A variety of other frames and tables that fulfill the same function are commercially available. The basic principle of patient positioning is to achieve abdominal decompression and, at the same time, maintain lumbar lordosis. With the legs extended at the hip, the patient's posture is maintained in the correct lordosis and in the appropriate sacral inclination. Tribus and associates have recently discussed the importance of proper surgical positioning during lumbosacral fusion and have found the kneeling position to be suboptimal for posterior fusion techniques, particularly when multiple-level fusions are performed.[57]

Prior to placement of the bone graft, the fusion bed must be thoroughly prepared by decortication of the bony surface to expose the underlying cancellous core. This should include the transverse processes, the facet joints, and the pars interarticularis. Decortication of the transverse processes can be achieved easily with a variety of instruments such as a burr or a curette. The authors prefer creating a curl of bone in the transverse process, using a large curette. This doubles the surface area for engraftment and, at the same time, creates a well-vascularized pedicle of bone. This can be accomplished by initially drilling a hole in the distal portion of the transverse process (Figure 7-1). A large curette is then placed in the hole and gently wiggled medially to create a corticocancellous strip that should remain attached medially (Figure 7-2).

Equally important, the lateral surface of the facet joint must also be prepared with a burr or curette. The adjacent surfaces of the facet joints can be removed with a narrow tipped rongeur and then packed with bone graft to enhance the likelihood of fusion. Although any exposed bony surface should be decorticated prior to bone grafting, decortication should not

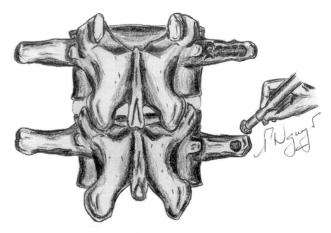

Figure 7-1 ■ **Artist illustration of a surgical view of lumbar spine.** Fusion bed is prepared by first making a hole in the lateral aspect of the transverse process using a drill. A well-vascularized bony curl is created using a large curette and deposited medially to increase graft surface area *(arrowhead).*

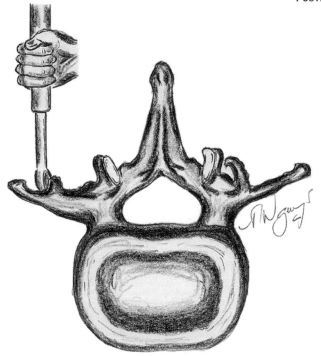

FIGURE 7-2 ■ **Artist illustration of the axial view of lumbar spine.** After the hole is drilled, a large curette is used with gentle wiggle motion to create a cortico-cancellous bony strip. A bony curl, created on the right, is ready for additional graft placement *(arrowhead).*

be so aggressive that it would compromise the integrity of the spine or of the instrumentation used. In order to optimize the chance for fusion to occur, generous quantity and quality of bone graft must be used, especially for PLF. Autograft should be used for onlay grafts, whereas allograft may be sufficient for interbody fusions, especially when used under compression. Autograft can be harvested from either one or both of the iliac crests and from the bony decompression.

For a short segment fusion, unilateral posterior iliac crest harvesting will provide adequate bone for grafting. For a longer, complex fusion, bilateral iliac crest bone harvesting may be necessary. In addition, autograft may be used alone or in combination with allograft and/or demineralized bone matrix if an adequate supply of autograft is unobtainable. Any extra bone obtained from the initial decompression should be cleaned free of soft tissue and broken down into small match-head size pieces. Once again, the authors emphasize the importance of an adequate bone graft, because this has been shown to be one of the factors that can influence fusion outcome.[2,3] The bone graft is carefully applied to the decorticated surfaces in a continuous fashion, forming a bridge from one segment to the next (Figure 7-3).

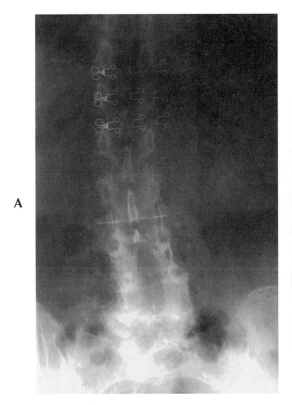
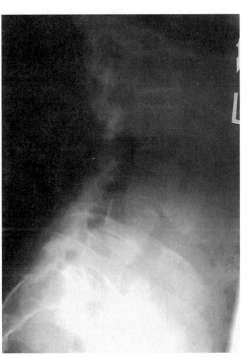

FIGURE 7-3 ■ **A, AP; and B, lateral lumbosacral spine x-rays.** Noninstrumented PLF in an 82-year-old patient with history of chronic low back pain resulting from lumbar stenosis and concomitant degenerative spondylolisthesis. Evidence of solid intertransverse processes bony fusion on AP view *(arrowheads).* Patient's symptoms resolved following fusion surgery.

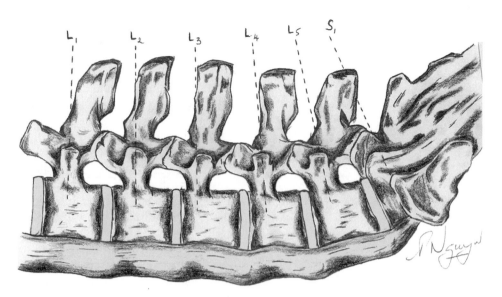

FIGURE 7-4 ■ **Artist illustration of the lateral view of lumbosacral spine.**
Demonstration of the rostrocaudal angle of each pedicle from L1 to S1. This
should serve as the trajectory for intra-operative pedicle screw placement.

For instrumented fusion, a thorough knowledge of the anatomy of the lumbosacral spine is mandatory if safe and accurate placement of pedicle screws is to be accomplished. Since pedicle screws are used as the primary anchoring device in lumbosacral fusions, preoperative assessment of the anatomy on imaging studies and a familiarity with the pertinent instrumentation system will ensure a smooth operation and will increase the likelihood of a good outcome.

Because of possible complications with pedicle screw placement, one must familiarize oneself with each individual lumbar and sacral pedicle size, as well as the potential variations. The width of each pedicle varies and is slightly increased in size rostrocaudally. In addition, there is a more caudal trajectory through the pedicles of lower lumbar and sacral levels (Figure 7-4). Therefore, the appropriate screw trajectory through a pedicle must be precise in order to avoid any compromise of the spinal canal or neural foramen. Similarly, the angle of pedicle placement is also varied from one level to another. A general rule of thumb is that there is an increasing angle of screw trajectory for lower lumbar and sacral pedicles. For each level descending along the lumbosacral spine, the angle of screw placement should be 5 degrees more medially (Figure 7-5).

A variety of methods have been described to place pedicle screws. The authors prefer to first determine the intersection between the mid-point of the base of the transverse process and between the superior articular facet as the entry point for screw placement. The bony surface is then decorticated with a drill until the cancellous appearance of the pedicular core is encountered. The pedicle is carefully probed with a gentle twisting to-and-fro motion applied with firm advancing pressure in the planned trajectory until the anterior

vertebral cortex is felt. The distinctive resistance of the pedicle to the probe is unique and can be easily appreciated with experience.

Nevertheless, ultimate control of the probing device must be maintained at all times to prevent plunging of

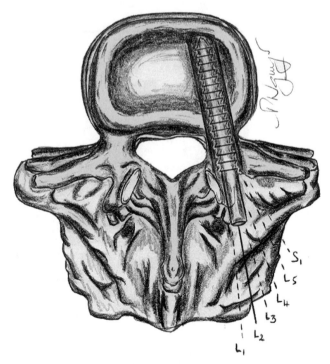

FIGURE 7-5 ■ **Artist illustration (in axial view) demonstrating the angle and trajectory of pedicle screw placement.** Entry site is at the junction between mid-point of the base of transverse process and superior articular facet. The further down the lumbosacral spine, the more medial angle of the trajectory.

the instrument beyond the anterior cortex of the vertebral body. In osteoporotic patients, great caution is needed because of the soft, poor quality of the bone, making a through-and-through probing a heightened risk. The pedicle is sounded to assess inadvertent penetration of the cortical wall. Once all the pedicles have been probed, radiographs should be obtained, with markers placed in each hole to document correct location and appropriate trajectories. Any additional adjustments of the trajectories must be performed prior to the placement of screws. Final screw placement is confirmed with a final lateral radiograph (Figure 7-6).

Frameless stereotactic image-guided technology can be used as an adjunct to safe and accurate screw placement. This new technology has been received with great enthusiasm and has been shown to be safe and effective. Pre-operative imaging data can be used prior to surgery to help in planning screw trajectory and to determine screw diameter and length. All of this information is subsequently mated to the actual intra-operative anatomy through registration. Image-guided tools are then used to locate and create pilot holes for pedicle screws.

The surgeon must be completely familiar with the particular instrumentation system that is to be used. Most commercially available systems come with standard screws ranging in diameter from 5.0 or 5.5 mm to as wide as 7.5 to 8.5 mm. Custom-made screws with a smaller diameter of 4.5 mm are also available. Standard screw lengths typically range from 30 to 75 mm. Furthermore, pedicle screws are available with fixed heads or multiaxial heads. The coupling devices also vary from system to system. The intricacies of each particular system are beyond the scope of this chapter; therefore, each surgeon must have a good understanding of the advantages and shortcomings of the system to be used.

COMPLICATION AVOIDANCE AND MANAGEMENT

Posterolateral fusion of the lumbosacral spine can be a formidable undertaking associated with a variety of complications. The surgeon must be aware of the pitfalls at each stage of the procedure. Thus, careful planning and meticulous execution of the procedure must be carried out in order to minimize such complications.

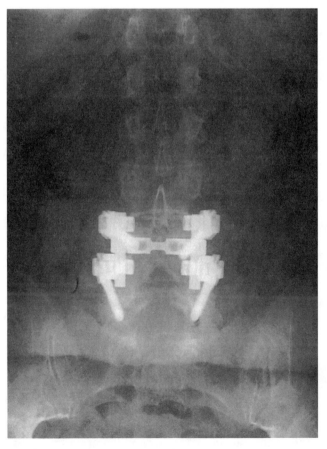
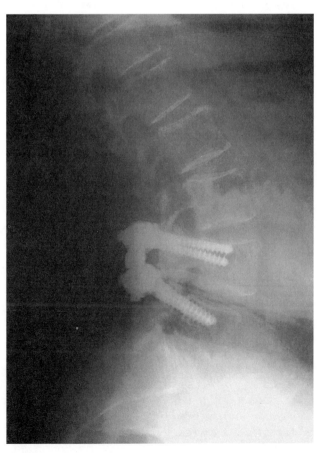

A   B

FIGURE 7-6 ■ A, AP; and B, lateral lumbosacral spine x-rays. Instrumented PLF in a 56-year-old patient with history of persistent low back pain resulting from postoperative spondylolisthesis following decompressive laminectomy. PLF with pedicle screw fixation using Texas Scottish Rite Hospital (TSRH) system. Symptoms resolved following fusion surgery.

It is apparent to many that PLF requires an extensive exposure of musculoskeletal components and can lead to considerable blood loss. Meticulous hemostatic control throughout the operation will greatly reduce the amount of blood loss. Bleeding points should be controlled at the time of discovery with monopolar or bipolar cautery. Though liberal utilization of electrocautery can decrease blood loss, thermal injury to areas where bone grafting will take place can impede fusion; therefore, care must be taken to avoid excessive injury to exposed bone.

Various strategies in addition to hemostatic techniques are available to limit the use of blood transfusion. These strategies include the following:

1. Autologous blood donation is an option that is available in most centers throughout the United States. In general, prior to surgery, a unit of blood may be donated every week, and the saved cells can be used within six weeks from the time of donation.
2. Cell-saver suction systems are also available in many institutions to allow blood collected during the course of the operation to be transfused back to the patient. This method should not, however, be used in patients with active infection or with spinal tumors that are undergoing surgery. Using this method, significant quantities of blood may be salvaged and can help to reduce the need for blood transfusion.

The infection rate for spinal fusion surgery has been reported to range from 1% to 14% in multiple retrospective series. No specific statistics for infection rate following PLF are available in the literature. However, avoidance of infection is of paramount importance. Strict adherence to sterile technique throughout the procedure is mandatory. A consistent operative team will shorten the operating time to reduce the risk of infection. If an infection were to occur, there are a variety of strategies available to treat it, and removal of hardware is not always necessary. The authors recommend re-exploring the wound, debridement of infected tissues, and copious irrigation using pulsatile lavage containing antibiotics. The wound can then be sewn over drains that allow instillation of antibiotics with simultaneous suction. Aerobic and anaerobic cultures should be obtained intra-operatively to confirm the pre-operative diagnosis, to check for other pathogens, and to guide the antibiotic choice.

Irrigation and suction drainage should be continued for at least one week. Irrigation should be discontinued 24 hours prior to removal of suction. Prolonged intravenous antibiotics must be administered. Discontinuation can be determined by clinical findings and by laboratory indicators, including white blood (cell) count (WBC), sedimentation rate, and C-reactive protein. The authors find that occasional consultation with infectious disease specialists may also be of benefit. If the patient continues to fail to respond to the treatment, wound re-exploration and removal of the hardware is inevitable. In the event that hardware removal is necessary, it is recommended that removal be delayed until after fusion has occurred, if possible.

Incorrect identification of the fusion level can occur in patients who have had previous surgery or in those who may require simultaneous decompressive surgery. Despite the familiarity of spinal anatomy, direct observation and palpation can sometimes be unreliable, and, therefore, an intra-operative lateral radiograph should be obtained routinely.[11] Malposition of hardware can often lead to complications involving the neural structures. Direct compromise of nerve roots can result in symptoms ranging from mild paresthesia to significant sensorimotor deficits. The appropriate guidelines for treatments of such complications depend solely on signs and symptoms presented. Treatment plans can vary from no immediate treatment to possible urgent removal of the offending device. Vascular and visceral injuries rarely occur during placement of posterior instrumentation, but their occurrence has been well documented in the literature. Again, these complications can be easily avoided if the surgeon pays meticulous attention to detail.

Pre-operative planning using imaging studies or information provided from frameless stereotactic systems can help reduce these risks by providing adequate information such as pedicle dimensions, trajectory, and screw length. One must keep in mind that instrumentation only serves as an adjunct to fusion. It is used to provide spinal rigidity to allow bony fusion to occur and has been shown to enhance fusion rates.[13,27,39,65,67] Without good solid bony fusion, all hardware will eventually fail. Treatment of hardware failure is usually dictated by symptoms.

Nonunion has been reported in the range of 35% to 58.6% in noninstrumented fusions and in the range of 0% to 14% of instrumented fusions.[39,65] Physiological properties of fusion have been studied thoroughly and have been shown to enhance or retard fusion via a variety of mechanisms.[2,15,16] Cigarette smoking has been implicated in increased risk of nonunion or pseudoarthrosis, as well as in risk of other systemic problems such as stroke, hypertension, cardiorespiratory-related problems, and cancers. Brown and associates reported a 40% incidence of pseudoarthrosis in smokers but only 8% in nonsmokers. Zdeblick and associates found the fusion rate in smokers reduced regardless of whether or not instrumentation was used. McGuire and Amundson reported 100% fusion rate with nonsmokers and 56% with smokers in their series.[42] Smoking cessation is therefore highly recommended in preparation for fusion procedure. The patient should be advised to cease smoking for at least two months preceding a fusion and for six months afterward. In addition, many have recently raised the issue of the effect on fusion rate of the use of NSAIDS following fusion surgery.[10,14] Because the initial phase of fusion is an inflammatory response, and because the use of NSAIDS has been shown to decrease fusion rates in animal models, the authors recommend that NSAIDs not be used for at least six weeks postoperatively.

Within the fusion bed, there are several factors that must be considered in order to optimize the fusion environment. The fusion mass receives its blood supply from the surrounding musculature. Necrotic or nonviable tissues should be debrided from the area surrounding the fusion bed prior to closure. As discussed earlier, thermal injury to the transverse processes through overzealous use of cauterization can impede fusion growth and should be avoided, if possible. Because nutrition undoubtedly plays a major role in the recuperation and healing process following fusion surgery, the patient's nutritional status should also be optimized.

Dural tear is not an uncommon occurrence in lumbar spine surgery. If feasible, primary closure is usually effective. Fibrin glue can be used as an adjunctive measure of security. Some surgeons recommend flat bedrest following the repair of a dural tear. The authors do not routinely use bedrest following repair unless patients have symptoms such as posture-related headaches (otherwise known as spinal headaches). In a few instances, spinal fluid leaks may not be reparable by primary closure and may require more complex treatment options. Patching with muscle, fascia lata, bovine pericardium, or Gortex (Gore, W.L.Gore & Associate, Inc.) has been used by many with reasonably good outcome. In these cases, however, cerebrospinal fluid (CSF) diversion and fibrin glue, in addition to patching, can be of great benefit.

Complications to structures adjacent to the graft site must also be taken into consideration. Because the cluneal nerve is located approximately 8 cm lateral to the posterior superior iliac spine, injury to these nerves can occur and can lead to pain at the harvest site. The sciatic nerve and superior gluteal vessels are positioned in the proximity of the sciatic notch and are, therefore, vulnerable to injury during the bone harvesting procedure. Stress fractures of the hip can occasionally occur following the removal of bone or in patients with severe osteoporosis.

Fusion operations are physiologically stressful operations. Thus, medical complications are not uncommon and can be minimized with vigilant treatment of the patient in the postoperative period. Ileus, deep venous thrombosis (DVT), fluid overload, and atelectasis are but a few of these complications.

CONCLUSION

Spinal arthrodesis has continued to claim an important position in the treatment of DSD and has been routinely performed in the treatment of many spinal degenerative conditions. With the exception of herniated disc condition, spinal fusion has been found to have reasonable success in the treatment of DSDs. PLF has been shown to be adequate, if not more superior, in comparison to other fusion techniques in the treatment of spinal stenosis with concomitant degenerative spondylolisthesis, isthmic spondylolisthesis, and other degenerative conditions. PLF, however, has not been shown to be successful in the treatment of discogenic pain.

Instrumentation has also been shown to improve both fusion outcome and postoperative clinical outcome. There remains difficulty in developing universal criteria for making a correct diagnosis of successful fusion versus failed fusion. Furthermore, the addition of instrumentation hardware must be carefully considered with a good understanding of both the potential benefits and the potential risks.

REFERENCES

1. Albee FH: Transplantation of a portion of the tibia into the spine for Pott's disease. **JAMA** 57:885-86, 1911.
2. Boden SD, Schimandle JH: Biologic enhancement of spinal fusion. **Spine** 20(24S):113S-23S, 1995.
3. Boden SD, Martin GJ, Borone M, et al: The use of coralline hydroxyapatite with bone marrow, autogenous bone graft, or osteoinductive bone protein extract for posterolateral lumbar spine fusion. **Spine** 24(4):320-27, 1999.
4. Boxall D, Bradford DS, Winter RB, et al: Management of severe spondylolisthesis in children and adolescents. **J Bone Joint Surg** 61:479-95, 1979.
5. Brantigan JW, Steffee AD: A carbon fiber implant to aid interbody lumbar fusion: two-year clinical results in the first 26 patients. **Spine** 18:2106-7, 1993.
6. Colhoun E, McCall IW, Williams L, et al: Provocative discography as a guide to planning operations of the spine. **J Bone Joint Surg** 70:267-71, 1988.
7. Crock HV: Internal disc disruption: a challenge to disc prolapse fifty years on. **Spine** 11:650-53, 1986.
8. Davis RA: A long-term outcome analysis of 984 surgically treated herniated lumbar discs. **J Neurosurg** 80:415, 1994.
9. Dean HG: Concise review for primary-care physicians. **Mayo Clin Proc** 71:283-87, 1996.
10. Deguchi M, Rapoff AJ, Zdeblick TA: Posterolateral fusion for isthmic spondylolisthesis in adults: analysis of fusion rate and clinical results. **J Spinal Disord** 11(6):459-64, 1998.
11. Ebraheim NA, Inzerillo C, Xu R: Are anatomic landmarks reliable in determination of fusion level in posterolateral lumbar fusion. **Spine** 24(10):973-74, 1999.

12. Feffer HL, Wiesel SW, Cuckler JM, et al: Degenerative spondylolisthesis: to fuse or not to fuse. **Spine** 10:287-89, 1985.

13. Fraser RF: Interbody, posterior, and combined lumbar fusions. **Spine** 20(Suppl):167S-77S, 1995.

14. Glassman SD, Rose SM, Dimar JR, et al: The effect of postoperative nonsteroidal anti-inflammatory drug administration on spinal fusion. **Spine** 23(7):834-38, 1998.

15. Glazer PA, Heilmann MR, Lotz JC, et al: Use of electromagnetic fields in a spinal fusion. A rabbit model. **Spine** 22(20):2351-6, 1997.

16. Goodwin CB, Brighton CT, Guyer RD, et al: A double blind study of capacitively coupled electrical stimulation as an adjunct to lumbar spinal fusions. **Spine** 24(13): 1349-56, 1999.

17. Hadra, B: Wiring of the vertebra as a means of immobilization in fracture and Pott's disease. **Am Orthop Assn Trans** 4:206, 1891.

18. Hanley EN: The indications for lumbar spinal fusion with and without instrumentation. **Spine** 20(Suppl):143S-53S, 1995.

19. Hanley EN, Levy JA: Surgical treatment of isthmic lumbosacral spondylolisthesis: analysis of variables influencing results. **Spine** 14:48-50, 1989.

20. Harrington PR, Dickson JH: Spinal instrumentation in treatment of severe progressive spondylolisthesis. **Clin Orthop** 117:157-63, 1976.

21. Harris IE, Weinstein SL: Long-term follow-up of patients with grade III and IV spondylolisthesis. treatment with and without posterior fusion. **J Bone Joint Surg** 69:960-69, 1987.

22. Herkowitz HN, Kurtz LT: Degenerative lumbar spondylolisthesis with spinal stenosis: a prospective study comparing decompression with decompression and intertransverse process arthrodesis. **J Bone Joint Surg** 73: 802-08, 1991.

23. Hibbs RA: Treatment of deformities of the spine caused by poliomyelitis. **JAMA** 69:787-96, 1917.

24. Hibbs RA, Swift WE: Developmental abnormalities at the lumbosacral juncture causing pain and disability. **Surg Gynecol Obstetric** 48:604-12, 1929.

25. Hodgson AR, Stock FE: Anterior spine fusion for the treatment of tuberculosis of the spine. **J Bone Joint Surg** 42: 295-310, 1960.

26. Howorth, MB: Evolution of spinal fusion. **Adv Surg** 117:278-89, 1943.

27. Kaneda K, Kazama H, Satoh S, et al: Follow-up study of medial facetectomies and PLF with instrumentation in unstable degenerative spondylolisthesis. **Clin Ortho & Related Research** 203:159-67, 1986.

28. Knox BD, Chapman TM: Anterior lumbar interbody fusion for discogram concordant pain. **J Spinal Disord** 6:242-44, 1993.

29. Knutsson F: The instability associated with disc degeneration in the lumbar spine. **Acta Radiol** 25:593-609, 1944.

30. Kuslich SD, Ulstrom CL, Griffith SL, et al: The Bagby and Kuslich method of lumbar interbody fusion: history, techniques, and 2-year follow-up results of a United States prospective, multicenter trial. **Spine** 23:1267-78, 1998.

31. Jacobs RR, Montesano PX, Jackson RP: Enhancement of lumbar spine fusion by use of translaminar facet joint screws. **Spine** 14:12-15, 1989.

32. Johnson JR, Kirwan EO: The long-term results of fusion in situ for severe spondylolisthesis. **J Bone Joint Surg** 65:43-46, 1983.

33. Lang F: Support for the spondylitic spine by means of buried steel bars, attached to the vertebra. **Clin Orthop** 203:3-6, 1986.

34. Lee CK, Vessa P, Lee JK: Chronic disabling low back pain syndrome caused by internal disc derangements. **Spine** 20(3):356-61, 1995.

35. Lehman TR, Spratt KF, Tozzi JE, et al: Long term follow-up of lower lumbar fusion patients. **Spine** 12:97-104, 1987.

36. Lenke LG, Bridwell KH, Bullis D, et al: Results of in-situ fusion for isthmic spondylolisthesis. **J Spinal Disord** 5:433-42, 1992.

37. Loeser J, Volinn E: Epidemiology of low back pain. **Neurosurg Clin N Am** 4:713-18, 1991.

38. Lombardi JS, Wiltse LL, Reynolds J, et al: Treatment of degenerative spondylolisthesis. **Spine** 10:821-27, 1985.

39. Lorenz M, Zindrick M, et al: A comparison of single-level fusions with and without hardware. **Spine** 16(8):455S-58S, 1991.

40. Martin GJ, Boden SD, et al: New formulations of demineralized bone matrix as a more effective graft alternative in experimental posterolateral lumbar spine arthrodesis. **Spine** 24(7):637-45, 1999.

41. McAfee PC, Farey ID, Sutterlin CE, et al: Device-related osteoporosis with spinal instrumentation. **Spine** 14:9, 1989.

42. McGuire RA, Amundson GM: The use of primary internal fixation in spondylolisthesis. **Spine** 18:1662-72, 1993.

43. Mixter WJ, Barr JS: Rupture of the intervertebral disc with involvement of the spinal canal. **N Engl J Med** 211: 210-15, 1934.

44. Modic MT, Pavliced W, Weinstein MA: Magnetic resonance imaging of the intervetebral disc disease. **Radiology** 152:103-11, 1984.

45. Modic MT, Steinberg PM, Ross JS, et al: Degenerative disc disease: assessment of changes in vertebral body marrow with MR imaging. **Radiology** 166:193-99, 1988.

46. Myers MA, Casciani T, et al: Vertebral body osteopenia associated with posterolateral spine fusion in humans. **Spine** 21:2368-71, 1996.

47. Nachemson A, Zdeblick TA, O'Brien JP: Controversy: lumbar disc disease with discogenic pain. What surgical treatment is most effective? **Spine** 21(15):1835-8, 1996.

48. Nashold BS, Hrubec Z: **Lumbar Disc Disease: A Twenty-Year Clinical Follow-up Study**. St. Louis: Mosby, 1971.

49. Pappas CT, Harrington T, Sonntag VK: Outcome analysis in 654 surgically treated lumbar disc herniations. **Neurosurgery** 30:862-66, 1992.

50. Reich SM, Kuflik P, Neuwirth M: Translaminar facet screw fixation in lumbar spine fusion. **Spine** 18(4):444-49, 1993.

51. Reynolds JB, Wiltse LL: Surgical treatment of degenerative spondylolisthesis. **Spine** 4:148-49, 1979.

52. Riley PM, Gillespie R, Koreska J: Severe spondylolisthesis: results of posterolateral fusion in children. **J Bone Joint Surg** 68:856, 1986.

53. Rosenberg NJ: Degenerative spondylolisthesis: predisposing factors. **J Bone Joint Surg** 57:467, 1975.

54. Roy-Camille R, Saillant G, Mazel C: Plating of thoracic, thoracolumbar and lumbar injuries with pedicle plates. **Orthop Clin North Am** 17:147, 1986.

55. Steffee A: Segmental spine plates with pedicle screw fixation. **Clin Orthop** 203:45, 1986.

56. Steiner ME, Micheli LJ: Treatment of symptomatic spondylolysis and spondylolisthesis with the modified Boston brace. **Spine** 10:937-43, 1985.

57. Tribus CB, Belanger TA, Zdeblick TA: The effect of operative position and short-segment fusion on maintenance of sagittal alignment of the lumbar spine. **Spine** 24(1):58-61, 1999.

58. Turner RH, Bianco AJ Jr: Spondylolysis and spondylolisthesis in children and teen-agers. **J Bone Joint Surg** 53:1298-306.

59. Watkins MB: Posterior fusion of the lumbar and lumbosacral spine. **J Bone Joint Surg** 35A:1014-8, 1953.

60. Weatherley CR, Prickett CF, O'Brien JP: Discogenic pain persisting despite solid posterior fusion. **J Bone Joint Surg** 68B (1):142-43, 1986.

61. White AH, Wiltse LL: Spondylolisthesis after extensive lumbar laminectory. **J Bone Joint Surg** 58:727-28, 1975.

62. Wiltse LL, Hutchinson RH: Surgical treatment of spondylolisthesis. **Clin Orthop** 35:116-35, 1967.

63. Witzel FT, LaRocca SH, Lowery GL, et al: The treatment of lumbar spinal pain syndromes diagnosed by discography. Lumbar arthrodesis. **Spine** 19(7):792-800, 1994.

64. Zdeblick TA, Smith GR, Warden KE, et al: Two-point fixation of the lumbar spine. Differential stability in rotation. **Spine** 16(6S):298S-301S, 1991.

65. Zdeblick TA: A prospective, randomized study of lumbar fusion. Preliminary results. **Spine** 18:983-91, 1993.

66. Zdeblick TA: The treatment of degenerative lumbar disorders. A critical review of the literature. **Spine** 20(Suppl): 126S-37S, 1995.

67. Zdeblick TA. Introduction of discogenic back pain. 13th Annual Meeting of the North American Spine Society. Oct. 1998.

68. Zucherman J, Hsu K, Picetti G, et al: Clinical efficacy of spinal instrumentation in lumbar degenerative disc disease. **Spine** 17(7):834-37, 1992.

CHAPTER 8

Posterior Lumbar Interbody Fusion

DANIEL K. RESNICK, M.D., M.S.

Based on 45 years' experience in the surgical treatment of lumbar disc disease, it is recommended that the following operations be eliminated: the simple discectomy, which may cure the sciatica but not the back pain; the "decompressive laminectomy," which leaves the patient with painful instability and nerve root scarring; and chemonucleolysis, which does not provide permanent relief of either low back or leg pain. The PLIF technique is the answer to treatment of the lumbar spine and may be the operation of the future.

RB CLOWARD, 1985[6]

INTRODUCTION

Since Dr. Cloward first described the PLIF (posterior lumbar interbody fusion) technique in 1945, the PLIF has been alternatively hailed and reviled as a treatment for low back pain and sciatica. Some of the techniques and principles described by Dr. Cloward, however, persist as a foundation upon which much of modern spine surgery rests. Dr. Cloward stressed the importance of placing bone grafts in the load-bearing portion of the spine (anterior and middle columns), described a surgical technique used to place such grafts from a posterior approach, and developed a bone banking system for the acquisition, processing, and storage of allograft bone material.[5,6,7,8] The PLIF technique has evolved over time, and it currently has regained favor in its latest forms. Several procedures that use streamlined instrumentation and preformed grafts (made of bone, titanium, or carbon fiber) to achieve similar biomechanical end results to the traditional PLIF technique are now popular. These constructs are usually combined with some sort of posterior instrumentation system (i.e., pedicle screws or facet screws) in order to restore the dorsal tension band. Whereas the new PLIF techniques make the operation more simple, and the addition of posterior instrumentation systems certainly results in a more rigid construct, the final outcome achieved may or may not differ substantially from that obtained using

the original PLIF technique. Certainly, these systems result in an increased cost of fusion. The purpose of this chapter is to review the surgical indications and patient selection criteria for PLIF (instrumented as well as noninstrumented), the surgical techniques used to perform the operation, commonly encountered complications, and the outcome obtained in a number of clinical series.

SURGICAL INDICATIONS

The indications used to justify a PLIF procedure vary widely among authors, and it is likely that the relatively indiscriminate use of the procedure has contributed to a perception that the PLIF operation may be a "bad" or "dangerous" operation. Every surgical procedure has attendant risks that must be balanced against the expected natural history of the disease process and other potentially therapeutic maneuvers. As such, despite Dr. Cloward's assertions, the use of a PLIF for radiculopathy caused by a simple disc herniation is considered inappropriate by most surgeons. Simple discectomy and microdiscectomy have been shown to provide excellent long-term results without the need for or attendant risks of a fusion.[12,23] The role of PLIF in the treatment of spinal stenosis is also limited, because decompression alone is an effective and certainly less invasive procedure for the majority of patients.[16] Similarly, there may be a role for "minimally invasive" percutaneous procedures such as chemonucleolysis and intradiscal electrotherapy (covered in separate chapters) for the treatment of back and radicular pain. The use of dorsal column stimulation for the treatment of low back and leg pain is also discussed in a separate chapter.

There exists a population of patients who may benefit from the PLIF procedure, with or without posterior instrumentation. These patients have disabling back pain with painful degenerative changes localized to one or two levels. Many of these patients would also be considered candidates for anterior lumbar interbody fusion (ALIF). PLIF provides an opportunity for an extraforaminal decompression of the nerve roots or cauda equina (i.e., within the spinal canal) (Figure 8-1), which ALIF does not, and allows anterior graft placement without the need for mobilization of the great vessels or manipulation of the sympathetic chain. Furthermore, the ability to use posterior fixation in combination with anterior column support allows for the creation of more rigid constructs. This is especially important when considering interbody fusion in a patient with a well-maintained disc space height. Patients with well-maintained disc space height are generally not candidates for anterior implants alone because these implants rely on the tension of the annulus to provide stability to the spine. It may not be possible to obtain adequate tension of the annulus with anterior implants without over-distracting a space with well-maintained height (this is usually the younger patient with a painful spondylolisthesis). The ability to use concomitant pedicle screw fixation makes the PLIF an attractive alternative in this population.

The most clear cut indication for a PLIF is disabling back pain and leg pain with extra-foraminal neural element compression. Relative indications for a PLIF, as opposed to ALIF, include unfavorable vascular anatomy at the L4-L5 level and fusion above the L4-L5 level (although a lateral approach to these levels via a retroperitoneal exposure is certainly an option as well). The PLIF is well suited to the patient with a well-maintained disc space height in whom posterior instrumentation is contemplated. Patients with contraindications to anterior approaches (previous abdominal or pelvic surgery) may also be treated with PLIF. Finally, the PLIF does not require the assistance of an "approach" surgeon, avoiding the associated scheduling and coding difficulties associated with a multiple surgeon procedure.

PATIENT SELECTION

The ideal patient for any lumbar interbody fusion operation is relatively young (25–45 years of age) and has suffered debilitating back pain (and possible upper thigh and buttock pain) for at least 12 months despite adequate trials of physical therapy, chiropractic manipulation, and medical therapy. The ideal patient has few, if any, secondary gain issues (Workers' Compensation, ongoing litigation, drug-seeking behavior), does not smoke, and is not obese. This patient may or may not have radicular signs on examination, will not demonstrate "Waddell Signs," and will generally not be seen accompanied by a "caseworker" or lawyer.[32] Plain films will reveal degenerative changes at a single (or possibly two) levels. Magnetic resonance imaging (MRI) will reveal typical signs of disc degeneration (i.e., Modic changes) limited to a single level, and discography will confirm painful disc degeneration at that level, with anatomical abnormalities noted in conjunction with the elicitation of concordant pain at a single level.[22]

The author only rarely sees the ideal patient and recognizes the difficulties encountered with patients who are "ideal patients" with the exception of one or two issues (i.e., a smoker, or a Workers' Compensation case). The author also freely acknowledges the limitations of discography.[3,4] All patients operated upon have had debilitating back pain and have all failed physical therapy and medical management. Patients are always encouraged to lose weight and to stop smoking (when applicable), but surgery is not withheld if the patient makes a sincere effort and has failed. We refer patients to both a dietician and a local smoking cessation center when applicable, with mixed results (about one half of patients are able to stop smoking completely for a month prior to surgery and three months after; most of the rest are able to cut down somewhat). Patients with three or more positive Waddell signs, with ongoing litigation, or with more than two-level involvement are not usually operated upon. Patients with three or more positive Waddell signs are referred to a comprehensive pain center for psychological counseling and further physical and medical therapy. Litigants are encouraged to settle lawsuits prior to surgery. Patients who do not anticipate timely resolution of ongoing litigation are encouraged to seek other surgical and nonsurgical opinions. Those with Workers' Compensation claims are operated upon if they are good candidates by other criteria; however, pre-operative discussions with the patient include a discussion of the effect of Workers' Compensation claims on ultimate outcome. These discussions are carefully documented in the patient record. A patient with more than two-level involvement (usually an older patient) usually requires a different (operative or nonoperative) approach, depending upon the levels of involvement and the severity of symptoms.

The choice of a posterior approach to lumbar interbody fusion, as opposed to an anterior or lateral

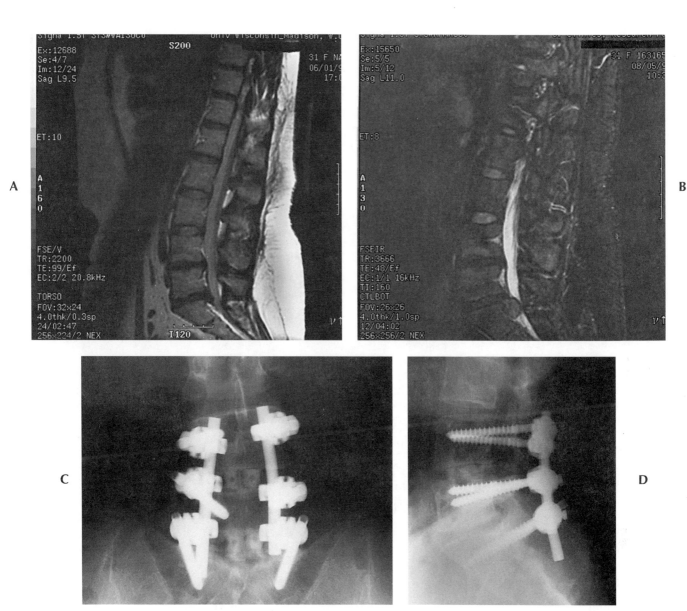

FIGURE 8-1 ■ **Case Example.** The patient is a 34-year-old woman who presented with a two-year history of worsening back pain. She had undergone over six months of supervised physical therapy and was doing home exercises on a regular basis. She did not smoke or drink and continued to work as a clerical worker despite her pain. Her neurological examination was normal, and she had no leg pain. Her initial MRI is shown in (**A**). The MRI demonstrates degenerative changes at both the L4-L5 and the L5-S1 level, with a small midline herniation at L5-S1. She underwent a discogram (not shown), which revealed internal disc disruption at both levels and normal anatomy at L3-L4. More importantly, injection at both levels reproduced her back pain, although the pain was more severe with injection of the L4-L5 level. There was no pain with injection at L3-L4. Three days prior to a planned two-level ALIF, she presented for her pre-operative work up (blood work, consent forms, etc.). Conversation in the office led her to relate several episodes of incontinence during the previous week. She also had some pain radiating down both legs, but this was not as severe as her back pain. She had not called the office, but wanted to mention it to us prior to her procedure "just in case." Her physical examination now revealed some sensory loss in the S1 distribution bilaterally but normal muscle strength and rectal tone; **B,** An MRI was repeated that day. This MRI reveals a large free fragment of disc material behind the L5 vertebral body. A laminectomy of L5, removal of the free fragment, and a two-level PLIF (supplemented with pedicle screw instrumentation) was performed on her originally scheduled surgery date (**C** and **D**). She is now nine months postoperative and is free of back pain.

approach, is dependent on several factors. First of all, the relevant pathology may dictate an approach. For example, the author has encountered patients with severe back pain as well as symptomatic nerve root or cauda equina compression. Although foraminal stenosis can be relieved by indirect decompression through anterior approaches, and a limited discectomy can be performed anteriorly, free fragments of disc (see Figure 8-1) cannot be addressed, nor can central stenosis. In these cases, a posterior approach is ideal. Another potential use for a posterior approach is the patient with degenerative disease at L4-L5 with unfavorable vascular anatomy. The author has been occasionally frustrated with an inability to adequately access the anterior surface of the L4-L5 disc space with anterior approaches (open as well as laparoscopic) and has had one significant venous injury resulting from an attempt to get adequate exposure at this level. A lateral or a posterior approach avoids this limitation. The author has also had two male patients who wanted to have children in the future. One of these patients donated sperm to a bank prior to an anterior procedure, the other elected for a posterior procedure in order to minimize the risk of retrograde ejaculation.

BIOMECHANICAL CONSIDERATIONS OF PLIF

Interbody fusion procedures place the bone graft in a load-bearing position within the anterior and middle columns of Denis (Figure 8-2).[11] Wolff's law indicates that placement of the grafts in an environment of compression enhances fusion potential.[33] Furthermore, restoration of anterior lumbar disc space height helps to restore the normal lumbar lordosis and to restore "sagittal balance" to the spine. Posterior approaches to interbody fusion, however, do disrupt the dorsal tension band and may leave the spine with a tendency towards kyphosis (see Figure 8-2). It is for this reason that many authors recommend posterior instrumentation for restoration of the dorsal tension band. Obviously, choice of technique and choice of implant may significantly alter the biomechanical properties of the construct. For example, safe and effective placement of certain interbody implants through a posterior approach may require the destruction of the facet complexes bilaterally. This maneuver obviously destabilizes the spine to some extent. Although placement of interbody grafts does restore significant stability to the spine, spinal stability may not return to normal.[31] Interestingly, the use of threaded cages as implants does not result in reduced rigidity to flexion loads in cadaveric spines, as might be anticipated.[25] Clinical experience has led several authors to recommend against the use of posteriorly placed cages as stand-alone devices because of a high rate of failure (see Chapter 10 for more discussion of this topic). Further

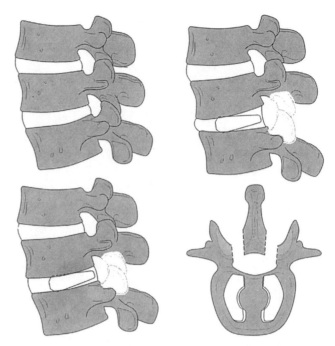

FIGURE 8-2 ■ **Biomechanics of PLIF.** The normal lumbar spine, at upper left, assumes a lordotic posture that is promoted by insertion of a wedge-shaped interbody graft (as shown at lower left). If the posterior elements are disrupted (as indicated by ghosting), the spine is rendered less able to resist both flexion and torsion. This may lead to a progressive loss of lordosis or even kyphosis (upper right figure). Minimalization of posterior element disruption through the use of newer techniques (as shown in the lower right illustration) may not lead to the same degree of destabilization.

complicating the picture is the development of new implant systems (such as the Tangent system marketed by Sofamor Danek) that do not require the extensive exposure needed for the traditional (as described by Cloward) PLIF or the implantation of threaded cylindrical cages. These new systems allow for placement of grafts through exposures not much greater than those needed for simple discectomy and allow for preservation of the facets to a great extent. As biomechanical testing of the new implant systems progresses, and as clinical experience with existent and emerging systems grows, we will learn more about the importance of the restoration of the dorsal tension band.

SURGICAL TECHNIQUE

The PLIF procedure has evolved significantly over time. The original procedure, described by Cloward in 1953, was described as a three-step procedure. The first step involves harvesting two full thickness (tricortical) bone plugs (1.5 × 3 cm) and a sufficient quantity of cancellous bone from the iliac crest. Next, a midline incision is made, and the spinous processes of the adjacent vertebral bodies are removed. A full laminectomy is not performed, although the intralaminar space is expanded by bone removal from the inferior edge of the rostral lamina and the inferior edge of the caudal lamina. The bone dissection is carried out far laterally, and at least half of the articular facets are removed. A self-retaining retractor is used to retract the nerve root and thecal sac medially; however, retraction should not be past midline. The lateral annulus is thus exposed, and a large rectangular annulotomy is made with a #11 blade. The disc is removed in its entirety, up to the anterior annulus. The cortical surfaces are then chiseled off, exposing raw, bleeding cancellous bone. The vertebral body spreader is used to assist visualization during the complete discectomy and during preparation of the end-plates. The spreader is then used to distract the disc space so that the bone grafts can be impacted into place. As many grafts as possible are inserted and then tamped towards the midline with specially designed chisels. Usually three or four plugs can be inserted at a single level. The bleeding from the interspace usually stops once the grafts are in place and the vertebral spreader is removed. Gelfoam is placed over the exposed dura, and cancellous chips are placed between the lamina (Cloward later stopped doing the posterior fusion).[6] A closed suction drain is left in the deep space to prevent hematoma accumulation, and the wound is closed in multiple layers.[8]

Since Cloward's original report, numerous modifications have been reported. Significant modifications used to eliminate the graft harvest include the use of allograft bone and the use of autograft spinous process and laminar bone as a "keystone" graft.[1,5,10] Although several authors have stressed the importance of patient positioning, significant disagreement exists as to the optimal position for the procedure.[8,9,18] All authors do stress the importance of decompressing the chest and abdomen to decrease venous bleeding. Transverse incisions, bilateral paraspinal approaches, and other technical modifications have been described over the years.[9,18] The concomitant use of posterior instrumentation and the use of preformed titanium and carbon fiber implants have significantly changed the procedure.[28,29] The use of these adjuncts are discussed in more detail in other chapters.

The author currently favors the use of commercially available preformed allograft implants that are placed with specially designed instrumentation. The use of these implants significantly decreases the amount of posterior element removal necessary for the placement of reasonably sized allografts and morselized autograft. The technique is usually combined with pedicle screw instrumentation. The clinical results obtained with the technique are described in a separate chapter. The author's technique is as follows. The patient is intubated supine on the stretcher, and a Foley catheter and pneumatic compression hose are placed. The eyes are lubricated and taped shut with hypoallergenic tape. The patient is then rolled onto a Jackson table with pads supporting the chest (just below the manubrium) and hips, allowing the abdomen to hang free. All bony prominences are inspected (especially the elbows) and adequately padded, the breasts and genitalia are inspected and adjusted to hang freely, and the orbital rims are inspected and padded to avoid undo intraocular pressure. The back is prepped and draped, and a localizing film with two spinal needles is obtained (in single-level cases; this step is eliminated in double-level cases because its only purpose is to limit the size of the incision used in a single-level case). An incision is made, and a second film is obtained with a marker on an easily identifiable bony landmark to verify level.

Soft tissue dissection is performed using monopolar electrocautery, and the soft tissue dissection continues until the lateral edge of the facet joint and the base of the transverse processes above and below the effected level are identified. The caudal edge of the rostral lamina is skeletonized with a curette, and a high-speed drill and kerrison rongeurs are used to create a laminotomy similar to (but slightly larger than) that used to perform a simple discectomy (Figure 8-3). Bone from the laminotomy is saved and used for graft material. The ligamentum flavum is opened with an angled curette, and the thecal sac and traversing root are exposed. A limited medial facetectomy is also performed, allowing exposure of the lateral annulus. It is not usually necessary to expose out to the level of the pedicle, and the exiting root may be left alone because it is protected by the remaining bone of the superior articulating facet of the caudal vertebral body. This is substantially different from the exposure used to place cylindrical cages. Implantation of adequately sized cylindrical cages requires more extensive bone removal and definitive identification, dissection, and retraction of the exiting root. Epidural hemostasis is meticulously preserved using bipolar electrocautery. The nerve root and thecal sac are retracted medially (rarely to midline, never beyond), and a rectangular annulotomy is made with a #15 blade.

Standard rongeurs and curettes are used to remove as much disc material as possible bilaterally. The annulus is generally not opened medially. Distraction plugs are then placed into the annulotomy defect and used to sequentially distract the space; usually a 10 or 11 mm distraction is possible in collapsed disc spaces without too much difficulty. It is important to get a good distraction of the interspace, as graft migration and failure of fusion are associated with inadequate distraction.[30]

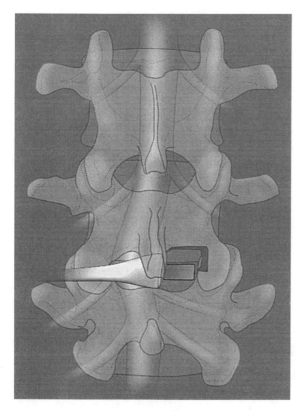

FIGURE 8-3 ■ Surgical exposure. This line drawing demonstrates the amount of soft tissue exposure and bony removal needed for placement of rectangular implants from a posterior approach. Note the relative preservation of the pars interarticularis and facet, which both preserves the structural integrity of the spine (to some extent) and protects the exiting nerve root.

Once a distraction plug is placed on one side, a more aggressive discectomy can be performed on the other side. As soon as a final distraction is complete, appropriately sized implants are prepared (by soaking in saline). It is important to get the implant soaking as soon as possible, as bleeding from the cut edges of vertebral body bone can be substantial. If the implants are used before reconstitution, there is a greater chance of fracturing the implant during placement. It is important, however, to wait until the disc space has been distracted prior to reconstituting the implants in order to select an appropriately sized implant. The author usually waits until the implants are soaking prior to proceeding with the final end-plate preparation.

Specially designed end-plate curettes and chisels are used to remove the entire cartilagenous end-plate and parts of the bony end-plate. This is a crucial part of the operation. It is important to completely visualize all corners of the curettes as they are placed into the space to avoid injury to the traversing or exiting root. It is important to scrape away all of the cartilagenous

end-plate prior to using the final chisel, which cuts away some of the bony end-plate in preparation for the allograft implant. Once site preparation is complete, an implant is placed on one side by impacting it into the prepared channel. The end-plate preparation procedure is then repeated on the other side. Autograft bone (from the laminotomy and facetectomy, or from the iliac crest if enough bone is not harvested from the decompression) is packed into the space and moved medially, using a small distraction plug. This bone will fill the space medial to the two crescentic allografts. The second implant is then placed in a similar fashion.

The wound is copiously irrigated with antibiotics and saline. Pedicle screw instrumentation placed in a compression mode or translaminar facet screws are placed to restore the dorsal tension band. Any remaining bone is placed over the lateral masses, and the wound is closed in multiple layers. A closed system subfascial drain is occasionally used if epidural oozing has not stopped completely. The wound is closed in multiple layers. The patient is allowed to ambulate as soon as possible after surgery. An elastic LSO brace is used for patient comfort, and the Foley catheter is removed the next morning. Patients are usually ready for discharge home within three to four days after surgery. Follow-up clinical evaluation and radiographs are obtained at six weeks, three months, six months, and one year following surgery.

COMPLICATIONS

In his 1953 report, Cloward reported astonishingly few complications in his series of 321 cases. He reported six failures of fusion, two of which went on to heal spontaneously and four of which required re-operation (a 98.8% fusion rate). He noted "occasional" and "usually transient" numbness of the foot and ankle, with weakness of the anterior tibial muscle, two cases of arachnoiditis (attributed to lipiodol), and 14 wound infections (of which only two required extensive debridement).[8] Cloward stressed that close adherence to his surgical technique and the use of his specialized instruments resulted in his clinical success (Cloward, comment following Lin paper).[18]

Hutter reported his results and complications in a series of 500 patients operated upon for various disorders over a 25-year period. He reported "technical difficulties in 24 patients." Complications included dislodgement of the bone graft in three cases, residual partial paralysis of the muscles supplied by the affected nerve in 18 cases, and 8 cases of the "cluneal syndrome" related to harvesting of the bone graft. There were also three cases of operation at the wrong level, five cases of deep venous thrombosis, and five wound infections.[14] Hutter dedicated a relatively large portion of his manuscript to the description of techniques for complication avoidance. He (as did Cloward) stressed the importance of decompression of the abdomen and also recommended intra-operative hypotension as a useful hemorrhage-limiting maneuver. He also stressed the utility of bipolar coagulation of the epidural veins, routine bladder catheterization, and the use of intra-operative lateral radiographs as other complication-avoidance techniques.[14]

Collis reported an approximately 4% complication rate in his series of 750 cases reported in 1984. His complications included four dural tears, four graft extrusions requiring corrective surgery, three graft extrusions not requiring surgery, six cases of new neurologic deficits (all transient), and several medical complications.[9] In 1987, Branch and Branch described the complications that occurred in their series of 172 patients. They reported an overall complication rate of 4%, with two patients each suffering a wound infection or graft extrusion, and single cases of broken drain, sterile discitis, and persistent pain requiring re-exploration.[1] Two years later, Rish described his experience with 250 cases accrued over 12 years. He described complications occurring in 13 patients (5.2%). Eight patients developed a new neurological deficit after surgery. Three patients developed phlebitis, and one suffered a pulmonary embolism. Rish stressed the importance of gentle retraction of the nerve root in order to reduce the likelihood of a new postoperative deficit.[26]

RESULTS

We have found too many examples of how enthusiasts can be deceived in their appreciation of their own success and how accomplishments are far removed from hopes-desires from realities. It is hard in such a case to recognize that one has deceived himself, but it is a sacrifice of the ego that the greatest have not blushed to make for science.

J. MALGAIGNE, 1843[21]

The majority of authors have reported excellent results with PLIF without instrumentation. For example, Cloward reported a greater than 85% rate of long-term cures in his first 321 patients.[8] In a follow-up paper, he reported an overall long-term cure rate of 87% to 92%.[6] He divided his series up somewhat and reported that patients with stenosis had a near 100% cure rate, patients with spondylolisthesis had a 95% cure rate, and that patients with failed back (multiply operated) syndrome had a better than 80% long-term cure with PLIF.[6,7] Lin reported a 94% fusion rate in an early series of 75 patients reported in 1977.[18] Lin later reported an 82% satisfactory outcome in a larger series of patients and a satisfaction rate of 74% in 143 patients who underwent PLIF for recurrent disc herniations.[17,19] Hutter, who used PLIF to treat 500 patients over a 25-year study, reported a 90% fusion rate and an 82% rate of excellent or good functional outcomes. Of note, 75% of Hutter's patients underwent operation for a herniated nucleus pulposus.[14] In a separate report dealing specifically with the results of PLIF in patients with lumbar stenosis, Hutter reported excellent or good results in 78%.[15] Following a review of 50 of his 750 cases, Collis reported "successful" results in 92% of patients.[9] Ma reported a good or excellent outcome in 74% of his 342 patients (35% excellent and 39% good), and Simmons reported a 79% rate of "objectively good results" with a modified PLIF procedure.[17,20,27] Branch and Branch reported an excellent or good clinical outcome in 75% of their 172 patients. This series, although heavily weighted towards patients with herniated discs (77%), is remarkable for the high percentage of Workers' Compensation patients included (48%).[1]

Other authors report less favorable results with the PLIF. For example, Rish reported a 60% rate of excellent or satisfactory results in his series of 250 patients who underwent PLIF for herniated discs. This was in spite of an 85.6% rate of fusion. He did note an imperfect association between nonunion and poor clinical outcome.[26] In a more recent series of patients with back pain and grade 1 spondylolisthesis, Verlooy and colleagues reported 45% good or excellent outcomes and 55% fair or poor outcomes.[30]

Interpreting the results of these series is difficult because of the variety of indications used to justify the procedure and the variety of outcome measures used to assess the results. Patient outcomes for patients with simple herniated discs are frequently combined with those with stenosis, failed back syndrome, and spondylolisthesis. Also, these studies all suffer, to some extent, from false endpoint reporting. For example, the occurrence of a solid bony fusion may not be the optimal outcome measure for a patient operated upon for radiculopathy related to a herniated nucleus pulposus.

Further difficulty arises when one considers that different authors have presented results with different definitions of fusion as well as different definitions of excellent/good/satisfactory outcomes. For example, Cloward used the appearance of trabecular bridging on static plain radiographs to define fusion. Hutter used the absence of motion on flexion/extension radiographs to define fusion, and Lin used tomograms to demonstrate "a viable graft with active osteosynthesis between the graft and the adjoining vertebral bodies."[8,14,18]

In an effort to standardize result reporting, and also to establish the relevance of the reported data, Prolo developed an outcome measure designed for patients undergoing back surgery. The measure is called the anatomic-economic-functional (AEF) rating system and includes factors related to the occurrence of a fusion, the patient's pre- and postoperative ability to work, and the patient's reported level of low back pain.[24] Prolo applied this rating system to 36 patients who underwent PLIF for a limited number of indications, all associated with lumbar instability. The use of PLIF for a simple disc herniation was not studied. Prolo reported an overall favorable response rate (functional and economic scores of 7 or greater; no patient scored higher than 5 pre-operatively) of 85% and a fusion rate of 94% in this group of patients.[24]

In 1988, Steffee reported his results with the PLIF supplemented by posterior pedicle screw instrumentation.[28] The ability to achieve immediate rigid fixation of the spine, to restore the dorsal tension band, and perhaps to enhance fusion rates was enthusiastically received by the spine community. Several series detailing the results of PLIF in conjunction with pedicle screw fixation or transfacet screw fixation have been published.[2,13,29] In some cases, the addition of posterior instrumentation appears to improve fusion rates and clinical outcome, but no randomized, controlled study has been performed. Further modifications of technique have followed, the most significant being the evolution of new interbody implants that allow for the use of autograft bone without the need for the harvest of large tricortical iliac crest grafts. These new implants are placed with specially designed instrumentation and require varying degrees of posterior element exposure (threaded cylindrical cages, rectangular cages, trapezoidal allograft, etc.). It remains to be seen if these new systems do in fact reduce operative morbidity and improve functional outcome when compared to the original PLIF.

Despite the difficulty encountered when attempting to condense the available literature regarding PLIF, there are several conclusions that can be drawn from the early series. It can be said with some certainty that a high rate of fusion has been achieved by some authors using the PLIF procedure. It is likely that significant differences in reported fusion rates are the result of technical factors related to graft and graft site preparation and insertion, as well as different definitions of fusion used by various authors. Patients with compensation related issues tend to do worse than others, and multiply operated patients tend to do somewhat worse than patients whose first operation is the PLIF. It is also clear that although the PLIF operation is technically demanding, it can be performed safely by experienced surgeons.

CONCLUSIONS

1. The PLIF procedure represents an effective procedure for the treatment of some patients with low back pain with or without radiculopathy.

2. The use of PLIF by experienced surgeons is associated with rates of fusion and rates of high patient satisfaction ranging from 60% to 90%.

3. Complications do occur and can be significant. Careful attention to patient positioning, hemostasis, and gentle handling of the neural elements are necessary to reduce the incidence of such complications.

4. The evolution of new implants and the addition of posterior instrumentation have significantly altered the original techniques and may allow for better patient satisfaction and fewer operative complications.

REFERENCES

1. Branch C, Branch CB, Jr: Posterior lumbar interbody fusion with the keystone graft: technique and results. **Surg Neurol** 27:449-54, 1987.
2. Brantigan J: Pseudarthrosis rate after allograft posterior lumbar interbody fusion with pedicle screw and plate fixation. **Spine** 19:1271-9, 1994.
3. Carragee E, Chen Y, Tanner C, et al: Provocative discography in patients after limited lumbar discectomy. A controlled, randomized study of pain response in symptomatic and asymptomatic subjects. North American Spine Society. Chicago: **North American Spine Society** 1999.
4. Carragee E, Tanner C, Yang B, et al: Reliability of subjective concordancy assessment during provocative disc injection. North American Spine Society. Chicago: **North American Spine Society** 1999, p. 74.
5. Cloward R: Gas sterilized cadaver bone grafts for spinal fusion operations. A simplified bone bank. **Spine** 5:4-9, 1980.
6. Cloward R: Posterior lumbar interbody fusion updated. **Clin Orthop** 193:16-19, 1985.
7. Cloward R: Spondylolisthesis: treatment by laminectomy and posterior interbody fusion. **Clin Orthop** 154:74-82, 1981.
8. Cloward R: The treatment of ruptured intervertebral discs by vertebral body fusion. 1. Indications, operative technique, after care. **J Neurosurg** 10:154-68, 1953.
9. Collis J: Total disc replacement: a modified posterior lumbar interbody fusion. Report of 750 cases. **Clin Orthop** 193:64-67, 1985.
10. Csecsei G, Klekner A, Sikula J: Posterior lumbar interbody fusion using the bony elements of the dorsal spinal segment. **Acta Chirurgica Hungarica** 36:54-56, 1997.
11. Denis F: Spinal instability as defined by the three-column spine concept in acute spine trauma. **Clin Orthop** 189:65-76, 1984.
12. Findlay G, Hall B, Musa B, et al: A 10-year follow-up of the outcome of lumbar microdiscectomy. **Spine** 23:1168-71, 1998.
13. Gill K, Blumenthal S: Posterior lumbar interbody fusion. A 2 year follow-up of 238 patients. **Acta Orthop Scand** 251:108-10, 1993.

14. Hutter C: Posterior intervertebral body fusion. A 25 year study. **Clin Orthop** 179:86-96, 1983.
15. Hutter C: Spinal stenosis and posterior lumbar interbody fusion. **Clin Orthop** 193:103-14, 1985.
16. Javid M, Hadar E: Long-term follow-up review of patients who underwent laminectomy for lumbar stenosis: a prospective study. **J Neurosurg** 89:1-7, 1998.
17. Lin P: Posterior lumbar interbody fusion technique: complications and pitfalls. **Clin Orthop** 193:90-102, 1985.
18. Lin P: A technical modification of Cloward's posterior lumbar interbody fusion. **Neurosurgery** 1:118-24, 1977.
19. Lin P, Cautilli R, Joyce M: Posterior lumbar interbody fusion. **Clin Orthop** 180:154-68, 1983.
20. Ma GW: Posterior lumbar interbody fusion with specialized instruments. **Clin Orthop** 193:57-63, 1985.
20. Malgaigne J: De quelques illusions orthopediques, a l'occasion du releve general du service orthopedique de M.J. Guerin. **J Chir** (Paris) 1:256-65, 1843.
21. Modic M: Degenerative disc disease and back pain. **Magn Reson Imaging Clin N Am** 7:481-91, 1999.
22. Moore A, Chilton J, Uttley D: Long term results of lumbar microdiscectomy. **Br J Neurosurg** 8:319-26, 1994.
23. Prolo D, Oklund S, Butcher M: Toward uniformity in evaluating the results of lumbar spine operations. A paradigm applied to posterior lumbar interbody fusions. **Spine** 11:601-06, 1986.
24. Rapoff A, Ghanayem A, Zdeblick T: Biomechanical comparison of posterior lumbar interbody fusion cages. **Spine** 22:2375-9, 1997.
25. Rish B: A critique of posterior lumbar interbody fusion: 12 year experience with 250 patients. **Surg Neurol** 31:281-89, 1989.
26. Simmons J: Posterior lumbar interbody fusion with posterior elements as chip grafts. **Clin Orthop** 193:85-89, 1985.
27. Steffee A, Sitkowski D: Posterior lumbar interbody fusion and plates. **Clin Orthop** 227:99-102, 1988.
28. Stonecipher T, Wright S: Posterior lumbar interbody fusion with facet screw fixation. **Spine** 14:468-71, 1989.
29. Verlooy J, De Smedt K, Selosse P: Failure of a modified posterior lumbar interbody fusion technique to produce adequate pain relief in isthmic spondylolytic grade 1 spondylolisthesis patients. A prospective study in 20 patients. **Spine** 18:1491-5, 1993.
30. Voor M, Mehta S, Wang M, et al: Biomechanical evaluation of posterior and anterior interbody fusion techniques. **J Spinal Disord** 11:328-34, 1998.
31. Waddell G, McCulloch J, Kummel E, et al: Nonorganic physical signs in low back pain. **Spine** 5:117-25, 1980.
32. Wolff J: **Des Gesetz der Transformation der Knocken**. Berlin: A. Hirschwald, 1884.

CHAPTER 9

PLIF and Impacted PLIF

■

BRYAN BARNES, M.D.

MARK MCLAUGHLIN, M.D.

GERALD RODTS, M.D.

REGIS W. HAID, JR., M.D.

HISTORICAL CONSIDERATIONS

Hadra and Lange first used posterior lumbar interbody fusion (PLIF) in the late 1800's as a treatment for Pott's disease, using primitive wires and rods. Eventually, Albee and Hibbs refined this procedure, using a technique that consisted of an interlaminar fusion using primitive autogenous bone grafts. Albee and Hibbs reported their method in JAMA in 1911, and until the World War II era, their techniques remained the mainstay of posterior spinal stabilization, predominantly for treatment of infectious diseases of the spine. The use of lumbar fusion expanded during the post-WWII era to include stabilization of trauma, postdiscectomy stabilization, and treatment of lumbar spondylitic disease. Subsequently, extremely low fusion rates and frequent overgrowth of interlaminar grafts were encountered, and surgeons began to pioneer more effective and innovative techniques.

In 1936, Mercer hypothesized that interbody fusion was the ideal theoretical operation for stabilization of the lumbar spine.[10] The first report of posterior lumbar interbody fusion was made by Jaslow in 1946, but many consider Cloward's 1953 report in the Journal of Neurosurgery to be the landmark description of PLIF.[3,7] Both Jaslow and Cloward used PLIF for lumbar stabilization following discectomy, using a small plug of autogenous bone (Figure 9-1). Remarkably, Cloward reported a 95% fusion rate in over 250 patients who underwent single-level PLIF following discectomy (Figure 9-2). In the latter portion of the 20th century, both Lin and Branch refined interbody fusion techniques, making a transition to current methods of PLIF.[2,9]

INDICATIONS

The indications for PLIF in recent years have ranged from universally accepted criteria such as gross instability to more controversial criteria such as significant low back pain following single-level discectomy. In general, current indications for PLIF are based on an understanding of the pathophysiology of the degenerative cascade and a clinical measure of the patient's disability. Correlation of objective diagnostic imaging with clinical symptomatology is the mainstay of an acceptable standard of care for the patient.

Patients with clinical histories of mechanical low back pain may present with or without leg pain. When imaging patients with known mechanical low back pain, the most common magnetic resonance imaging (MRI) findings include degenerative disc disease characterized by segmental disc degeneration with Modic changes. Foraminal stenosis is often found but is not required as an indication for fusion. Plain films should demonstrate disc space collapse. If computerized tomography (CT) imaging or CT myelography is used, parasagittal reconstructions frequently show impingement of the neural foramen by the superior facet of the inferior vertebrae. Traditional discography has focused on disc morphology, but recent application is based on the reproduction of the patient's typical pain at the appropriate clinical level combined with a negative control at a nonsymptomatic level. At a minimum, good candidates for PLIF demonstrate mechanical low back pain with or without leg pain and concordant radiographic evidence of degenerative disc disease.

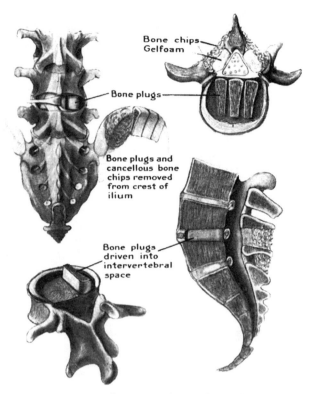

FIGURE 9-1 ■ Illustration from Cloward's 1953 Journal of Neurosurgery manuscript, showing the use of autologous bone plugs for interbody fusion.

Other indications for PLIF have been delineated by Fessler, and include the following:

1. Discectomy with concomitantly unstable lesions such as spondylolysis.
2. Iatrogenic instability caused by discectomy or laminectomy.
3. Pseudoarthrosis.
4. Degenerative scoliosis.
5. Postfusion instability at the first mobile segment above and below the fusion site.
6. Segmental instability.
7. Degenerative spondylolisthesis.[4]

The authors feel that the following conditions are contraindications to either anterior or posterior approach lumbar interbody fusion:

1. Multilevel disc disease with a nondiagnostic discogram.
2. Single-level disc disease and radicular pain without symptoms of instability (little or no mechanical back pain).
3. Patients with severe osteoporosis.

Relative contraindications to interbody fusion include active smokers, patients with multilevel disease with more than two levels testing positive on discogram, and those patients with significant comorbid illness.

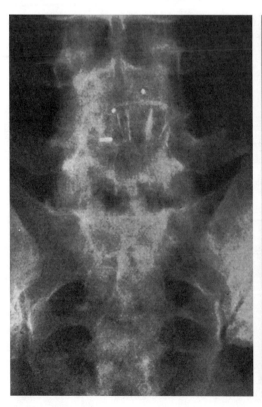
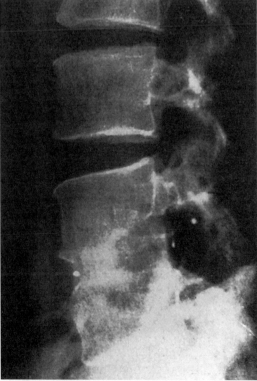

FIGURE 9-2 ■ Plain radiographs showing results from Cloward's first series of lumbar interbody fusions.

CHOICE OF ANTERIOR VERSUS POSTERIOR FUSION

When attempting to determine the optimal approach for a lumbar interbody fusion (i.e., anterior vs. posterior), it is important to consider evidence of posterior pathology such as a disc fragment in the canal, facet hypertrophy, lateral recess stenosis, or central spinal stenosis. Contraindications to anterior approaches may include multiple prior abdominal procedures or severe arteriosclerosis, which may preclude mobilization of the aorta and iliac vessels in fusions above the L5-S1 level. Relative contraindications to posterior procedures include patients with multiple prior posterior surgeries suggesting significant scar formation. With continuing advances in technology, it is possible that some posterior pathology, such as free fragments, may eventually be addressed by an anterior approach similar to anterior cervical discectomy.

CURRENT OPTIONS FOR PLIF

Over the past 10 years, techniques for PLIF have undergone a remarkably fast evolution. The introduction of pedicle screw fixation by Roy-Camille for posterior stabilization stimulated a resurgence of posterolateral fusions and was followed by the development of better instrumentation systems for reconstructing the stability of the intervertebral disc space.[12,13] Placement of threaded cylindrical titanium cages became more popular than standard posterolateral fusion techniques with pedicle screw fixation because the cages provided better biomechanical, biological, and functional advantages.[10,11] The improved instrumentation systems stimulated an explosion of interbody procedures because of reduced risk of neurologic injury. After initial reports of good success with threaded cylindrical titanium cages, various modifications of this prosthesis were created.[10,11] The authors' experiences have produced an evolution of philosophy regarding instrumentation for patients undergoing PLIF and, by means of relaying our experiences, we intend to illustrate the benefits and disadvantages of several types of commonly used implants. Several years ago we began using stand-alone threaded titanium cages packed with morselized autograft as our front line PLIF procedure. Using this technique, we began to find similar stability rates (91%) and clinical outcomes compared to our previous posterolateral fusion techniques.[5,6] *Stability* is defined as no movement on dynamic plain films and an absence of lucency around the implant.

However, we were concerned about the extensive disruption of the posterior tension band required to place these devices. Because of this, we began to supplement cages with pedicle screw fixation in a theoretical attempt to restore the posterior tension band. As a result of pedicle screw supplementation, our stability rate increased to 100%. Further evidence of the efficacy of supplemental pedicle screw fixation is provided by Zdeblick, who, in 1993, determined that supplemental pedicle screw fixation significantly increased posterolateral fusions.[14]

Despite increasing stability rates with supplemental pedicle screw fixation, it was difficult to determine fusion rates because of heavy metallic artifacts from the cages. In addition, there was concern about the implication of implanting a device with a different modulus of elasticity compared to native bone. As a result, we began to use threaded cortical bone dowels with morselized autograft in an attempt to more accurately determine fusion and to provide patients with a more physiological implant. Our results with threaded cortical bone dowels supplemented with pedicle screw fixation have shown a 95% fusion rate at one-year follow-up, with a 70% satisfactory outcome. More disappointing have been the results with "stand-alone" threaded cortical bone dowels. at one-year follow-up. With all "stand-alone" dowels implanted via anterior approach, our fusion rate was 16%, and our patient satisfaction rate was less than 50%.[5] As a result, we have abandoned the use of threaded cortical bone dowels as "stand-alone" devices.

During the period of using both metallic and cylindrical cages, we noted a significant number of nerve root injuries and cerebrospinal fluid (CSF) leaks. Cylindrical devices present technical difficulties because they are as wide as they are tall, and in implanting these devices, extensive dural and nerve root retraction are required (Figure 9-3).

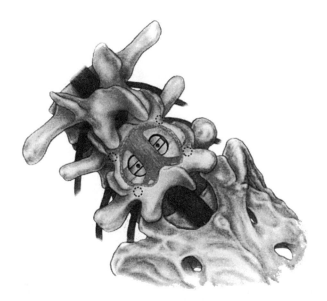

FIGURE 9-3 ■ Posterior view of implanted allograft bone dowels, demonstrating proximity of nerve roots to implant trajectory.

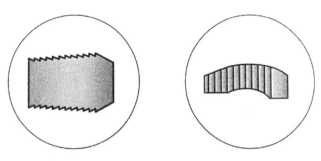

FIGURE 9-4 ■ Sagittal view of rectangular impacted wedges.

The development of rectangular implants has, in our preliminary experience, dramatically reduced the incidence of nerve root injuries and CSF leaks. Rectangular implants are considerably easier to navigate through the window of the superior and inferior nerve roots because of their slender profile in the sagittal plane (Figure 9-4). Although width is decreased, height is not sacrificed, preserving the distractive capability of the implant with less nerve root retraction (Figure 9-5).

The most common rectangular devices include carbon fiber, titanium, and allograft bone. Metallic rectangular devices are predominantly used in Europe. Our

group prefers using allograft bone implants because they offer structural stability under compression with a similar modulus of elasticity to the vertebral bodies. Remarkably, currently available implantable allograft bone wedges are similar to the bone plugs used by Cloward for his single-level fusions in the early '50s (Figure 9-6). Metallic artifact is eliminated, allowing for better assessment of fusion, and osseous integration is initiated. The allograft implants are lordotically shaped in the axial plane, allowing the surgeon to restore lumbar lordosis when the construct is supplemented with pedicle screw fixation. The implant is placed in the posterior one half to one third of the disc space. Thus, with posterior pedicle screw compression, the graft is "loaded," aiding arthrodesis. The posterior compression also uses the implant as a fulcrum, helping to re-establish lordosis and sagittal balance.

TECHNICAL ASPECTS OF PLIF AND "IMPACTED PLIF" WITH SUPPLEMENTAL PEDICLE SCREW FIXATION

Despite recent advances in technology and instrumentation, PLIF is still a difficult and technically demanding procedure. We present the current methods we use for the implantation of both rectangular allograft

FIGURE 9-5 ■ Illustration of minimal nerve root retraction requirements for implantation of impacted wedges.

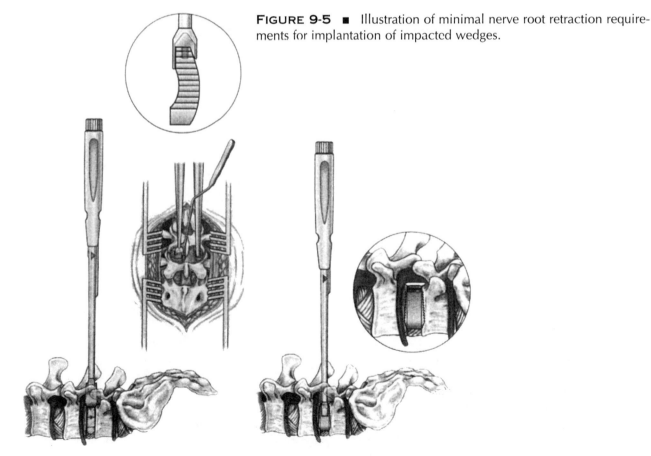

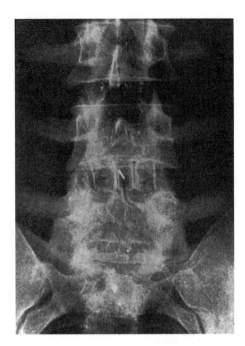

FIGURE 9-6 ■ AP view of bone plugs used by Cloward for interbody fusion in the '50s.

wedges ("impacted PLIF") and standard PLIF using threaded cortical bone dowels.

Impacted PLIF

In general, wide exposure and a generous skin incision with deep muscle relaxation offers the best visualization for the surgeon and the least amount of postoperative pain for the patient. Routinely, we use one twitch in a train of four paralyses to achieve muscular relaxation. Prior to skin incision, the proper size of the implant is determined by templating an adjacent normal level to determine optimal distraction. Pedicle screw length is also determined by measuring the length of the pedicles on axial CT scans and should incorporate 80% of the vertebral body.

1. *Harvest autologous bone:* After the initial midline incision is made, a suprafascial plane is dissected through the same incision to identify the posterior superior iliac spine (PSIS). The fascia over the PSIS is opened, and the roof of the PSIS is exposed, taking care not to dissect the gluteus off the ileum to avoid postoperative graft pain. The cortical bone of the PSIS is chipped off with an osteotome, and a gouge is used to harvest cancellous graft without violating the cortex. The graft is then morselized, the graft site is irrigated and packed with Gelfoam, and the fascial opening is closed. The dead space created by the suprafascial approach is then closed.

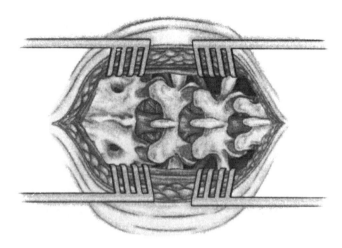

FIGURE 9-7 ■ Initial exposure requirement for PLIF.

2. *Obtain wide bony exposure* (Figure 9-7): The midline incision is deepened and the spinous processes are identified. The muscle is dissected laterally to the base of the transverse processes. The pars interarticularis is identified and clearly dissected from the soft tissues. The intersection of the pars interarticularis and the base of the transverse process will mark the pedicle screw entry site, and the pars interarticularis also serves as a landmark of the exiting nerve root. Before proceeding to the next step, the surgeon should be able to visualize the base of the transverse process and the pars interarticularis of the superior and inferior vertebrae.

3. *Decompression* (Figure 9-8): At this point, the spinous processes and the lamina are removed to decompress the spinal canal and to give the surgeon an intracanal view of the pedicles. A complete laminectomy of the superior and inferior vertebrae is the best method of visualizing the

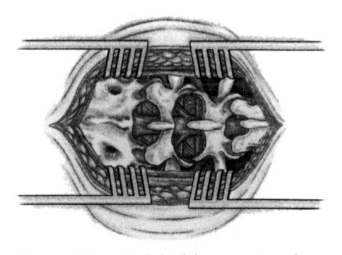

FIGURE 9-8 ■ Single level decompression and exposure in preparation for PLIF.

nerve roots. A high-speed drill (Midas Rex, AM-35 bit; Medtronic Sofamor Danek, Memphis, TN) is the best instrument to thin the posterior elements and the lateral bony overhang, paving the way for smoother bony removal with a Kerrison rongeur. After achieving laminectomy, a one-quarter inch bone chisel may be used to perform a medial facetectomy.

4. *Follow the nerve roots:* After a wide decompression and medial facetectomy is performed, the pedicles of the superior and inferior vertebrae can be visualized and palpated. Using a Woodson or dental dissector, the surgeon must follow the course of the nerve root laterally into the foramen. A generous foraminotomy is then made one centimeter lateral to the origin of the nerve root at the superior and inferior level. This allows for good exposure of the true axilla of the superior nerve root in subsequent steps and also decompresses symptomatic nerve roots.

5. *Find the true axilla of the superior nerve root* (Figure 9-9): After completion of the foraminotomy,

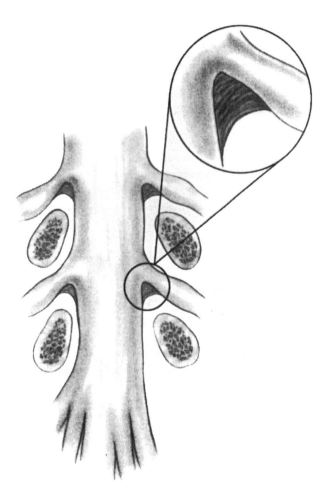

FIGURE 9-9 ■ Schematic illustration of the true axilla of the nerve root.

it is important to remove the lateral bony overhang comprised by the inferior facet of the superior vertebrae. The epidural veins within the lateral gutter are coagulated and cut, and the remaining ligamentum flavum is removed, taking care to visualize both the superior and inferior nerve roots. Using careful bipolar cautery, the veins located in the axilla of the superior nerve root can be cauterized, and the tethering venous plexus is divided. This dissection affords a large portal of entry for the interbody prosthesis, allows for more laxity of the superior nerve root during dural retraction, and minimizes the chance for dural and nerve root injury.

6. *Placement of pedicle screws:* Preliminary pedicle screw entry sites are checked and verified with c-arm fluoroscopy. The pedicles are then probed, tapped, and screwed, using fluoroscopic guidance. If the pedicle screw entry site has been well chosen, the tap will almost guide itself down the pedicle. Pedicle screw depth can be estimated by lateral fluoroscopy and should incorporate 80% of the vertebral body. Our rationale for placing pedicle screws prior to performing a PLIF is that after PLIF epidural bleeding can be difficult to control because of loss of thecal sac turgor.

7. *Perform the discectomy:* The discectomy is performed using standard annulotomy, curettage, and pituitary rongeur removal of the nucleus pulposis. Although modern PLIF instrumentation can be used to perform a significant discectomy using reamers and scrapers, we have found that a prior standard discectomy enhances the effectiveness of scrapers and reamers. A vigorous, effective discectomy is completed.

8. *Perform the PLIF:* Standard steps for performing the "impacted PLIF" are outlined below.
   a. Disc space "distractors" are hammered into place using direct fluoroscopy, and sequentially larger size distractors are used on both the right and left sides until the desired distraction is achieved (Figure 9-10). One distractor is left in place, and a rotating cutter is inserted on the contralateral side of the thecal sac and hammered into position, using fluoroscopic guidance, to a typical depth of 26 to 30 mm. The remaining loose disc material is then removed from the interspace. An endplate scraper is then placed in the disc space, and the end plates are denuded of their cartilage. As we have gained experience, we are much more aggressive with end-plate removal and preparation.

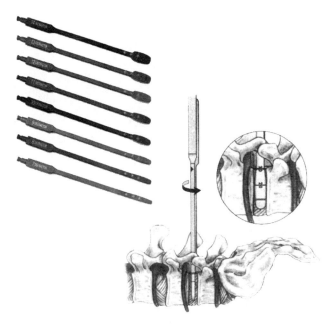

FIGURE 9-10 ■ Sequential use of distractors is required to restore disc space height.

b. A channel cutter is inserted under fluoroscopic guidance, and a channel of bone 1 to 2 mm into the end-plates of both the superior and inferior vertebral bodies is cut (Figure 9-11). It is important to use a correct trajectory with the channel cutter in order to ensure that the implant is not partially placed in the vertebral body. The preselected rectangular allograft is

placed in the space and tamped into place (Figure 9-12). Ideal countersinking depth is usually 3 mm.

c. Steps "a" and "b" are repeated on the contralateral side. Prior to implantation of the wedge, at least 10 cc of morselized autologous allograft is packed within the interspace and medially toward the contralateral implant (Figure 9-13). We pack as much autograft iliac crest bone into the interspace as possible, placing bone anterior, medial, and lateral to the graft. The wedge is then implanted.

9. Remaining bone surfaces are then decorticated, and the rod connector construct is placed onto the pedicle screws and tightened. We feel that compression of the graft increases chances for fusion because the graft is placed under stress, a necessary component for bone growth. We do not routinely perform posterolateral fusion, although bone is placed over the decorticated facet joints and the base of the transverse processes. In patients with a high risk for nonunion, we often do perform a concomitant lateral transverse process fusion. Prior to closure, all nerve roots are checked to verify decompression and to identify any loose autograft segments in the foramen. Figure 9-14 represents ideal postoperative radiographic confirmation of allograft wedges.

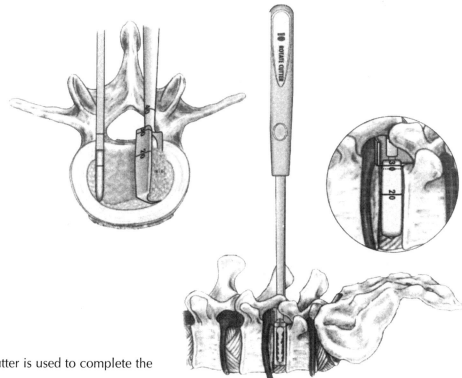

FIGURE 9-11 ■ A channel cutter is used to complete the discectomy.

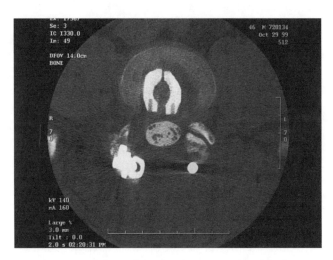

FIGURE 9-12 ■ CT scan demonstrating ideal placement of wedges in the interspace.

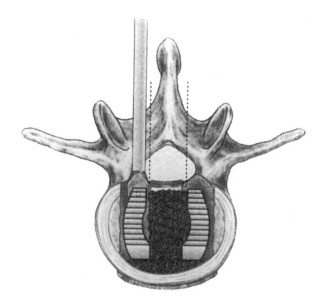

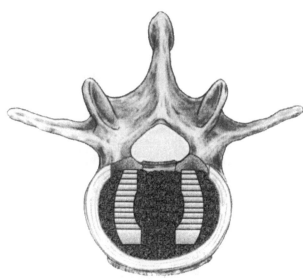

FIGURE 9-13 ■ Axial view of implants in the disc space.

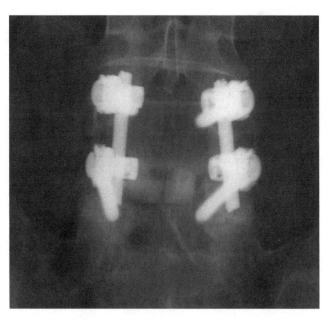

FIGURE 9-14 ■ AP plain films showing ideal placement of wedges in the disc space.

Standard PLIF with Threaded Cortical Bone Dowels

Steps 1 through 7, outlined previously in the description of impacted PLIF, are utilized in the placement of threaded cortical bone dowels, including pedicle screw placement.

Additional steps in standard PLIF with threaded cortical bone dowels are as follows:

1. Distraction of exiting and neighboring nerve roots with working channel.
   a. *Distraction* (Figure 9-15): Dura and nerve roots are retracted with a nerve root retractor, while fluoroscopy is used to impact the distractor. Fluoroscopy is used to confirm distractor depth.
   b. *Working channel insertion:* A working channel is inserted over the distractor, using tang-style blades for stabilization. When inserting the working channel, care should be taken to protect the exiting root (Figure 9-16). Fluoroscopy is used to confirm that the blades are of equal distance into the superior and inferior vertebral bodies.
   c. *Reaming/tapping:* The distractor is removed, and using fluoroscopy, the disc space is prepared for the implant, using a reamer and a tapping device.
   d. *Threaded construct placement* (Figure 9-17): Using fluoroscopy, the implant is placed in the interspace. Steps "a" through "d" are then repeated on the contralateral side.

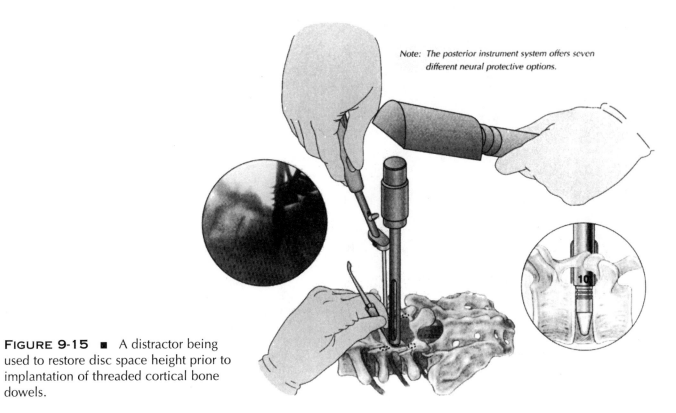

Note: *The posterior instrument system offers seven different neural protective options.*

FIGURE 9-15 ■ A distractor being used to restore disc space height prior to implantation of threaded cortical bone dowels.

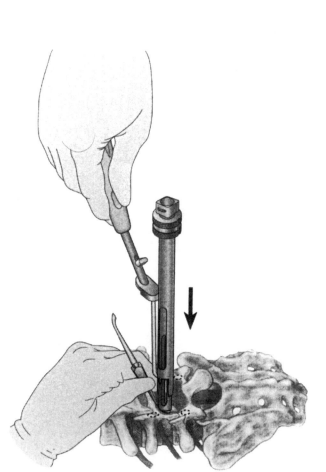

FIGURE 9-16 ■ Working channel with tang-style blades.

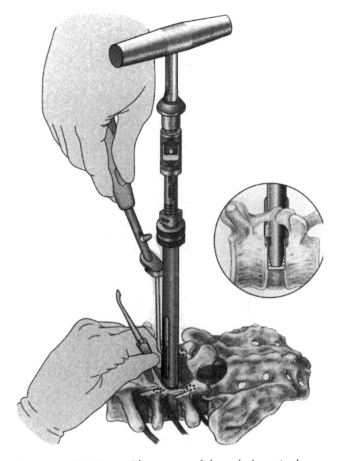

FIGURE 9-17 ■ Placement of threaded cortical bone dowel construct.

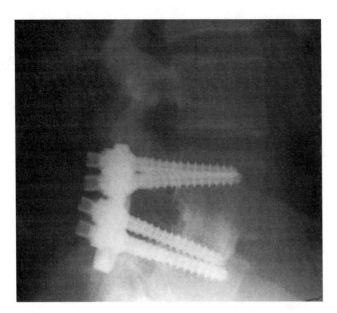

FIGURE 9-18 ■ Lateral radiograph showing mature lumbar fusion after placement of threaded cortical bone dowels and pedicle screws.

2. Compress the pedicle screws, as in step 9 for the impacted PLIF, in order to load the graft, restore lumbar lordosis, and restore sagittal balance.

Figure 9-18 radiographically illustrates ideal postoperative placement of threaded cortical bone dowels.

SUMMARY

Techniques for posterior lumbar interbody fusion have evolved rapidly over the last 10 years and now include metallic and allograft bone implants with the option of pedicle screw supplementation. We have described the indications and techniques currently used by our group to secure consistently high rates of radiographically confirmed fusion with concordantly high rates of clinically satisfactory outcomes.[1] Options for PLIF continue to expand and will undoubtedly lead to intriguing developments in procedures available for posterior lumbar interbody fusion.

REFERENCES

1. Barnes B, McLaughlin MR, Birch B, et al: Threaded cortical bone dowels for lumbar interbody fusion: 1 year follow-up in 28 patients. **J. Neurosurgery-Spine**, in press.
2. Branch CL: The case for posterior lumbar interbody fusion. **Clin Neurosurg** 1996 43:252-67.
3. Cloward RB: The treatment of ruptured intervertebral discs by vertebral body fusion. **J Neurosurg** 10:154, 1953.
4. Fessler RG, Locantro J: Indications and techniques for stabilization in degenerative disease of the lumbar spine. In **The Practice of Neurosurgery**, editors, Tindell GT, Cooper PR, Barrow DL. Baltimore: Lippincott-Williams & Wilkins, 1996.
5. Haid RW, Dickman CA: Instrumentation and fusion for discogenic disease of the lumbosacral spine. **Neurosurg Clinic N Am** 4:135-48, 1993.
6. Haid RW, Morone MA: Spondylolisthesis and spondylolysis. **The Practice of Neurosurgery** 2541-60.
7. Jaslow IA: Intercorporeal bone graft in spinal fusion after disc removal. **Surg Gynecol Obst** 82:215, 1946.
8. Kuslich SD, Ulstrom CL, Griffith SL, et al: The Bagby and Kuslich method of lumbar interbody fusion: history, techniques, and 2-year follow-up results in United States prospective, multicenter trial. **Spine** 23 :1267-78, 1998..
9. Lin PM: Posterior lumbar interbody fusion technique: complications and pitfalls. **Clin Orthop** 193:90-102, 1985.
10. Mercer RW, Spondylolisthesis with a description of a new method of operative treatment and notes of ten cases. **Edinb Med J** 43"545-72, 1936.
11. Ray CD: Threaded titanium cages for lumbar interbody fusion. **Spine** 22:667-80, 1997.
12. Roy-Camille R, Saillant G, Mazel C: Internal fixation of the lumbar spine with pedicle screw plating. **Clin Orthop** 203:7-17, 1986.
13. Steffe A, Biscup R, Sitkowski D: Segmental spine plates with pedicle screw fixation: a new internal fixation device for the lumbar and thoracic spine. **Clin Orthop** 203:45-54, 1986.
14. Zdeblick TA: A prospective, randomized study of lumbar fusion: preliminary results. **Spine** 18:983-91, 1993.

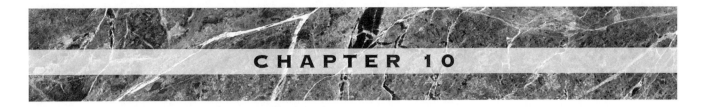

CHAPTER 10

Anterior Lumbar Interbody Fusion: Threaded Bone Dowels Versus Titanium Cages

■

RICK C. SASSO, M.D.

THOMAS M. REILLY, M.D.

HISTORY

Spinal fusion has become a widely used option in the treatment of degenerative conditions of the lumbar spine. Posterior, posterolateral, and interbody fusions, both anterior and posterior, have been used successfully, alone or in combination. The earliest reports of anterior interbody arthrodesis were in association with the treatment of tuberculosis and lumbar spondylolisthesis, initially with transperitoneal approaches and, later, retroperitoneal approaches.[9,48,49,66,68] The first description of an anterior transperitoneal approach occurred in 1906 by Mueller, with Iwahara[50,68] reporting the first lumbar arthrodesis performed through a retroperitoneal approach. In 1948, Lane and Moore, in a classic description, were the first to report anterior lumbar interbody fusion (ALIF) for the treatment of lumbar degenerative disc disease.[60] In 1950, Harmon described a retroperitoneal transabdominal approach for cases of acute intervertebral disc prolapse caused by disc degeneration.[41]

Capener considered fusion of the lumbar spine by an anterior approach biomechanically ideal but technically impossible in 1932; however, over the ensuing decades, surgical technical advances allowed ALIF to become a common procedure.[12] The anterior approach to the lumbar spine was increasingly used in the management of a variety of spinal pathologies, using a number of different grafting materials, including corticocancellous blocks, corticocancellous dowels, and femoral ring allografts.[40,43,44,71,85] Hodgson pioneered the anterior approach for spinal tuberculosis, using corticocancellous blocks.[43,44] Cylindrically shaped corticocancellous dowels were first used for an anterior lumbar fusion in 1963 by Harmon and in 1965 by Sacks.[40,85] Ralph Cloward pioneered the dowel technique in 1953.[16,17,18] Although he used a posterior

approach, his methods for disc removal, end-plate preparation, and grafting came to be used extensively. Later, Henry Crock adapted Cloward's dowel technique for use with an anterior approach to the lumbar spine using cylindrical allograft.[21] O'Brien devised a hybrid interbody graft using a biological fusion cage (femoral cortical allograft ring) packed with autogenous cancellous bone graft.[71] The concept of this hybrid is that the femoral allograft ring provides the acute stability of the construct, whereas the autogenous iliac crest graft provides for long-term stability.

Although the technical feat of exposing the anterior lumbar spine safely was reliable in the 1970s to 1980s, stand-alone ALIF fell out of favor because of low fusion rates. Despite initial reports encompassing a heterogeneous group of patients and surgical techniques indicating fusion rates of 95% by Harmon, 70% by Hoover, 90% by Crock, and 96% by Fujimaki, other reports demonstrated significantly poorer fusion rates.[21,31,40,45] Calandruccio, Nisbet, Raney, and Flynn, cited fusion rates of 19%, 40%, 45%, and 56%, respectively, but the 1972 study from the Mayo Clinic authored by Stauffer and Coventry drove the final nail in the coffin of stand-alone ALIF.[11,27,70,78,89] They reported on 83 patients who had anterior lumbar interbody arthrodesis without instrumentation between 1959 and 1967. They found an alarmingly low success rate, with pseudarthrosis occurring in a discouraging 44%, and concluded that the only justification for this procedure was as salvage for failed posterolateral fusions. These outcomes resulted in a reassessment of ALIF as a stand-alone procedure and a gradual decline in its popularity, particularly for the indication of lumbar degenerative disc disease and lumbar axial back pain.

The combination of anterior interbody fusion with a posterior fusion technique was developed with the aim of obtaining higher rates of fusion and improved outcome. Because of the significant drop in the fusion rate, especially over multiple levels, combined anterior interbody fusion with posterior fusion and internal fixation became common.[57] The advantage of a very high fusion rate with these circumferential (360°) procedures, however, must be balanced against the increased risk of morbidity related to the increased magnitude of the procedure.

Techniques to increase the fusion rate of ALIF with an anterior-only approach to approximate the success of circumferential constructs began with anterior lumbar instrumentation, which was first reported by Humphries and Hawk in 1961.[46] They developed a slotted, contoured plate to be placed over the anterior lumbar spine in an attempt to enhance arthrodesis; however, it was the threaded cylindrical cage that brought stand-alone anterior interbody fusion back as an option for the treatment of discogenic pain.

During the mid-1970s and early 1980s, Bagby and colleagues began treating "Wobbler Syndrome," a chronic cervical instability causing myelopathy in thoroughbred horses, by means of a smooth, stainless steel, fenestrated cylinder (Bagby Basket) placed through an anterior approach.[2] The standard Cloward technique had resulted in unacceptable morbidity resulting from the necessity of autogenous iliac bone graft harvest.[22] Bagby eliminated the need for autograft harvest by packing his cage with cancellous bone chips obtained from the reaming of the cervical decompression. This novel device was designed with perforations in its walls to allow bone in-growth and to enhance arthrodesis. They coined the term *distraction-compression stabilization*, referring to their technique of distraction of the cervical interspace with this implant, achieving early stability while improving arthrodesis. Animal studies demonstrated excellent clinical results, particularly in comparison to previous techniques using interbody allografts or xenografts, with up to 88% fusion success.[2,20,22,94] This stand-alone interbody fusion technique continued to evolve with material changes and the design of threaded cages to increase stability and decrease displacement rates.[73,82] Similar to the method of Wiltberger, bilateral, parallel implants were designed for use in the lumbar spine.[20,99] This ultimately resulted in the current Bagby and Kuslich design (BAK, Spine-Tech, Minneapolis, MN) (BAK), with the first human implantation occurring in 1992.[59] This cylindrical titanium cage has threads to screw into the end-plates, thereby stabilizing the device and allowing for increased fusion rates with a stand-alone anterior device. Ray developed a similar titanium interbody fusion device (Ray TFC, Surgical Dynamics, Norwalk, CT) (RTFC), which was initially used in posterior lumbar interbody fusions (PLIF) but expanded to include ALIF procedures.[82] In 1985, Otero-Vich reported using threaded bone dowels for

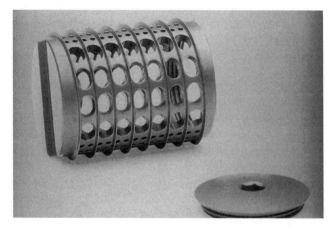

FIGURE 10-1 ■ Inter Fix threaded interbody fusion device. (Sofamor Danek Group, Memphis, TN.)

anterior cervical arthrodesis, and femoral ring allograft bone has subsequently been fashioned into cylindrical threaded dowels for lumbar application.[73]

Currently, there are a wide number of interbody fusion devices of varying design and material available, not all of which have gained Food and Drug Administration (FDA) approval for anterior application in the setting of a stand-alone device. These include the following:

1. Cylindrical threaded titanium interbody cages (BAK, Spine-Tech, Minneapolis, MN; RTFC, Surgical Dynamics, Norwalk, CT; and Inter Fix, Sofamor Danek Group, Memphis, TN) (Figure 10-1).
2. Cylindrical threaded cortical bone dowels (MD II, MD III, MD IV) (Sofamor Danek Group, Memphis, TN) (Figure 10-2).

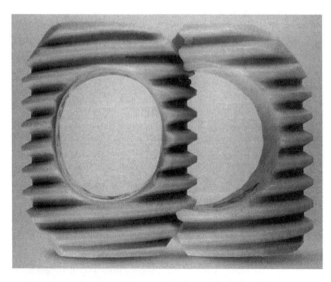

FIGURE 10-2 ■ MD II (left) and MD IV (right) threaded bone dowels. (Sofamor Danek Group, Memphis, TN.)

3. Vertical interbody rings or boxes (Harms titanium-mesh cage, DePuy-Acromed, Cleveland, OH; Brantigan carbon fiber cages, DePuy-Acromed, Cleveland, OH; and Femoral Ring Allograft–FRA Spacer, Synthes, Paoli, PA).

As a result of the improved clinical results associated with the use of many of these interbody fusion devices in stand-alone anterior procedures, avoiding many of the problems associated with instrumented posterolateral arthrodesis, their use has become more widespread, both in the United States and internationally. Approximately 80,000 lumbar interbody fusion cages have been implanted internationally over the past five years, with the United States accounting for 5000 implants per month.[63] In the United States, it is estimated that in 1999 alone, sales of interbody fusion cages will have reached approximately 224 million dollars, 15% of which represents bone dowel products (Merrill Lynch personal communication, August 2, 1999). According to McAfee, the recent interest in performing lumbar interbody arthrodesis with use of cages is attributable to three factors.[63] First, the rate of failure associated with the use of bone graft alone is high. Second, the rate of failure associated with the use of posterior pedicle-screw instrumentation is high. Finally, the rate of success associated with the use of stand-alone anterior fusion cages and autogenous bone graft is high. This obviates the need to perform a 360° (combined anterior and posterior) lumbar arthrodesis with the use of posterior instrumentation. Interbody fusion cages have had a tremendous effect on anterior fusion. The rates of fusion after anterior interbody arthrodesis have improved from Stauffer and Coventry's 56% to 93% with the use of the BAK titanium cage.[59,89]

BIOMECHANICS

The greatest strength of the vertebral body is present in the subchondral bone of the cortical end-plate. The maximal end-plate strength is peripheral near the ring apophysis. Two techniques of end-plate preparation during interbody fusion are practiced. One involves purposeful end-plate cavitation to provide an optimal bleeding bed of cancellous bone. This chapter deals with this technique in which two cylindrical grafts are screwed into adjacent circular holes oriented parasagittally across a disc space prepared by a reamer that partially removes the subchondral bone, and at the apex of the cavity, exposes weak but very vascular cancellous bone. The outer portion of the perforated, cylindrical cage has a continuous threadform that engages the adjacent vertebral bodies and end-plates. This threaded design permits insertion by screwing the device into the disc space, which provides resistance to device migration and stabilization to the vertebral bodies. This facilitates spinal fusion. The intervertebral disc space is predrilled so that a hole is created. The hole spans the entire height of the disc and includes semicircular concavities in the vertebral bodies above and below the disc space. The cages, packed with autogenous bone graft, screw into the predrilled holes.

The second technique of end-plate preparation involves preservation of the subchondral bone. The advantage of preserving much of the end-plate and filling the disc space with a greater quantity of bone graft should reduce the risk of graft collapse and increase the fusion rate. This leaves the strongest bone adjacent to the implanted graft and requires a precisely cut graft to match the interspace exactly. The disadvantage, however, is that the end-plate is minimally vascularized, and the recipient bed is less vascular. Technically, the dowel technique is easier to perform and consistently allows accurate fitting of the cage to the prepared graft bed. By reaming a cavity, the recipient bed is reliably created for the cylinders. The disadvantage with this technique is that the strong trabeculae adjacent to the end-plates are breached, increasing the risk of graft settling. The second technique is much more difficult because a perfect fit between host and graft is mandatory, and the graft must be perfectly cut to match the subchondral bone surfaces. The accurate insertion of individual blocks is less reproducible than with the dowel technique.

During daily activity, the lumbar spine is exposed to significant biomechanical forces. Studies indicate that a motion segment may experience axial compressive loads ranging from 400 N during quiet standing to more than 7000 N during heavy lifting.[69,98] The ultimate compressive strength of a nonosteoporotic vertebral body has been reported to be slightly over 10,000 N.[25] Corticocancellous autografts demonstrate inadequate initial mechanical strength for lumbar interbody loading, often leading to collapse or extrusion.[23,73,82] The compressive forces across the grafted interspace should be less than that required to induce failure of the graft construct. The graft should be able to transmit force without significant motion so that immediate mechanical load transfer is achieved, and the technique should induce arthrodesis as quickly as possible with minimal to no morbidity associated with its use. Threaded titanium alloy (Ti-6Al-4V) interbody fusion cages have undergone extensive in vitro and in vivo biomechanical testing, demonstrating rigidity sufficient to withstand lumbar spinal loading forces without fracture or deformation.[50,59,80,91] Long-term clinical studies have reported no cases of structural cage failures, and cages have been shown to impart increased stiffness as compared to the intact spine.[7,33,34,59,82,91] One study comparing biomechanical stability performance among three interbody devices (Threaded Bone Dowels, BAK, and RTFC) found no significant difference under physiological loading conditions.[39] Bone dowels performed as well as titanium cages. In flexion, bone dowels increased stiffness by 970%, Ray increased by 253%, and BAK increased by 96%. Under extension, bone dowels increased local stiffness by 166%, BAK by 71%, and Ray by 56%. In torsion, bone dowels increased intact stiffness by 20%. BAK also increased global intact stiffness by 20%, whereas Ray decreased intact stiffness by 5%. Bone dowels increased intact stiffness by 91% under lateral bending, whereas Ray cages and BAK cages maintained the intact stiffness under lateral bending. None of the implants fractured during failure tests. The vertebral end-plate and the sacroiliac joint were found to be the most common failure sites. All devices withstood load to failure, with the vertebral body end-plate failing before the implant.[39] Threaded cortical bone dowels (Sofamor Danek MD II and MD III) provide an increase in construct stiffness of 68% to 334% over the intact motion segment.[90] Additionally, the threaded cortical bone dowels demonstrated static compressive strengths of over 24,000 N, well above maximal physiological loads.

Several biomechanical studies have shown that these threaded anterior interbody devices improve overall stiffness but are least rigid in extension and axial rotation.[62,74,86,91] Oxland and associates compared the stability of a traditionally paired anterior implantation with that of a lateral implantation technique (preserving the anterior longitudinal ligament [ALL] and the anterior annulus).[74] The purpose was to test whether this decreased extension rigidity was to the result of resection of the ALL and the anterior annulus during cage insertion. They found no significant improvement in extension stability with lateral insertion, leading them to conclude this lack of rigidity was associated with distraction of the facet joints after interbody cage placement. Additional posterior instrumentation can provide the added stability required in extension and axial rotation. Supplemental translaminar facet screws that can be placed in a minimally invasive fashion significantly reduce the motion of a BAK biomechanical model in extension and axial rotation. Rathonyi and associates found that using translaminar screw fixation can substantially stabilize the problematic loading directions of extension and axial rotation.[81] Volkman also demonstrated in a cadaveric biomechanical model that motion segment stiffness of an anteriorly placed threaded spine cage was increased, especially in extension, with transfacet screws.[93]

The ideal interbody graft combines a strong mechanical construct to withstand compressive loads across the disc space while providing an osteogenic, osteoinductive, and osteoconductive matrix. The gold standard for this matrix is autogenous cancellous bone. The com-

pressive strength of this bone, however, is very poor. Combining this with a strong titanium or cortical allograft shell (cage) is sensible. The cancellous autograft iliac crest bone is packed into the cylindrical screw-in cages with the goal that the cage provides mechanical strength to prevent collapse, subsidence, shear, and torsional forces. This produces an optimum stable environment while the autogenous graft grows through the cages into the vertebral bodies above and below. The mechanical strength of the cage is combined with the biological strength of the autograft. This graft, however, is not biomechanically loaded while it is inside the cage, and the surface area available for the graft to grow through the cage is not large and varies between cage types. Optimally, graft should be packed around and between the cages to maximize the surface area of bone available for fusion and to allow bone graft to undergo physiological loading. Maximally packing the interspace with bone graft also ensures removal of all disc material and cartilaginous end-plate that is avascular and that inhibits fusion. With this concept in mind, performing a subtotal "channel discectomy" (only removing a cylindrical channel of disk material using a drill) that occurs in the laparoscopic technique, is not optimal.[65] This partial "reamed channel" discectomy results in a limited fusion confined to a small cross-sectional area (the fenestrations in the cage). In a prospective, randomized study of BAK cages packed with autogenous iliac bone graft, a complete discectomy versus partial reamed channel discectomy was performed in 100 patients.[65] All 50 patients in the complete discectomy group achieved a solid arthrodesis at a mean follow-up of 25 months, with no revision surgical procedures. In contrast, seven patients in the partial reamed channel discectomy group had a pseudarthrosis, and eight patients required revision surgery. The difference between the groups was significant (p = 0.019).

One conceptual problem associated with cylindrical interbody fusion devices, both titanium cages and threaded cortical bone dowels, is their geometric shape. The volume available for bone graft in cylinders is less than that in vertical ring devices, such as the femoral ring allograft.[97] A tapered device, as opposed to a cylindrical shape, which has identical anterior and posterior height, better restores lordosis and sagittal balance.[91] The segmental lordosis and wedge-shaped anatomy present in the human intervertebral disc space results in nonuniform implant contact, anterior to posterior.[4] Additionally, it has been calculated that the BAK cage allowed a maximum interface with only 10% of the total surface area of the end-plate.[97] Some authors have concluded that the interbody bone graft area should be significantly greater than 30% of the total end-plate area to prevent failure.[15] However, to increase interbody graft contact with high quality bony bed, greater amounts of subchondral bone need to be removed, increasing the risk of subsidence.[86] In a sheep in vivo model, a threaded titanium interbody fusion device was compared to an anterior fusion using autogenous iliac crest dowel graft. After surgery, interbody distraction successfully occurred in cage and autograft sites. Loss of interbody height ensued in both groups during the first two months. Percentage loss of height was lowest in the cage sites. Both techniques effectively distracted the intervertebral spaces beyond their baseline measures. The cylindrical cages nearly doubled the normal vertical span of the disc spaces. All, however, experienced subsidence of disc height during the first two months. Although the absolute reduction in intervertebral height was similar between the groups, the cage sites lost a smaller fraction of their initial distraction. At final measure, the cage-implanted sites had lost 19.6% of their postoperative height but remained well above the normal disc height.[86]

Unlike titanium interbody cages, threaded cortical bone dowels are subject to supply shortages and processing problems. Presently, the majority of threaded cortical allograft bone dowels are obtained through aseptic harvest techniques with subsequent processing steps occurring in "class 10 certified" clean rooms. After appropriate donor screening tests and chemical processing with hydrogen peroxide and 70% ethanol, the bone dowels are freeze-dried or frozen. This often avoids the need for terminal sterilization by high-dose gamma irradiation or ethylene oxide methods that can impair the mechanical and physiological properties of the allograft.[26] The biomechanical properties of allograft bone can be altered by the methods chosen for its preservation and storage. These effects are minimal with deep-freezing or low-level radiation. Freeze-drying, however, markedly diminishes the torsional and bending strength of bone allografts but does not deleteriously affect the compressive or tensile strength. Irradiation of bone with more than 3.0 megarad, or irradiation combined with freeze-drying, appears to cause a significant reduction in breaking strength.[76]

There have been no documented cases of human immunodeficiency virus (HIV) transmission from musculoskeletal allografts since 1985, although there have been over seven million bone and soft tissue transplants performed since that time. Using current-generation PCR (polymerase chain reaction) screening tools, the risk of HIV transmission is estimated to be approximately one in eight million.[8]

PATIENT SELECTION

While the overwhelming majority of patients with mechanical low back pain secondary to lumbar degenerative disc disease have only transient, self-limiting episodes, up to 5% do not respond to appropriate non-operative treatment.[24,30] ALIF procedures have been used in an increasing fashion for the management of these failures.[21,27,57,82,89] The actual pathophysiology of such "discogenic" pain patients is poorly understood, involving a combination of degenerating intervertebral discs and social and psychological factors.[24,36] Magnetic resonance imaging (MRI) has proven to be of value in the assessment of such patients, demonstrating excellent sensitivity and specificity in the diagnosis of discal pathology.[28] However, even among 20-to 39-year-olds, the rate of asymptomatic disc degeneration is as high as 34%, with up to 21% having asymptomatic disc herniations.[6] Because of this, discography is a useful tool in the assessment of patients with MRI-documented "black disc disease."[13,31,55,57] To date, discography is the sole procedure capable of correlating pathoanatomy and symptomatology in patients with primary discogenic pain, and several studies have suggested improved surgical outcomes among interbody fusion patients with concordant discography pre-operatively.[19,32,88]

Appropriate patient selection is critical to the clinical success of ALIF. Indications for interbody fusion procedures include degenerative disc disease of one or two contiguous levels of the lumbar spine, with chronic, severe, disabling, intractable low back pain of at least six months' duration in patients unresponsive to an adequate and extensive trial of nonoperative treatment.[59, 82] Although some series have included patients undergoing up to three-level stand-alone ALIFs, it has been clearly shown that with each additional level fused, the interbody pseudarthrosis rate increases, and the clinical success rate declines.[13,35,57] Ray stressed the importance of disc height and mobility loss.[82] Patients who had a disc space height of more than 12 mm were excluded from his series. Interbody fusion may also be indicated in selected patients with failed prior posterior fusion attempts.[10,27,35,57,71] Certainly, under these circumstances, avoiding the peridural fibrosis is a major advantage of these devices in an anterior application.

Contraindications for ALIF include active systemic or local disc space infection; osteopenia; the presence of degenerative changes at adjacent, neighboring disc spaces; symptomatic peripheral vascular disease; malignancy; gross obesity; spondylolisthesis greater than grade 1; pregnancy; neural compression secondary to stenosis; and previous retroperitoneal surgery.[59,82] Kuslich limited his procedure to patients between the ages of 21 and 65 years.[59] Although these devices have been FDA approved for grade I spondylolisthesis, caution should be used with isthmic pathology rather than a degenerative etiology. The pars defect leads to increased posterior column instability (particularly in axial rotation) and potentially could lead to an increased failure rate (Figure 10-3).[67, 98]

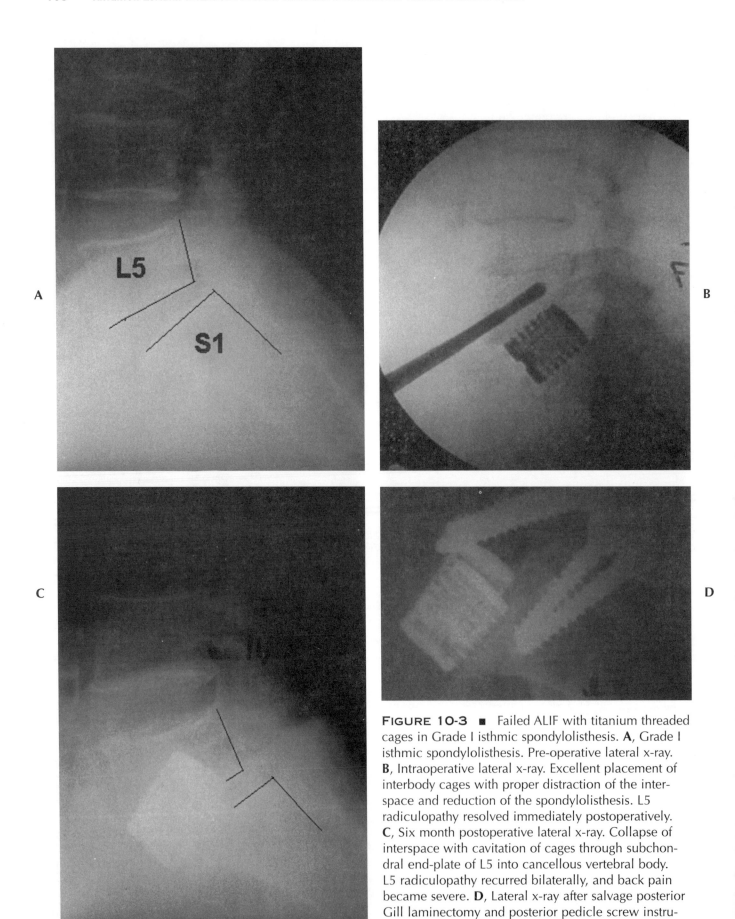

FIGURE 10-3 ■ Failed ALIF with titanium threaded cages in Grade I isthmic spondylolisthesis. **A,** Grade I isthmic spondylolisthesis. Pre-operative lateral x-ray. **B,** Intraoperative lateral x-ray. Excellent placement of interbody cages with proper distraction of the interspace and reduction of the spondylolisthesis. L5 radiculopathy resolved immediately postoperatively. **C,** Six month postoperative lateral x-ray. Collapse of interspace with cavitation of cages through subchondral end-plate of L5 into cancellous vertebral body. L5 radiculopathy recurred bilaterally, and back pain became severe. **D,** Lateral x-ray after salvage posterior Gill laminectomy and posterior pedicle screw instrumentation and fusion.

McAfee believes the use of cages should be limited to patients who have postlaminectomy syndrome or disc space collapse with neuroforaminal narrowing.[63] Optimally, only patients who have involvement of one disc level should be treated with stand-alone cages, and patients who require more than a two-level fusion should undergo a posterior procedure.

CLINICAL STUDIES

Many authors have reported excellent clinical results with the use of threaded cylindrical devices for ALIF. In a prospective, multicenter trial of the BAK device, Kuslich and associates reviewed 947 patients.[59] An anterior approach was used in 591 operations, with 93% obtaining fusion at 24 months postoperatively. Pain was eliminated or reduced in 84%. Function was improved in 91%. Major complications occurred in 2%. Implant migration occurred in 1.2%, with all requiring re-operation. Vessel damage or iliac vein tears (1.2%) were all repaired without apparent long-term problems. The overall rate of device-related re-operation was 4.4%, with most requiring additional posterior instrumentation to relieve ongoing pain. There were no instances of implant fracture or other forms of structural failure. There were no deaths, major paralyses, or deep infections. Fusion rate at 12 months after ALIF was 88.3%. At 24 months, the fusion rate increased to 93% of ALIF procedures, and at three years after surgery (118 patients), 98.3% of patients had fused operative segments.

Blumenthal and associates also found a low revision surgery rate (3.3%) among their series of 130 consecutive stand-alone open and laparoscopic threaded interbody cage patients.[5] However, in a prospective nonrandomized study of 51 stand-alone open and laparoscopic BAK patients, O'Dowd and associates recently reported an overall failure rate requiring revision of 31% resulting from clinical failures at a mean of 15 months.[72] Furthermore, 75% of their patients had residual symptoms at two years postoperatively, and 47% had the same or poor self-assessment. The authors believe the unacceptable failure rate and poor clinical results were the result of the use of the cage as a stand-alone device. Based on these findings, in order to avoid such poor outcomes, the authors recommend supplemental posterior stabilization for all threaded interbody ALIF patients.[72,74]

In the only direct comparison of threaded bone dowels and titanium cages to date, 100 anterior interbody fusion patients were randomized in a prospective study comparing titanium interbody cages (BAK) with threaded cortical bone dowels (MD II).[87] At 12 months, there were no significant differences in clinical outcome or radiographic evaluations.

Ray reported a large series (236) treated with his threaded cages through a posterior approach. Of 208 followed for a minimum of 24 months, 203 (96%) had radiographic evidence of fusion.[82] Clinical outcome as described by Prolo was excellent for 84 (40%), good for 53 (25%), fair for 44 (21%), and poor for 30 (14%). Unlike traditional posterolateral fusion or posterior lumbar interbody fusion (PLIF) techniques, ALIF avoids *fusion disease* (resultant postoperative muscle fibrosis, as well as muscle and facet joint denervation). Posterior fusion disease causes severe damage to the posterior spinal musculature, not only by the direct dissection but also by the denervation that must occur as the result of the destruction of its nerve supply during the exposure.

Posterior lumbar muscles are injured after posterior lumbar spine surgery, as demonstrated by findings on histology, computed tomography (CT), and magnetic resonance imaging (MRI). These pathological changes likely contribute to poor clinical outcome. Degeneration of the back muscle occurs just after surgery, and the muscle in most re-operated patients shows severe histologic damage, including denervation, re-innervation, and early aging. External compression by a retractor increases the intramuscular pressure and decreases local muscle blood flow. The pathological condition of the back muscle beneath the retractor blade is similar to that of skeletal muscle beneath a tourniquet. Metabolic changes and microvascular abnormalities occur. A pathogenic mechanism for the muscle injury is based on compression and ischemia of the affected muscle. Two hours of continuous retraction caused significant histologic changes and neurogenic damage, including degeneration of the neuromuscular junction and atrophy of the muscle.[51] In an animal model, muscle injury after surgery was related to the retraction time and the pressure load generated by the retractor.[52] Posterior surgical intervention to the lumbar spine always produces a risk of back muscle injury. Degeneration of the multifidus muscle was found after surgery, and human back muscle in patients who underwent repeat surgery showed severe neurogenic damage.[53,54] This muscle injury after posterior surgery might cause postoperative low back pain and compromise the functional integrity of the muscle.[79] Rantanen and associates also found selective type 2 muscle fiber atrophy and pathological structural changes in the back muscles of the patients who had severe handicap after posterior lumbar surgery.[79]

Furthermore, an ALIF procedure does not significantly alter the rate of development of adjacent level degenerative changes over that of natural history.[29] In one study with 16-year follow-up after ALIF, the rate of adjacent level degenerative changes was similar to an age-matched control population.[92] Luk and associates found no increased compensatory motion in the transition zone immediately above an ALIF.[61] Penta and associates concluded that the rate of degenerative changes adjacent to an ALIF at 10 years, as assessed by MRI, was not significantly increased.[77]

The advantages of anterior lumbar fusion in comparison to PLIF are many, including ease of dissection, reduced operative time and blood loss, noninterference with the potentially painful posterior elements of the lumbar spine, and avoidance of scarring within the spinal canal. In addition, the disc can be resected in its entirety, which is advantageous from a structural and biochemical perspective. Pain from a degenerative disc can remain, despite a solid posterolateral fusion, which may be resolved with an anterior discectomy and fusion.[96]

In an independent review of a prospective comparative series of anterior interbody fusions and posterolateral fusions with pedicle screw and plate fixation, ALIFs did better despite a lower fusion rate.[37] Although the fusion rate for anterior interbody fusion was less than that for posterolateral fusion with internal fixation, there was no difference in the subjective opinion of fusion between the two groups. Patients treated with ALIF were statistically significantly better in terms of functional outcome as assessed by the Low Back Outcome Score. One surgeon performed all of the procedures, and there was a minimum follow-up period of two years. Posterolateral lumbar fusion with pedicle screw instrumentation (135 patients) was compared to a group of 151 patients who underwent ALIF. The improved outcome in the anterior fusion group, despite the higher pseudarthrosis rate, supports the concept that part of the benefit with anterior fusion is removal of the pain source itself. Another possible explanation is that some of the patients' continuing pain and disability is related to the effects of posterior surgery on the spinal musculature and the presence of a rigid pedicle screw fixation system.

COMPLICATIONS

The majority of complications associated with cylindrical anterior interbody fusion devices are a result of the operative approach, as opposed to specific device-related problems.[63, 83] These include autograft harvest morbidity, postoperative hernias, bowel obstruction (which can occur after violation of the peritoneum during a retroperitoneal approach), postoperative ileus, iliac venous thrombosis, urological injury (1.4%), and retrograde ejaculation.[11,13,35,46,47,59] The latter has been reported to occur in 0.4% to 2.0% of male patients.[13,59,89] It is to the result of injury of the autonomic superior hypogastric plexus in the retroperitoneal space, which normally mediates closure of the

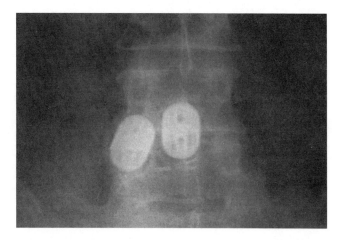

FIGURE 10-4 ■ AP x-ray of a laterally positioned titanium cage.

bladder neck during ejaculation. Major vascular (venous or arterial) complications have been reported in 0.5% to 4.0% of ALIF procedures.[56,59,83,84] Particularly at risk is the left iliolumbar vein, which can be avulsed during mobilization of the left common iliac vein, in procedures at the L4-L5 interspace.[3]

Device-related complications of anterior interbody fusion procedures consist primarily of cage malposition, migration, and iatrogenic disc herniation. Laterally positioned titanium cages (Figure 10-4) or threaded cortical bone dowels can cause direct foraminal nerve root compression and radiculopathy.[38,63,64,72] Often, this can be a result of the surgeon failing to accurately identify the anterior vertebral anatomic midline prior to inserting the paired interbody devices. Similarly, placement of the threaded interbody device into the interspace too far lateral can result in an iatrogenic disc herniation, causing compression of the exiting root in the manner of a "far lateral" disc herniation.[64] Ante-

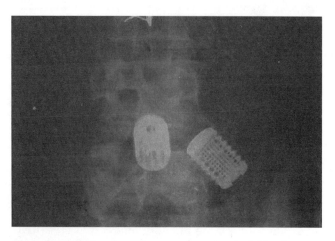

FIGURE 10-5 ■ AP x-ray of a migrated titanium cage.

rior interbody implant migration (Figure 10-5) has been reported in 2.3% of patients, with 1.2% of the total requiring re-operation.[59] Dural complications associated with the anterior placement of threaded interbody devices have not been reported.[59,63,82] The PLIF technique, however, by the very nature of its dorsal approach, is associated with a 10% incidence of dural injury and can lead to paresthesia from nerve root retraction.[59]

Laparoscopic anterior interbody cage insertion has been associated with a higher rate of device-related complications as compared to the open technique, largely because of postoperative disc herniation.[83] Using laparoscopic transperitoneal techniques, some authors have reported somewhat longer operative times, but significantly less blood loss and shorter hospital stays, as compared to open ALIF procedures with threaded interbody fusion devices.[83,84] Usually, the L5-S1 interspace is caudal to the bifurcation of the common iliac vessels, requiring minimal mobilization (except in instances of lumbosacral transitional vertebrae). A recent prospective study of threaded interbody device procedures performed at the L4-L5 level found no difference in operative time, blood loss, or length of stay when comparing laparoscopic transperitoneal ALIF to mini-open ALIF.[101] The authors, however, found a significantly higher rate of complications in the laparoscopic ALIF group (25% vs. 4%). Furthermore, adequate exposure was attained in only 84% of the laparoscopic cases, whereas in 100% of the mini-open ALIFs, two cages could be inserted.

IMAGING

The assessment of a successful interbody arthrodesis is difficult and controversial.[14,29,63] The rates of "successful" fusion are approximately 20% higher when fusion is based solely on assessment of motion on plain film radiographs, as compared to methods that also require other criteria, such as the complete absence of peri-implant lucencies.[38,63] Many studies also differ in the amount of motion permissible in a "successful" fusion, ranging from 1 to 5 degrees.[58,59,63,65,82,100] Some suggest that the best indication of fusion with threaded interbody implants is the presence of a "sentinel sign," radiographically evident bridging trabecular bone anterior to the interbody device.[63,65] In order to improve clinical results and assist in fusion determination, the concept of "ream long, fuse short" has been proposed. The threaded cylindrical interbody device is placed at the far posterior portion of the reamed and tapped channel, allowing room in the interspace anterior to the device for the packing of cancellous bone graft. When using this method of cylindrical interbody device placement, the surgeon

must ream to a sufficient depth prior to cage placement. Otherwise, attempts to seat the cage more posteriorly can result in "stripping" of the threads, a factor that has been associated with failure and implant migration.[59] In the case of threaded cortical bone dowels, this can exceed the insertional torque threshold of the implant-driver interface and cause device fracture. On the other hand, the periphery of the endplate is stronger than it is centrally; thus, for biomechanical purposes, the cage is best placed in the anterior aspect of the interspace.

Traditional methods of radiographically detecting pseudarthrosis are plain x-ray and CT. The standard criteria for pseudarthrosis are lucency around the cages, motion at the fused segment, and lack of viable bone extending through the cage into the vertebral marrow on reconstructed thin section, high resolution CT. High resolution CT scans, however, have been unreliable in fusion status assessment.[14,42,65,97] One recent report reviewed patients with postoperative persistent low back pain and surgically confirmed interbody pseudarthrosis.[42] The standard criteria failed to accurately predict pseudarthrosis proven at surgery. Six out of 7 patients who underwent prerevision CT scanning had no identifiable peri-implant lucencies, and seven out of eight patients who had prerevision plain films showed no evidence of loosening. Because of the metal artifact at the periphery of titanium interbody cages, fusion assessment has been found to be more difficult (both on CT scans and plain films) than with threaded cortical bone dowels.[14,97] It is clear that CT and plain films do not reliably detect pseudarthrosis pre-operatively. CT as well as plain films may be falsely reassuring in the evaluation of patients with titanium intervertebral lumbar spine fusion cages.

A very interesting cadaveric study on the imaging pitfalls of interbody spinal implants was reported by Cizek and Boyd.[14] They compared titanium threaded cylindrical cages, threaded bone dowels, and carbon fiber trapezoidal cages. They found the presence of bone seen extending through the cage from end-plate to end-plate on x-ray and CT could not be differentiated from a fusion. One may see lucencies on either plain film or CT but not the other. Bone within the dowel and titanium cage devices could not be discerned by plain film. Most importantly, CT artifact was not present with the bone cage but was seen with titanium and carbon fiber. The artifact was more prominent anteriorly and posteriorly, as was the implant/end-plate interface, which may obscure thin lucencies (Figure 10-6). In conclusion, current imaging techniques are suboptimal for evaluating spinal interbody implants. Errors may arise in interpreting the presence of bridging bone, lucencies, and obstruction

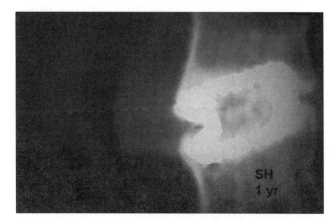

FIGURE 10-6 ■ Sagittal high resolution CT scan through titanium threaded cylindrical cage. Because of the metallic artifact at the cage-host junction, lucencies are extremely difficult to detect.

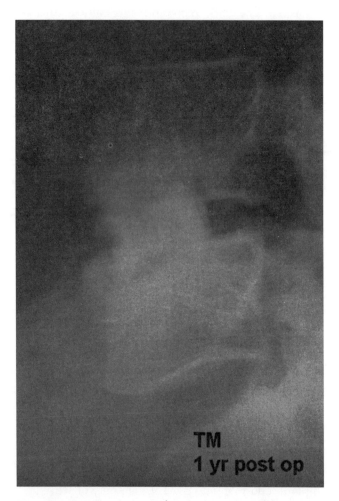

FIGURE 10-7 ■ Lateral x-ray one year after threaded bone dowel insertion. Radiolucency at the graft-host junction is easily detected, signifying pseudarthrosis.

by metallic artifact. Bridging bone may be misinterpreted as fusion, and radiolucency was better seen in threaded bone dowels compared to titanium cages (Figure 10-7).

REVISION

According to Weiner and Fraser, interbody cage devices have the following four goals: to correct the existing mechanical deformation, to provide stability to the segment until arthrodesis is obtained, to provide the best possible environment for successful arthrodesis, and to achieve this with limited morbidity associated with their use.[97] As previously discussed, clinical failures and morbidity are usually to the result of factors such as surgical technique or patient selection rather than an actual material failure of the threaded cylindrical interbody device, be it titanium or cortical bone dowel. Clinical failure has been associated with undersized cages, which fail to achieve adequate distraction of the annulus fibrosis. This is less problematic in ALIFs than PLIFs, where size is constrained by neurologic structures and the facet joints. Failure is also higher with the use of local bone graft instead of iliac crest cancellous bone and excessive lateral placement of the threaded interbody fusion device (as a result of failing to correctly identify the midline).[59,64]

Postoperatively, approximately 20% of the initially distracted disc space height is lost, largely because of bony subsidence.[86] In a biomechanical study examining the effect of cyclical loading on threaded interbody cages (simulating patient activity), one group found a gradual loss of stability resulting from local trabecular bone failure and subsequent loss of annular tension.[75] Ahrens and associates reported that anterior interbody cage subsidence occurred throughout the first 12 months after surgery but found no correlation with vertebral bone mineral density on dual energy x-ray absorptiometry (DEXA) evaluation.[1] Conversely, others have reported that vertebral body bone mineral density is a significant factor in threaded interbody device stability and is correlated with failure rates.[50,62]

ALIF pseudarthrosis can lead to continued lumbar axial back pain and, rarely, interbody device migration. In this setting, one theoretical disadvantage of titanium devices (vs. threaded cortical bone dowels) is the potential for the generation of titanium debris. Although not well-studied, significant concentrations have been identified in the paraspinous soft tissues of pseudarthrosis patients with more traditional titanium spinal implants.[95] Titanium debris has been shown to stimulate a macrophage cellular response and cytokine release, which could possibly have a deleterious effect on spinal tissues.[95,97] The most compelling theoretical advantage of threaded bone dowels over titanium cages, however, is the fact that they are much easier to revise.

REFERENCES

———————————◼———————————

1. Ahrens JE, Risk DE: Correlation of fusion cage subsidence and preoperative bone mineral density. **13ᵗʰ Annual Meeting North American Spine Society**, San Francisco, 1998.

2. Bagby GW: Arthrodesis by the distraction-compression method using a stainless steel implant. **Orthop** 11:931-34, 1988.

3. Baker JK, Reardon PR, Reardon MJ, et al: Vascular injury in anterior lumbar surgery. **Spine** 18:2227-30, 1993.

4. Benzel EC, Ferrara L, Baldwin N: Multidirectional stabilizing potential of BAK interbody spinal fusion system for anterior surgery (letter). **J Spinal Dis** 11:454-55, 1998.

5. Blumenthal SL, Regan JJ, Hisey MS, et al: Can threaded fusion cages be used effectively as stand-alone devices? **14ᵗʰ Annual Meeting North American Spine Society**, Chicago, 1999.

6. Boden SD, Davis DO, Diaz TS, et al: Abnormal magnetic resonance scans of the lumbar spine in asymptomatic subjects: a prospective investigation. **JBJS** 72A:403-08, 1990.

7. Brodke DS, Dick JC, Kunz DN, et al: Posterior lumbar interbody fusion. A biomechanical comparison including a new threaded cage. **Spine** 22:26-31, 1997.

8. Buck BE, Malinin TI: Bone transplantation and human immunodeficiency virus: an estimate of risk of AIDS. **Clin Orthop** 303:8-17, 1994.

9. Burns BH: An operation for spondylolisthesis. **Lancet** 224:1233-9, 1933.

10. Buttermann GR, Glazer PA, Hu SS, et al: Revision of failed lumbar fusions: a comparison of anterior autograft and allograft. **Spine** 22:2748-55, 1997.

11. Calandruccio RA, Benton BF: Anterior lumbar fusion. **Clin Orthop** 35:63-68, 1964.

12. Capener, N: Spondylolisthesis. **British Journal of Surgery** 19:374-86, 1932.

13. Chow SP, Leong JC, Ma A, et al: Anterior spinal fusion for deranged lumbar intervertebral disc. **Spine** 5:452-58, 1980.

14. Cizek GR, Boyd LM: Imaging pitfalls of interbody spinal implants. **14ᵗʰ Annual Meeting North American Spine Society**, Chicago, 1999.

15. Closkey RF, Parsons R, Lee CK, et al: Mechanics of interbody fusion. **Spine** 18:1011-5, 1993.

16. Cloward RB: Lesions of the intervertebral disks and their treatment by interbody fusion methods. **Clin Orthop** 27:51-77, 1963.

17. Cloward RB: Spondylolisthesis: Treatment by laminectomy and posterior interbody fusion. **Clin Orthop** 154:76-82, 1981.

18. Cloward RB: The treatment of ruptured lumbar intervertebral discs by vertebral body fusion. **J Neurosurg** 10:154-68, 1953.

19. Colhoun E, McCall IW, Williams L, et al: Provocation discography as a guide to planning operation on the spine. **JBJS** 70B:267-71, 1989.

20. Crawley GR, Grant BD, White KK: A modified Cloward's technique for arthrodesis of the normal metacarpophalangeal joint in the horse. **J Vet Surg** 17:117-127, 1988.

21. Crock HV: Anterior lumbar interbody fusion: indications for its use and notes on surgical technique. **Clin Orthop** 165:157-63, 1982.

22. DeBowes RM, Grant BD, Bagby GW, et al: Cervical vertebral interbody fusion in the horse. **Am J Vet Res** 45:141-56, 1984.

23. Dennis S, Watkins R, Landaker S, et al: Comparison of disc space heights after anterior lumbar interbody fusion. **Spine** 14:876-78, 1989.

24. Deyo RA, Cherkins D, Conrad D, et al: Cost, controversy, crisis: low back pain and the health of the public. **Ann Rev Pub Health** 12:141-56, 1991.

25. Dolan P, Earley M, Adams MA: Bending and compressive stresses acting on the lumbar spine during lifting activities. **J Biomech** 27:1237-48, 1994.

26. Fernyhough JC, White JF, LaRocca H: Fusion rates in multilevel cervical spondylosis comparing allograft fibula with autograft fibula. **Spine** 16:561-64, 1991.

27. Flynn JC, Hoquema MA: Anterior fusion of the lumbar spine. End result study with long-term follow-up. **JBJS** 61A:1143-50, 1979.

28. Forristall RM, Marsh HO, Pay NT: MRI and contrast CT of the lumbar spine: comparison of diagnostic methods and correlation with surgical findings. **Spine** 13:1049-154, 1988.

29. Fraser RD: Interbody, posterior, and combined lumbar fusions. **Spine** 20:167S-77S, 1995.

30. Frymoyer JW, Pope MH, Clemens JH, et al: Risk factors in low back pain. **JBJS** 65A:213-18, 1983.

31. Fujimaki A, Crock HV, Bedbrook GM: The results of 150 anterior lumbar interbody fusion operations performed by two surgeons in Australia. **Clin Orthop** 165:164-67, 1982.

32. Gill K, Blumenthal S: Functional results after anterior lumbar fusions at L5-S1 in patients with normal and abnormal MRI scans. **Spine** 17:940-42, 1992.

33. Glazer PA, Colliou O, Klisch SM: Biomechanical analysis of multilevel fixation methods in the lumbar spine. **Spine** 22:171-82, 1997.

34. Glazer PA, Colliou O, Lotz JC, et al: Biomechanical analysis of lumbosacral fixation. **Spine** 21:1211-22, 1996.

35. Goldner JL, Urbaniak JR, McCollum DE: Anterior disc excision and interbody spinal fusion for chronic low back pain. **Ortho Clin North Am** 2:543-68, 1971.

36. Greenough CG, Fraser RD: The effects of compensation on recovery from low back injury. **Spine** 14:947-55, 1989.

37. Greenough CG, Peterson MD, Hadlow S, et al: Instrumented posterolateral lumbar fusion: Results and com-

parison with anterior interbody fusion. **Spine** 23:479-86. 1998.

38. Hacker RJ: Comparison of interbody fusion approaches for disabling low back pain. **Spine** 22:660-66, 1997.

39. Haher TR, Yeung AW, Merola AA, et al: An in vitro biomechanical investigation of spinal interbody fusion devices. **14ᵗʰ Annual Meeting North American Spine Society,** Chicago, 1999.

40. Harmon PH: Anterior excision and vertebral body fusion operation for intervertebral disc syndromes of the lower lumbar spine. **Clin Orthop** 26:107-27, 1963.

41. Harmon PH: Results from the treatment of sciatica due to lumbar disc protrusion. **American Journal of Surgery** 80:829, 1950.

42. Heithoff KB, Mullin JW, Holte D, et al: Failure of radiographic detection of pseudarthrosis in patients with titanium lumbar interbody fusion cages. **14ᵗʰ Annual Meeting North American Spine Society**, Chicago, 1999.

43. Hodgson AR, Stock FE: Anterior spinal fusion. **Br J Surg** 44:226-75, 1956.

44. Hodgson AR, Stock FE: Anterior spine fusion for the treatment of tuberculosis of the spine. **JBJS** 42:295-310. 1960.

45. Hoover NW: Methods of lumbar spine fusion. **JBJS** 50A:194-210, 1968.

46. Humphries AW, Hawk WA, Berndt AL: Anterior interbody fusion of lumbar vertebrae. **Surg Clin North Am** 41:1685-1700, 1961.

47. Inoue SJ, Watanabe T, Hirose A, et al: Anterior discectomy and interbody fusion for lumbar disc herniation: a review of 350 cases. **Clin Orthop** 183:22-31, 1984.

48. Ito H, Tsuchiya J, Asami G: A new radical operation for Pott's disease. **JBJS** 16B:499-515, 1934.

49. Iwahara T: A new method of vertebral body fusion. **Surgery** (Japan) 8:271-87, 1944.

50. Jost B, Cripton PA, Lund T, et al: Compressive strength of interbody cages in the lumbar spine. **Euro Spine J** 7:132-141, 1998.

51. Kawaguchi Y, Matsui H, Gejo R, et al: Preventive measures of back muscle injury after posterior lumbar spine surgery in rats. **Spine** 23:2282-8. 1998.

52. Kawaguchi Y, Matsui H, Tsuji H: Back muscle injury after posterior lumbar spine surgery: part 1. Histologic and histochemical analyses in rats. **Spine** 19:2590-7, 1994.

53. Kawaguchi Y, Matsui H, Tsuji H: Back muscle injury after posterior lumbar spine surgery: part 2. Histologic and histochemical analyses in humans. **Spine** 19:2598-602, 1994.

54. Kawaguchi Y, Matsui H, Tsuji H: Back muscle injury after posterior lumbar spine surgery: A histologic and enzymatic analysis. **Spine** 21:941-44, 1996.

55. Knox BD, Chapman TM: Anterior lumbar interbody fusion for discogram concordant pain. **J Spinal Dis** 6:242-44, 1993.

56. Kozak JA, Heilman AE, O'Brien JP: Anterior lumbar fusion options: technique and graft materials. **Clin Orthop** 300:45-51, 1994.

57. Kozak JA, O'Brien JP: Simultaneous combined anterior and posterior fusion: an independent analysis of a

58. Kumar A, Kozak JA, Doherty BJ, et al: Interspace distraction and graft subsidence after anterior lumbar fusion with femoral strut allograft. **Spine** 18:2393-400, 1993.

59. Kuslich SD, Ulstrom CL, Griffith SL, et al: The Bagby and Kuslich method of lumbar interbody fusion. **Spine** 23:1267-79, 1998.

60. Lane JD, Moore ES: Transperitoneal approach to the intervertebral disc in the lumbar area. **Annals Surg** 127:537-51, 1948.

61. Luk KL, Chow DH, Evans JH, et al: Lumbar spine mobility after short anterior interbody fusion. **Spine** 20: 813-18, 1995.

62. Lund T, Oxland TR, Jost B, et al: Interbody cage stabilization in the lumbar spine: Biomechanical evaluation of cage design, posterior instrumentation and bone density. **JBJS** 80B:351-59, 1998.

63. McAfee PC: Interbody fusion cages in reconstructive operations on the spine. **JBJS** 81A:859-80, 1999.

64. McAfee PC, Cunningham, Lee GA, et al: Revision strategies for salvaging or improving failed cylindrical cages. **Spine** 24:2147-53, 1999.

65. McAfee PC, Lee GA, Fedder IL, et al: A prospective randomized study of 100 anterior interbody cage arthrodeses: complete versus partial discectomy. **14ᵗʰ Annual Meeting North American Spine Society**, Chicago, 1999.

66. Mercer W: Spondylolisthesis with a description of a new method of operative treatment and notes of ten cases. **Edinburg Med** J 43:545-72, 1936.

67. Miahara H, Cheng BC, Orr RD, et al: Tapered interbody fixation cage for lumbar spondylolysis: A biomechanical study. **14ᵗʰ Annual Meeting North American Spine Society,** Chicago, 1999.

68. Muller W: Transperitoneale freilegung der wirbelsaule bei tuberkuloser spondylitis. **Deutsch Z Chiro** 85:128-37, 1906.

69. Nachemson AL, Schultz AB, Berkson MH: Mechanical properties of human lumbar spine motion segments: influence of age, sex, disc level and degeneration. **Spine** 4:1-8, 1979.

70. Nisbet NW, James A: Results of intervertebral bony fusions. **JBJS** 38B:952-53, 1956.

71. O'Brien JP, Dawson MH, Heard CW, et al: Simultaneous combined anterior and posterior fusion. **Clin Orthop** 203:191-95, 1986.

72. O'Dowd JK, Lam K, Mulholland RC, et al: BAK cage: Nottingham results. **13ᵗʰ Annual Meeting North American Spine Society**, San Francisco, 1998.

73. Otero-Vich JM: Anterior cervical interbody fusion with threaded cylindrical bone. **J Neurosurg** 63:750-53, 1985.

74. Oxland TR, Hoffer Z, Nydegger T: Comparative biomechanical investigation of anterior lumbar interbody cages: entral and bilateral insertion. **Ortho Trans** 22: 728-29, 1999.

75. Oxland TR, Hoffer Z, Nydegger T, et al: Compressive loading affects interbody cage stabilization in the lumbar spine. **13ᵗʰ Annual Meeting North American Spine Society**, San Francisco, 1998.

76. Pelker RR, Friedlaender GE, Markham TC: Biomechanical properties of bone allografts. **Clin Orthop** 174:54-57, 1983.

77. Penta M, Sandhu A, Fraser RB: Magnetic resonance imaging assessment of disc degeneration 10 years after anterior lumbar interbody fusion. **Spine** 20:743-47, 1995.

78. Raney FL, Adams JE: Anterior lumbar disc excision and interbody fusion used as a salvage procedure. **JBJS** 45A:667-68, 1963.

79. Rantanen J, Hurme M, Falck B, et al: The lumbar multifidus muscle five years after surgery for a lumbar intervertebral disc herniation. **Spine** 18:568-74, 1993.

80. Rapoff AJ, Ghanayem AJ, Zdeblick TA: Biomechanical comparison of posterior lumbar interbody fusion cages. **Spine** 22:2375-9, 1997.

81. Rathonyi GC, Oxland TR, Gerich U, et al: The role of supplemental translaminar screws in anterior lumbar interbody fixation: a biomechanical study. **Eur Spine J** 7: 400-7. 1998.

82. Ray CD: Threaded titanium cages for lumbar interbody fusions. **Spine** 22:667-80, 1997.

83. Regan JJ, Yuan H, McAfee PC: Laparoscopic fusion of the lumbar spine: minimally invasive spine surgery. **Spine** 24:402-411, 1999.

84. Regan JJ, Aronoff RJ, Ohnmeiss DD, et al: Laparoscopic approach to L4-L5 for interbody fusion using BAK cages: experience in first 58 cases. **Spine** 24:2171-4, 1999.

85. Sacks S: Anterior interbody fusion of the lumbar spine. **JBJS** 47B:211-23, 1965.

86. Sandhu HS, Turner S, Kabo JM, et al: Distractive properties of a threaded interbody fusion device: an in vivo model. **Spine** 21:1201-10, 1996.

87. Schofferman J, Slosar P, Reynolds J, et al: Anterior lumbar interbody fusion: Comparison of titanium threaded cages with threaded bone dowels. **14th Annual Meeting North American Spine Society**, Chicago, 1999

88. Schwarzer A, Aprill C, Derby R, et al: The prevalence and clinical features of internal disc disruption in patients with chronic low back pain. **Spine** 20:752-60, 1995.

89. Stauffer RN, Coventry MB: Anterior interbody lumbar spine fusion. Analysis of Mayo clinic series. **JBJS** 54A:756-68, 1972.

90. Sutterlin CE, Bianchi JR, Reilly TM: Threaded cortical dowel construct stiffness testing. **University of Florida Tissue Bank** 1:1-4, 1997.

91. Tencer AF, Hampton D, Eddy S: Biomechanical properties of threaded inserts for lumbar interbody spinal fusion. **Spine** 20: 2408-14, 1995.

92. Van Horn JR, Bohnen LM: The development of discopathy in lumbar discs adjacent to a lumbar anterior interbody spondylodesis. A retrospective matched-pair study with a postoperative follow-up of 16 years. **Acta Orthop Belg** 58:280-86, 1992.

93. Volkman T, Horton WC, Hutton WC: Transfacet screws with lumbar interbody reconstruction: biomechanical study of motion segment stiffness. **J Spinal Disord** 9:425-32. 1996.

94. Wagner PC, Grant BD, Bagby GW, et al: Evaluation of spine fusion as treatment in the equine wobbler syndrome. **J Vet Surg** 8:84-88, 1979.

95. Wang JC, Yu WD, Sandhu HS, et al: Metal debris from titanium spinal implants. **Spine** 24:899-903, 1999.

96. Weatherley CR, Prickett CF, O'Brien JP: Discogenic pain persisting despite solid posterior fusion. **JBJS** 68B:142-43, 1986.

97. Weiner BK, Fraser RD: Spine update: lumbar interbody cages. **Spine** 23:634-40, 1998.

98. White AA, Panjabi MM: **Clinical Biomechanics of the Spine**, 2nd ed. Philadelphia: Lippincott, 1990.

99. Wiltberger BR: Intervertebral body fusion by the use of posterior bone dowels. **Clin Orthop** 35:69-79, 1964.

100. Zdeblick TA: A prospective randomized study of lumbar fusion: Preliminary results. **Spine** 18: 983-91, 1993.

101. Zdeblick TA, David S, Cheng B: A prospective comparison of surgical approach for anterior L4-5 fusion: laparoscopic versus mini-ALIF. **14th Annual Meeting North American Spine Society**, Chicago, 1999.

CHAPTER 11

Circumferential Fusion Techniques: The TLIF

CLIFFORD B. TRIBUS, M.D.

INTRODUCTION

The TLIF is a technically demanding yet viable surgical alternative in the spine surgeon's armamentarium for the treatment of lumbar disorders. Part of the problem in learning and teaching the TLIF is the lack of available information. The obvious example is the meaning of TLIF. TLIF has been characterized as both *transforaminal lumbar interbody fusion* as well as *transfacet lumbar interbody fusion*. The exact characterization of the TLIF is in evolution. Its most obvious predecessor is the posterior lumbar interbody fusion (PLIF), but the development of transpedicular fixation and increased biomechanical awareness of lumbar spine conditions was also required for TLIF to reach its current point of development. The goal of this chapter is to discuss briefly the historical evolution of the TLIF, to outline patient selection guidelines, to describe in detail the operative technique complete with avoidance of complications, and to discuss early results.

HISTORY OF THE TLIF

The history of interbody fusion techniques spans the last 50 years. Cloward is often credited with describing the PLIF technique in 1963, yet Wiltberger described a posteriorly placed interbody fusion using a bone dowel in 1957.[3,14] The PLIF is a technically demanding operation.[1,2,4, 9,-11] It requires wide exposure to the disc space, necessitating aggressive neural element mobilization while attempting to maintain the integrity of the facet joints. Need for additional exposure to the disc without the overt manipulation of the neural elements is one of the forces that led to the development of the TLIF. In "Posterior lumbar interbody fusion with specialized instruments," by Ma, the author describes the surgical technique for PLIF maintaining facet integrity.[8] The clinical drawings and radiographs

from that same article, however, demonstrate facet resection that apparently was necessary for adequate placement of the interbody fusion graft.[8] The aggressive lateral resection of facet joints has been a characteristic of the PLIF for many years.

Early noninstrumented PLIFs were completed by inadvertent retropulsion of the interbody graft material toward the neural elements. This has been mirrored more recently by reported experiences of posteriorly placed interbody fusion cages.[7] It was the development of transpedicular fixation that allowed the evolution of the modern TLIF. Transpedicular fixation allows compression to be applied to the fused segment, thus securing the interbody device, which is not otherwise inherently stable.

Whereas the modern TLIF is not currently formalized in the literature, Dr. Juergen Harms is frequently credited for its recent teaching. Patients with isthmic spondylolisthesis are treated by a posterior-only approach, using anterior column load-sharing principles placed by a TLIF approach supported by a posterior tension band using transpedicular fixation. Thus, with transpedicular fixation allowing intra-operative disc distraction to facilitate the surgeons' exposure of the disc space, and ultimately allowing the application of compression to stabilize the anterior interbody fusion, the maturation of the TLIF was facilitated.

PATIENT SELECTION GUIDELINES

The surgical criteria for a TLIF are similar to other lumbar fusion techniques. Patients must have severe incapacitating low back pain, with or without lower extremity symptoms that have been refractory to aggressive nonoperative treatment programs. The patient's outcome will be dependent upon these selection criteria, arguably as much as the technical expertise with which the surgery itself is performed. The TLIF is not presented in this chapter as a definitive way of managing intralumbar pathology, yet it is presented as a technique in the surgeon's armamentarium for dealing with a variety of pathologies. Once the patient has reached a surgical threshold, then ultimately the procedure of choice is dependent on the patient's pathology, the surgeon's expertise, and their mutual preference.

A TLIF is a reasonable technique to obtain the advantage of anterior column support without an anterior approach.[12] Diagnoses readily addressable by the TLIF the following:

1. Isthmic spondylolisthesis.
2. Degenerative disc disease.
3. Third time or greater recurrent herniated disc disease to be treated by fusion.
4. One- or two-level lumbar kyphosis.
5. Discogenic back pain warranting fusion treatment.

Other conditions for which the TLIF might be considered are the following:

1. Posterior treatment of pseudoarthrosis.
2. One- or two-level postlaminectomy kyphosis.

The TLIF is also useful for any patient considered for an anterior-posterior procedure where the anterior procedure is deemed more challenging because of previous abdominal or retroperitoneal surgery, or where there is a strong patient aversion to the possibility of retrograde ejaculation.

The only absolute contraindication to the TLIF is severe osteopenia. Severe osteopenia prevents the safe distraction of the intervertebral disc. Ultimately, anterior column support may not be enhanced by the interbody fusion device because of subsidence. Relative contraindications to the TLIF include the need for anterior column support over greater than two levels or the existence of severe bilateral epidural fibrosis.

In summary, the indications for the TLIF are quite similar to the indications for the PLIF. The TLIF does have several distinct advantages over the PLIF, but does so at the expense of facet joint resection and, therefore, decreased posterior bone mass. The advantages include significant decrease in the necessary neural element manipulation, with decreased epidural bleeding and, presumably, decreased epidural fibrosis.

SURGICAL TECHNIQUE OF THE TLIF

The patient is positioned on the operating table in a prone position. The abdomen should be well decompressed to reduce epidural bleeding. The author's preference is to use the Jackson table (Orthopedic Sys-

tems, Inc. Union City, CA) to allow maintenance of lumbar lordosis, particularly in multilevel lumbar procedures. A kneeling position for a one-level procedure is quite acceptable. After the lumbosacral spine is prepped and draped, a midline approach is performed, and the posterior elements are subperiosteally exposed. The facets at the levels to be fused are stripped of their facet capsule and the facet joint cartilage (Figure 11-1).

Upon completion of the exposure, bone graft is obtained. Next, the appropriate decompression procedure, if indicated, is performed. Transpedicular fixation is then placed bilaterally at the levels to be fused. Distraction is then applied across the construct, either through temporary placement of a unilateral rod or by a distraction device applied to the pedicle screws. A complete unilateral facet joint resection is then performed. This may be started with a large rongeur and completed with a Kerrison rongeur. The superior aspect of the inferior pedicle should be easily palpable, and the superiorly exiting nerve root should be visualized (Figure 11-2).

The bony resection will allow direct visualization and palpation of the posterolateral corner of the disc space. Epidural and foraminal fat and epidural vessels will be encountered. Occasional transforaminal ligaments will be encountered and should be resected.[5]

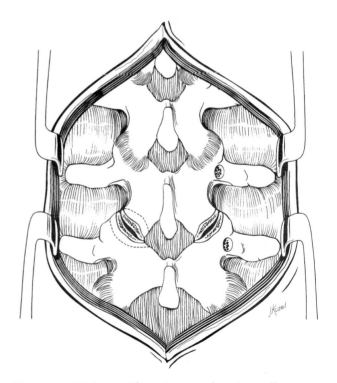

FIGURE 11-1 ■ The spine is subperiosteally exposed with the facet joints to be fused stripped of their respective capsules. The dotted lines reflect the facet joint to be resected to approach the posterolateral corner of the intervertebral disc.

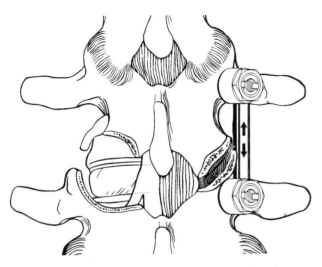

FIGURE 11-2 ■ Transpedicular fixation has been placed opposite the facet resection and distraction applied across the construct. Both the proximal and distal exiting nerve roots are exposed.

Electrocautery and blunt dissection should be used to mobilize the soft tissues and to visualize the disc space. Great care, particularly with the dorsal root ganglion of the superiorly exiting nerve, should be exercised. An annular window, rectangular in shape, should be created in the posterolateral corner of the disc. A medial hinge of the annulus may be retained and used as a soft tissue neural retractor, or, conversely, the annular window may be resected to facilitate wide exposure. Neural elements need to be protected during the discectomy. The lateral border of the thecal sac will be present medially, the superior nerve root rostrally, and the inferior exiting nerve root cau-

dally. A complete discectomy is performed with resection of the disc and preparation of the end-plates up to the surrounding annulus (Figure 11-3).

A variety of chisels and curettes are available to resect the disc and to prepare the respective end-plates. The posterior ridge of each end-plate should be resected to facilitate placement of the structural interbody devices. The interbody fusion is then performed. A variety of options are available to the surgeon. Structural corticocancellous autogenous bone graft, structural allograft, horizontal or vertical interbody fusion cages, and morsellized autogenous bone graft represent most of the available options. If a reduction maneuver is being performed, structural anterior support is preferable. If structural support is used, the rest of the disc space should be filled with impacted morsellized autogenous bone graft. The morsellized bone graft should be placed anteriorly in the disc space, with the structural support placed posteriorly to recreate load bearing through the middle column. The interbody grafting material should be recessed anterior to the posterior longitudinal ligament to avoid retropulsion. The transpedicular construct is then converted from distraction to compression, thus providing a lordotic moment arm while stabilizing the anterior column interbody fusion device (Figure 11-4).

A check of the neural elements at this stage is indicated to assure that there is no retropulsed material. A posterolateral intertransverse process fusion is completed with morsellized autogenous bone graft (Figure 11-5). The usefulness of a posterior intertransverse process fusion in addition to an interbody fusion has been debated, but a clinical study documenting the advantages of not performing a posterolateral fusion has not been reported. Intraoperative radiographs or

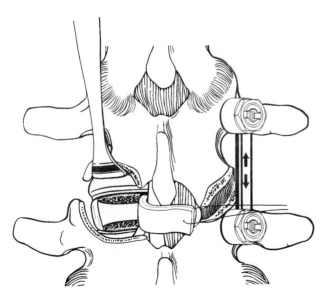

FIGURE 11-3 ■ The annular window with a medial hinge has been created and is used as a neural retractor. The superiorly exiting nerve root is protected with a retractor, and a complete discectomy is performed.

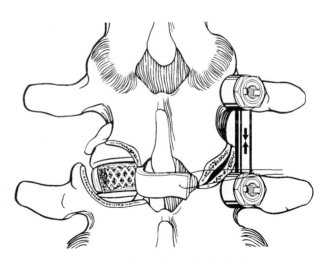

FIGURE 11-4 ■ Vertical interbody fusion cages are in place and are surrounded and packed with autogenous bone graft. The transpedicular fixation is converted from distraction to compression, thus securing the interbody fusion devices.

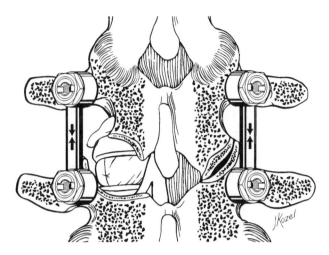

FIGURE 11-5 ■ The annular window has been repaired, and additional transpedicular fixation has been added with compression applied. The posterior elements are decorticated, and morsellized autogenous bone graft is to be added.

fluoroscopy should be used during the procedure to facilitate the discectomy and interbody fusion and to check hardware placement.

Postoperatively, the patient is mobilized on the first postoperative day, and a walking program is initiated. Adjunctive bracing is not necessary for structural support but may be used for patient comfort. Return to

normal activities is expected between months three and six. Radiographic and clinical follow-up should be at least until clinical and radiographic union has been obtained, with longer follow-up indicated based on the surgeon's preference (Figure 11-6).

RESULTS OF TLIF

Lowe and associates reported their results on 40 patients with a minimum of two-year follow-up at the Scoliosis Research Society Meeting in 1999. The diagnoses of their patient population included 23 patients with degenerative disc disease, 13 patients with spondylolisthesis, and four patients with recurrent herniated nucleus pulposus at L4-L5. One-level TLIFs were performed in 34 patients, whereas six patients underwent two-level TLIFs. Radiographic fusion indicated by bridging trabecular bone on plain radiographs and no motion on flexion extension radiographs was obtained in 38 out of 40 patients. Clinical outcome included good to excellent results in 88% of patients, as measured by greater than 50% reduction in pain levels, a return to high levels of activities, and a return to work. Complications included two patients suspected to have pseudoarthrosis and one patient with a transient neurapraxia.[6]

Whitecloud and associates reported on 80 patients undergoing anterior column reconstruction augmented with posterior transpedicular fixation. Half of these patients were approached anteriorly for their

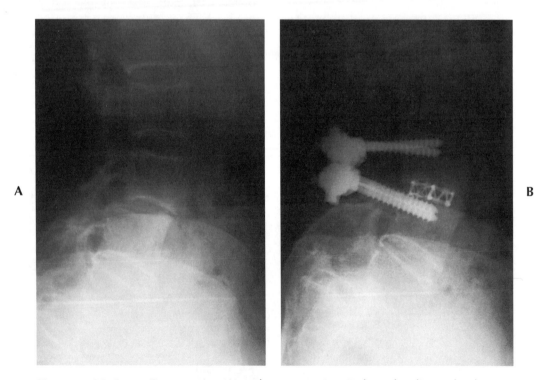

FIGURE 11-6 ■ Preoperative (**A**) and postoperative (**B**) lateral radiographs demonstrating appropriate hardware placement, reduction of spondylolisthesis, and healing anteriorly across the disc space.

interbody fusion. The other 40 patients were reconstructed through a posterior-only approach using a TLIF. The TLIF group demonstrated a shorter hospital stay with reduced blood loss and decreased operative time.[13] No comments were made as to the long-term follow-up of these two groups.

SUMMARY

The TLIF is an evolving surgical technique that is not yet well supported in the literature. Its theoretic benefits over posterior lumbar interbody fusion, however, are clear. With the use of adjunctive transpedicular fixation and the development of improved interbody fusion devices and instruments, its future as a viable alternative to anterior-posterior surgery and PLIF is assured.

REFERENCES

1. Aebi M: Adding posterior lumbar interbody fusion to pedicle screw fixation and posterolateral fusion after decompression in spondylolytic spondylolisthesis – point of view. **Spine** 22(2):219-20, 1997.
2. Brodke DS, Dick JC, Kunz DN, et al: Posterior lumbar interbody fusion. A biomechanical comparison, including a new threaded cage. **Spine** 22(1):26-31, 1997.
3. Cloward RB: Lesions of the tubervertebral disks and their treatment by interbody fusion methods. **Clin Orthop** 27:51-77, 1963.
4. Csecsei G, Klekner A, Sikula J: Posterior lumbar interbody fusion (PLIF) using the bony elements of the dorsal spinal segment. **Acta Chirurgica Hungarica** 36(1-4):54-56, 1997.
5. Golub BS, Silverman B: Transforaminal ligaments of the lumbar spine. **J Bone Joint Surg-Am Vol** 51(5):947-56, 1969.
6. Lowe T, Tahernia AD: Unilateral transforaminal posterior interbody fusion. Presented at Scoliosis Research Society Annual Meeting, San Diego, CA. September 1999.
7. McAffe PC, Cunningham BW, Lee GA, et al: Revision strategies for salvaging or improving failed cylindrical cages. **Spine** 24(20):2147-53, 1999.
8. Ma GWC: Posterior lumbar interbody fusion with specialized instruments, in Lin PM, Gill N (eds.): **Lumbar Interbody Fusion.** Rockville, Maryland: Aspen Publishers, 1989, pp. 243-49.
9. Nakai S, Yoshizawa H, Kobayashi S: Long-term follow-up study of posterior lumbar interbody fusion. **J Spinal Disord** 12(4):293-99, 1999.
10. Simmons JW: Posterior lumbar interbody fusion with posterior elements as graft. **Clin Orthop** 193:85-89, 1985.
11. Voor MJ, Mehta S, Wang M, et al: Biomechanical evaluation of posterior and anterior lumbar interbody fusion techniques. **J Spinal Disord** 11(4):328-34, 1998.
12. Weatherley CR, Prickett CF, O'Brien JP: Discogenic pain persisting despite solid posterior fusion. **J Bone Joint Surg Br** 68:142-3 , 1986.
13. Whitecloud T, Ricciardi J, Roesch W: Transforaminal interbody fusion versus anterior/posterior interbody fusion of the lumbar spine: a financial analysis. Poster presented at American Academy of Orthopaedic Surgeons® Annual Meeting, Orlando, FL. March 2000.
14. Wiltberger BR: The dowel intervertebral body fusion used in lumbar disc surgery. **J Bone Joint Surg** 39A:284-92, 1957.

CHAPTER 12

Failed Back Surgery Syndrome

■

SETH M. ZEIDMAN, M.D.

INTRODUCTION

Failed back surgery syndrome (FBSS), or the "failed back syndrome," is a clinical condition in which patients who undergo one or more surgical procedures for lumbosacral disease obtain unsatisfactory long-term relief of symptoms, with persistent or recurrent low back pain.[10,16,43]

Failed back syndrome is characterized by a constellation of pain, psychological disturbances, and incapacitation from low back and/or leg pain secondary to lumbar spinal disease. The major etiologies of FBSS include inappropriate patient selection, diagnosis, poor operative technique, iatrogenic instability, and surgical complications. Failed back syndrome most often occurs in those patients inappropriately selected for surgery who are left with residual pain and neurological deficits. Most FBSS patients have undergone multiple surgical procedures in attempts to relieve intractable and incapacitating sciatica and/or low back pain. Appropriate therapeutic decision-making in FBSS patients depends on the following two factors: the establishment of an accurate diagnosis that considers underlying medical problems and related comorbidities and a rational, individualized therapeutic regimen that addresses the diagnosed abnormalities.

Prevention of FBSS is more important than any available treatment. It requires an understanding of the history of spinal traumatic and degenerative disease as well as the complications from psychological, social, and economic factors. In this chapter, we define FBSS, detail the causes of failure in patients who have had lumbosacral spine surgery, and outline the clinical presentations of FBSS patients. We also delineate the therapeutic regimens available when specific failures have occurred, and provide an algorithm for the evaluation and treatment of this complex clinical entity (Table 12-1).

HISTORY/EPIDEMIOLOGY

Mixter and Barr first recognized lumbar disc herniation as a distinct surgical entity in 1934.[52] Operations to correct disc herniation rapidly gained acceptance, and by the early 1950s, reports of the first series of re-operations on the lumbar spine were published.[29] Each year more than 250,000 patients undergo lumbosacral operative procedures.[24,55] The responses of 207 patients to a questionnaire indicate that success rates from lumbosacral surgery depend on the design of the questionnaire, with satisfactory results ranging from 97% to 60%.[32] Experience shows that 10% of patients who undergo lumbar disc surgery are permanently disabled and unable to work, whereas 25% never return to their original occupations.

ETIOLOGY AND PATHOGENESIS

Multiple factors that contribute to the failure of lumbar surgery to relieve symptoms and to effect a favorable outcome from surgery include incorrect pre-operative diagnosis, improper patient selection, inadequate surgical decompression, complications from the procedure, and psychosocial factors. Biological and iatrogenic factors also contribute to FBSS. Spinal stenosis, recurrent disc herniation, fusion overgrowth, development of mechanical pain, pseudarthrosis, and neuropathic pain all may follow lumbar spine surgery. Neuropathic pain may result from nerve root injury, pseudomeningocele formation, adhesive arachnoiditis, epidural fibrosis, and reaction to a retained foreign body. Patient populations and author biases are often poorly defined, which increases the problem of identifying FBSS.

Complaints of pain are subjective phenomena, and clinicians can only observe pain-related behavior. Pain does not necessarily denote active tissue damage or

TABLE 12-1 ■ Algorithm for the Treatment of FBSS

I. Diagnosis: history and physical examination
  A. History
    1. Number of previous back operations
    2. Length of pain-free interval(s)
    3. Distribution of pain
    4. Exacerbating/relieving factors
  B. Physical examination
    1. Neurological examination
    2. Tension signs
    3. Functional signs
    4. Thorough general medical examination and review of systems
  C. Determine if pain has nonspinal cause (e.g., diabetes, abdominal aortic aneurysm, pancreatitis)
    1. Psychiatric evaluation (i.e., if any hint of psychosocial abnormality)
    2. Radiographic evaluation
  D. Plain radiographs
  E. Flexion/extension films
  F. CT myelogram
  G. MRI with gadolinium
II. Therapeutic intervention
  A. Nonsurgical
    1. Rehabilitation
    2. Detoxification as needed
    3. Multidisciplinary pain treatment center
  B. Surgery
    1. Re-operation (minority)
    2. Ablative procedures, other than facet denervations, are not helpful
    3. Spinal cord stimulation (particularly for radicular pain)

injury, and chronic pain behaviors rarely correlate with active tissue irritation or damage. In general, FBSS patients are not malingerers. Many of the factors that contribute to the chronicity and incapacity are on a subconscious level, and failure is likely when inadequate pre-operative assessment is combined with incomplete comprehension of the impact of psychosocial problems on outcome.

Most clinicians gain insight into a patient's psychological status during the history and physical examination. Personality dysfunction is the most common psychological problem complicating FBSS. Over 50% of patients referred to the Johns Hopkins chronic paint treatment center suffer from substantial personality dysfunction.[44] Questions relating to interactions with family and friends, marital history, military and vocational history, problems with the law, and substance abuse (including misuse of narcotics and psychotropics) often provide relevant information.

The role of psychological factors in FBSS is difficult to assess, but these factors, which include unresolved compensation issues, should be considered in patient selection. Many patients who present with intractable back pain are incapacitated by personality and psychosocial factors. The degree of incapacitation should reflect demonstrated pathology and the degree of physical impairment. During the history and physical examination, patients should be carefully observed for signs of exaggerated pain and disability. Skilled clinicians learn to recognize these behaviors, which other patients do not display and which are always related to psychosocial dysfunction. Several studies indicate that patients diagnosed with psychological problems have poor outcomes for re-operation.[10,27] Psychological testing may be affected by organic disease, reflecting the underlying diagnosis. Standardized psychological testing explains only a portion of the variance in treatment outcome and should be used as one of several patient selection criteria.

Before selection for any procedure, FBSS patients with drug habituation problems should undergo behavioral programs with an emphasis on detoxification. Patients with substance "addiction" should not be denied necessary therapy because of psychosocial symptomatology; however, they should be encouraged to seek assistance with their substance abuse before direct intervention is initiated.[44]

CLINICAL FINDINGS/CRITERIA

Criteria-AANS/AAOS

The American Association of Neurological Surgeons (AANS), and the American Academy of Orthopedic Surgeons (AAOS) developed the following criteria for the selection of patients for lumbosacral spine surgery:

1. Failure of extended conservative therapy.
2. An abnormal myelogram, computed tomography (CT) scan, and/or magnetic resonance imaging (MRI) study that demonstrates nerve root compression and/or segmental instability consistent with the patient's symptoms and signs.
3. Conformity of radicular pain complaints to physiological, dermatomal, or sclerotomal patterns.
4. One or more of the following: sensory loss, motor loss, and deep tendon reflex abnormalities in corresponding segment(s).

These criteria apply to both re-operation and primary procedures. Analyses of the initial pre-operative imaging studies of patients with FBSS commonly fail to meet standard criteria for surgical intervention.[11,55] The probability of a successful outcome is small in these circumstances, even if criteria for re-operation are met.

Patient History and Physical Examination

Clinical evaluation of FBSS patients does not differ substantially from that of other patients who suffer from intractable and incapacitating low back pain. It is important to obtain all of the details of the patient's original presentation, previous examinations, prior neurodiagnostic imaging studies, and reports of interventional therapy. These data should be reviewed before the patient's initial visit because these data provide technical details of which the patient may be unaware, as well as an overview of prior interactions with the health care system. They also make the initial appointment more directed and revealing. Pain behavior, postural abnormalities, impairment of range of motion, and elements of neurological deficit are often evident even before formal examination begins.

A general medical history and physical examination can rule out extraspinal causes of pain that include abdominal aortic aneurysm, gynecological disease, prostate tumor, renal disease, or rectosigmoid disease. Entities such as meralgia paresthetica, acetabular pain, and sacroiliac joint pain should form part of a working differential diagnosis. Patients should be examined for evidence of local myositis, fasciitis, or bursitis and for indications of arthritic or autoimmune disease. The possibility of undiagnosed disease, including Paget's disease, metastatic neoplasia, and rheumatoid/acromegalic spondylitis, should also be considered.

The combination of history and physical examination will often provide clues indicating the likelihood of both instability and nerve root compression. Straight leg raising can be useful to identify root compression. The interpretation of neurological findings may be difficult because of residual deficits from prior surgery. Long-term follow-up studies have shown that 40% to 50% of patients with prior successful disc excision have residual alterations in deep tendon reflexes and sensation corresponding to the original level of root involvement.[25,53] Fixed neurological deficits suggest root injury but may result from ongoing compression, although nerve root tension signs rarely persist after surgery and are very useful when positive.[26] It is unlikely that surgical intervention will be useful in the absence of symptoms suggesting nerve root compression or instability.

One goal of examination is to determine physical impairment and exaggeration of impairment. Waddell and associates proposed the use of clinical tests that provide a simple means of identifying patients who have inappropriate pain responses.[82]

DIAGNOSIS

The physician must distinguish between the patient with a mechanical lesion, such as recurrent disc herniation, spinal instability, or spinal stenosis, and one with nonmechanical conditions, including intradural scar tissue and systemic medical disease. Surgery benefits patients with mechanical lesions, but surgical intervention rarely helps patients with nonmechanical lesions.

The clinical history is critical to assessing the probable reasons for the patient's symptoms, particularly when radiculopathy is predominant, because surgical candidates have histories of radicular pain. The pain from instability is worsened by sitting, standing, and normal activity, and bracing often lessens the pain. Neurogenic claudication that is characterized by increasing lower extremity pain from walking even short distances continues for a brief period upon cessation of the activity. The pain is reduced by bending forward to expand the spinal canal.

The probability of a favorable outcome diminishes with each procedure, regardless of diagnosis. Finnegan and associates emphasized the importance of the postoperative pain-free interval and identified the following three typical syndromes[18]:

1. No initial relief or symptoms immediately worse.
2. Initial relief followed by increased numbness or weakness.
3. Patient receives complete relief but develops recurrent radiculopathy months or years later.

Persistent radicular pain in the immediate postoperative period suggests inadequate nerve root decompression, irreversible nerve root injury, or improper patient selection. If the pain-free interval is between one and six months, and the recurrent symptoms occur gradually, scar tissue may be responsible. Recurrent pain six months postoperatively may result from disc herniation at the same or at a different level. Frymoyer and associates stressed the importance of long-term failures, which are usually the manifestation of an ongoing degenerative process.[26] Predominant leg pain suggests disc herniation or spinal stenosis, although scar tissue can also produce this. Instability, infection, and scar tissue are all possible causes if back pain is the major component.

Physical examination should include attention to functional findings, which may have alternative explanations. Some apparently nonphysiological findings can result from arachnoid fibrosis, including nondermatomal sensory loss and nerve injury producing superficial lumbosacral spine tenderness with hyperalgesia. Such syndromes often predict a poor response to therapy on a physiological rather than a behavioral basis, suggesting the need for alternative treatments. New neurological deficits occurring after the last surgery or positive tension signs as on straight leg raising may indicate pressure on the neural elements, although these deficits are not pathognomonic.

Imaging and Diagnostic Studies

Precise correlation of clinical findings with diagnostic imaging studies is necessary because of the high incidence of clinically false positive myelograms, discograms, CT scans, and MRI scans in asymptomatic individuals or at asymptomatic levels.[1,2,4,7,18,25-27,44,53,56,81,82] Imaging studies of asymptomatic postoperative patients often reveal significant abnormalities. Frymoyer reported that 40% of CT scans, myelograms, and discograms show abnormalities in asymptomatic individuals.[26] The combination of clinical history, physical examination, and radiological imaging studies should provide an excellent correlation between anatomical abnormalities and the patient's complaints. Nonspecific spondylotic changes do not necessarily correlate with pain, and these changes do not always indicate the need for surgery. Anatomical abnormalities must be consistent with the patient's complaints and disabilities, and their relative importance must be assessed. The specificity of diagnostic imaging in FBSS is not yet established; in patients diagnosed with the latest imaging techniques, long-term clinical correlations with radiographic findings are unavailable.

Modern diagnostic imaging techniques have improved the definition of both primary and postsurgical lumbosacral spine disease. Radiological evaluation is particularly important in excluding surgically correctable lesions, including retained or recurrent disc herniation, spinal stenosis, instability, and pseudarthrosis. However, imaging studies should confirm the probable cause deduced from the history and physical examination rather than providing the dominant basis for diagnosis.

Plain Radiographs

Radiographic evaluation should begin with plain radiographs to determine the extent and level of previous surgery. Lateral flexion/extension radiographs may demonstrate abnormal motion and instability and may also detect the presence of primary bone tumors. The degree of disc degeneration, facet joint arthritis, spinal misalignment, and spondylolisthesis with or without motion can all be identified from plain radiographs. MRI and/or CT are usually satisfactory, and plain myelography is generally unnecessary for a patient who has had a single surgical procedure.

Myelographically Enhanced CT Scan

Oil-based myelography, which provided the only radiographs of the spinal cord available in the past,

showed large recurrent disc protrusions but frequently overlooked more subtle lesions. Myelography with water-soluble contrast media is a significant improvement but can miss a number of lesions, including far lateral disc herniations.[9,54,61]

The first improvement over conventional myelography was high resolution CT scanning and computed tomography with myelographic enhancement (CT myelography). CT myelography is perhaps the most important diagnostic technique for evaluating the patient with FBSS. Patients who have undergone previous operations are often difficult to evaluate without intrathecal contrast. However, CT myelography permits determination of canal size, bony defects, and hypertrophic bony changes as well as bony encroachment on the neural elements and evaluation of the lateral recesses and neural foramina. Contrast allows evaluation of the cauda equina by demonstrating the presence or absence of nerve root compression and the relationship of the nerve roots to the lateral recesses, foramina, and discs.

Myelography with enhanced multiplanar CT provides the most powerful modality to assess the possibility of lateral or central stenosis as a cause of continued nerve root symptomatology after lumbar decompression. CT with three-dimensional reconstruction is a significant advancement that benefits examinations of the neural foramina and the remainder of the bony anatomy.

MRI Scan

The enhanced MRI scan is very sensitive to inflammatory and neoplastic conditions and is the most sensitive technique for differentiating scar tissue from recurrent pathology. In the immediate postoperative period, the area of bone and ligament resection shows edematous soft tissues isointense to muscle on T1-weighted images that increases on T2-weighted images and replaces normal tissue signal. In the absence of postoperative hematoma, significant mass effect on the thecal sac is unusual. Gradual replacement of the immediate postoperative changes to scar tissue occur six months postsurgery.[11,12] The signal intensity of posterior scar tissue is variable on T2-weighted images.

Changes from discectomy are visible immediately after surgery. T1-weighted images show increased signal anterior to the thecal sac, with an indistinct posterior annular margin. This soft-tissue signal may blend smoothly into the disc space and may increase on T2-weighted images. Anterior epidural edema combined with posterior annular disruption caused by disc incision and curettage can mimic pre-operative disc herniation and produce mass effect. These changes within the anterior epidural space involute in the months after surgery, with a corresponding normalization of the thecal margin.

Sagittal T2-weighted images can define the site of annular disruption and disc curettage in the immediate postoperative period by high signal in the nucleus pulposus extending posteriorly in the area of annular disruption. Annular perforation, which is not clearly seen on T1-weighted images, resolves within six months.

The interpretation of MRI within the first six weeks postoperatively requires caution because of the tremendous changes in the epidural soft tissues and intervertebral disc after surgery. Tissue disruption and edema can impinge on the thecal sac. Magnetic resonance imaging in the immediate postoperative period provides a gross overview of the thecal sac and epidural space and can often exclude significant hemorrhage, pseudomeningocele, and disc space infection. Small posterior fluid collections are common after laminectomy. Signal intensities depend upon whether the collections are serous (cerebrospinal fluid [CSF]) or serosanguinous (increased signal on T-weighted images); MRI cannot distinguish between benign and infected collections on the basis of morphology or signal intensity.

Electrophysiology

Electromyography (EMG), thermography (TMG), and spinal evoked potentials are of limited use in the evaluation of the patient with FBSS. The major benefit of these diagnostic tools is in differentiating cauda equina compression from peripheral nerve entrapment syndromes. Electromyography will corroborate root injury but cannot differentiate injury from compression. Thermography may help diagnose a secondary sympathetic dystrophy syndrome and can be useful in differentiating root from peripheral nerve injury. Both electrophysiological studies and TMG have a role in certain clinical settings, although their sensitivity is limited. Equivocal neurological deficits may be objectively demonstrated and quantitated clinically. Paraspinous EMG typically demonstrates nonspecific postsurgical changes in the patient with FBSS.

Lumbar Discography

Lumbar discography has undergone a resurgence as a physiological rather than an anatomical study. Injection of fluid into the disc is postulated to reproduce pain originating in the same disc. Subsequent injection of local anesthetic provides relief. Pain provocation by injection and relief with local anesthetic constitutes a positive study. However, no controlled study has verified the hypothesis underlying this procedure.

CT discography may be useful when low back pain predominates, particularly in light of additional information derived from pain provocation. Although standard lumbar discography has been abandoned for diagnosing disc herniation, CT discography may have a role in the evaluation of recurrent disc herniations. Grenier and associates postulate that extravasation of contrast medium from the disc space three to six months after surgery indicates a persistent rent in the annulus, which may be consistent with a recurrent herniated disc.[44] Conversely, if dye does not escape, it suggests an intact annulus and that any epidural mass represents fibrosis. In Grenier's study, 21 of 23 patients with positive discograms had recurrent disc herniations at surgery, but two of three patients with negative discograms also had herniated discs.[44]

Facet and Nerve Blocks

Facet blockade has been unsatisfactory in defining the role of anatomical structures that cause pain, although in one series it did prove useful.[17] Selective nerve root injections under radiographic control are helpful in more difficult cases in which radiculopathy predominates.[39] No definitive scientific evidence exists that peripheral blockade that produces pain relief predicts a successful outcome from surgery. The role of blockade of the lumbar zygapophyseal joints remains unproven.

Some patients suffer from intractable back pain because of zygapophyseal joint arthritis. Specific blockade of these joints by intra-articular blockade, or blocking the medial branch of the posterior primary rami that supply the joint, relieves back pain in some individuals. It is less predictable whether percutaneous facet denervation can relieve pain for a prolonged period of time. Patients selected for facet blockade should have back pain exacerbated by rotation and lateral bending and improved with bracing. The block technique described by Bogduk and Long involves blocking the medial branch of the posterior primary ramus on the transverse process or the sacrum with a small amount of local anesthetic. A positive block provides total pain relief for the duration of the procedure. Patients with radicular pain and those with partial pain relief from blockade rarely respond satisfactorily to permanent neurotomy.[5]

INCORRECT DIAGNOSIS

Inappropriate Surgery

Incorrect diagnosis, which occurs with an incidence of 0.3%, may result in continued pain after discectomy.[5,55] Metastatic carcinoma, diabetic radiculopathy, neurofibroma, sacral cyst, and lumbar spondylosis can all mimic disc rupture. In the subset of patients with suspected lumbar disc herniations, neural tumors are reported to be present in 1%.[46]

Inappropriate surgery that results from inaccurate diagnosis or incomplete comprehension of the involved pathological processes is one of the major causes of FBSS. It is often difficult for the neurosurgeon experienced in the evaluation and management of these types of cases to find objective clinical data that support the initial decision for operative intervention. As many as 50% of patients with FBSS are found on review of their original history, physical examination, and diagnostic studies not to have met generally accepted criteria for the primary surgical procedure. Despite the absence of physical findings in 80% of patients with low back pain, in one large series, 30% of these patients underwent lumbar spine surgery.[56]

Inappropriate stabilization procedures in patients with mechanical etiology for their pain are another source of FBSS. Although inadequate surgery is often cited, inappropriate surgery is the major factor. Operations at the wrong level, on the wrong side, and for the wrong pathology are rare but often quite dramatic and memorable.

Psychosocial Causes

Psychogenic factors are the single most common cause of failure to relieve pain by discectomy. Long states that "patients suffering from failed back syndrome are incapacitated by psychiatric, psychologic and social/vocational factors which relate to the back complaint only indirectly."[43] In a study of 266 patients with FBSS, 15% of these patients were diagnosed with psychiatric disorders before the onset of low back pain.[43]

Data from Brown indicate that poor or fair results were twice as common in Workers' Compensation cases, whereas good to excellent results were one third more common in the non-Workers' Compensation group.[5] Sorenson and associates attempted to predict the outcome of disc surgery by pre-operative testing with a modification of the Minnesota Multiphasic Personality Inventory (MMPI).[83] Some patients can be expected to do poorly for reasons unrelated to the surgery. The important factors in predicting failure are Workers' Compensation, job dissatisfaction, low education and income, heavy job requirements, cigarette smoking, psychological disturbances, and litigation.[16,45,74]

Discogenic Pain/Internal Disc Disruption

Internal disc disruption (IDD) is a condition marked by alterations in the internal structure and metabolic functions of one or more discs, usually after significant trauma. The clinical syndrome includes axial and extremity pain exacerbated by any physical activity that compresses affected discs. The pain is typically deep, does not rapidly abate with rest, and worsens over time. Profound energy loss occurs, sometimes in conjunction with significant weight loss and psychological disturbances. It is not associated with herniation of the disc fragment. Disc degeneration with loss of disc height and osteophyte formation is rare.

Discography, which was the principal diagnostic tool for IDD, has been supplanted by MRI. Patients with IDD show changes in the signal generated from the affected intervertebral disc and often from adjacent vertebral levels. Once the diagnosis of disc disruption is made and surgical intervention is considered appropriate, disc excision with anterior interbody fusion is the most effective operation for persistent disabling symptoms. Disc excision is also indicated for patients who do not respond to nonoperative therapies, including analgesics, nonsteroidal anti-inflammatory drugs, and psychotropic agents.

Missed Level or Levels

Surgery on the wrong interspace may be discovered either intra-operatively or afterward when the patient has no relief from pain. The incidence from this rare surgical error ranges from 0.14% to 2.7%. The highest incidence was reported with a microsurgical series because the limited exposure used with microsurgery may increase the occurrence of the error. Intra-operative recognition permits redirection to the proper interspace. Neither nontraumatic exploration nor violation of a nonpathological interspace is associated with appreciable morbidity.

Wide exposure with identification of the sacrum and intra-operative radiographic localization are effective but not foolproof methods to avoid operating on the wrong interspace. Discovery of the disc herniation is the best way to identify the correct interspace and to avoid this complication. Obesity often prevents adequate intra-operative radiographic confirmation of the level of disc herniation.

Segmentation abnormalities can produce a neurological level of involvement different from the motion segment level. A sacralized L5 or lumbarized S1 can disorient even an experienced spine surgeon. Reviewing anteroposterior (AP) and lateral plain radiographs and correlating them with more sophisticated imaging modalities are essential to avoid surgery at the wrong level. The possibility that the wrong disc was operated upon should be considered if the patient complains of lower extremity pain that persists two days postsurgery. In a patient with a missed level or side, scarring is not a problem if re-operation is performed immediately.

INADEQUATE SURGERY

Inadequate surgery (i.e., inadequate decompression) has been suggested as a frequent cause of FBSS. Lateral recess stenosis and persistent disc herniation are usually cited as the responsible pathologies for inadequate decompression. One of the most common pitfalls is failure to recognize the contribution of lateral foraminal or extraforaminal compression to the patient's radiculopathy, with initial disc removal without adequate decompression of the bony component. Burton analyzed the data of 800 FBSS patients and reported that concomitant lateral recess and/or central stenosis account for 71% of failures.[11] MacNab concluded that lateral recess stenosis was the most common source of failure after lumbar disc surgery.[47] Spengler and associates reported a 30% incidence of lateral recess stenosis that required medial foraminotomy at surgery in his series of discectomy patients.[74] Nerve root decompression should provide an excursion of at least 5 mm so that a blunt probe can be easily passed into the foramen. Further bony decompression to uncover a laterally herniated disc or hypertrophic superior facet in the foramen should be necessary if nerve root decompression is not accomplished. In some cases, the entire joint or even the pedicle must be sacrificed. Fusion is indicated in patients with a destabilized spine.

Retained Disc Fragment

A retained disc fragment can cause continued postoperative pain. In one large series, 13 retained fragments accounted for 29 failures, representing an incidence of 0.2%. When the patient awakens from anesthesia with unrelieved lower extremity pain, the possibility should be considered that one or more fragments of disc has been left behind. The presence of multiple free fragments of disc at the initial surgery increases the chances that retained fragments were overlooked. Reexploration is indicated, provided that other causes of pain have been excluded. Adequate operative exposure provides the best means of avoiding the complication. The increased possibility of overlooking a retained fragment is one of the inherent problems with microsurgical discectomy.

Conjoined Nerve Root

A conjoined nerve root is present in 2% to 14% of patients. Surgical decompression in patients with a conjoined root is associated with a significant incidence of failure. Failure to recognize the conjoined nerve root at the time of the initial surgery may have the following three consequences:

1. The conjoined nerve root is avulsed, which produces a neurological deficit
2. The conjoined nerve root is battered, which causes increased perineural scarring.

3. The compressed portion of the nerve root is overlooked, which allows continued symptoms.

The first two conditions are more common than the third, which is the only one amenable to further surgical intervention.

TEMPORARY RELIEF (DAYS TO WEEKS) WITH EARLY FAILURE OF RELIEF/INFECTION

In 1936, Milward described the clinical and radiographic characteristics of interspace infection after the inadvertent introduction of microorganisms into a disc space during lumbar puncture.[51] Ramirez and Thisted reported infection rate of 0.3% in an analysis of 28,395 patients who underwent lumbar laminectomy for radiculopathy in the United States in 1980.[63] Patients with aseptic necrosis or interspace infection are typically asymptomatic immediately after surgery but within two weeks begin to experience excruciating spasms in the lower back, with or without radiation into the legs. The white blood cell count and temperature of these patients are often normal, but the sedimentation rate is elevated, often higher than 100 mm/h. Lumbosacral radiographs may reveal erosion of the cartilaginous plates as the disease progresses. Needle aspirations of the interspace may reveal the offending organisms, although such aspirations are often negative.[28] Patients with a clearcut infectious syndrome should be placed on intravenous antibiotics. The persistence of an elevated temperature for several days postoperatively may indicate an infection. The wound should be examined for erythema, swelling, tenderness, and drainage. Management of the infection should include Gram's stain and culture, with antibiotics if the clinical indication is strong. The patient should be returned to the operating room, and the wound should be reopened, thoroughly debrided, and irrigated if the infection continues despite antibiotic treatment. The wound may be managed open with frequent dressing changes.

Discitis

Postoperative intervertebral disc space infection (discitis) is uncommon, with reports of infection rates ranging from 0.1% to 3.8%.[3,20,33,49,63,64] The presence of the microscope over the open wound may account for the higher incidence of disc space infection from microsurgery. Postoperative discitis typically produces persistent intense back pain with unremarkable associated physical findings two weeks to three months after discectomy.

Patients with discitis often have elevated erythrocyte sedimentation rates. Bone scan, CT, and MRI are sensitive for detecting discitis and can identify changes associated with discitis earlier than plain radiographs can. CT is effective in the early diagnosis of discitis; hypodensity of the affected disc space may be detected as early as 10 days postoperatively. The responsible bacteria are identified in fewer than 50% of cases, with *Staphylococcus* species being the most common organisms cultured.[62]

Early diagnosis and prompt treatment are important to prevent chronic infection. Immobilization is often effective for pain relief, and four to six weeks of intravenous antibiotic therapy is recommended. Uncomplicated discitis should not require surgery, and most patients undergo spontaneous interbody fusion. Paresis may develop from lumbar epidural abscesses, which then require immediate decompressive laminectomy.

Postoperative Osteomyelitis

Infection may be introduced directly into the intervertebral disc space during surgery and can spread to the adjacent vertebral bodies, producing osteomyelitis. Surgery for protruding or herniated discs is the most frequent cause of infection introduced directly into the intervertebral disc space. This complication from disc surgery occurs in fewer than 1% of patients. Organisms may be inadvertently inoculated during surgery, and residual hematoma, necrotic tissue, and foreign bodies provide an environment conducive to bacterial proliferation. Weeks, months, or even years may elapse before the diagnosis of a disc space infection is established. Symptoms of an infection may not be apparent immediately after surgery, and often initial pain relief is followed by recurrence several days to weeks later. Fever may be transient, intermittent, or nonexistent, and frequently no evidence of infection exists when symptoms develop. The degree of pain may appear to be out of proportion to the objective findings and may erroneously be attributed to hysteria, malingering, or even psychoneurosis.

The typical radiological changes of vertebral osteomyelitis may not be apparent for several months. Radionuclide bone scans are sensitive and often demonstrate evidence of infection before plain films of the spine show any changes. However, they are not specific; surgical edema and disc changes may yield false positive results. The bone scan may be negative in a significant percentage of patients early in the course of disc space infection.[79] CT may show destructive changes of the vertebral bodies before these are evident on plain films. However, end-plate irregularities on CT are not specific for discitis, and normal curettage changes in vertebral end-plates may mimic erosions of discitis.[10] MRI may show changes of discitis long before any changes are present radiologically.[11] MRI and CT may be negative early in the course of

postoperative or posttraumatic discitis, and the risk of infection is always a possibility. Any patient with increasing back pain more than two weeks postoperatively and an erythrocyte sedimentation rate greater than 50 mm/h should be considered to have discitis until proven otherwise. Percutaneous disc biopsy can be helpful in the diagnosis of postoperative discitis but is often falsely negative. A recent study compared MRI, plain radiographs, and radionuclide studies in evaluation vertebral osteomyelitis. MRI and combined bone and gallium scans were equally accurate and sensitive, whereas MRI was more sensitive than plain films.[70] MRI is a rapid, noninvasive method for the detection of vertebral osteomyelitis and its complications, including epidural abscess, because of the characteristic appearance of pyogenic infection on MRI. Infected disc material on T1-weighted images shows decreased signal intensity from the intervertebral disc space and contiguous vertebral bodies relative to the normal vertebral signal, whereas on T2-weighted images, these infected tissues show increased signal. MRI provides more anatomical detail than radionuclide scanning and allows differentiation of neoplasm and degenerative disease from osteomyelitis. The disc space is nearly always spared in neoplastic disease, whereas degenerative disease with nucleus desiccation produces decreased disc signal on T2-weighted images. Gallium scans may be positive earlier in the course of infection than MRI and are more sensitive to changes resulting from treatment and decreasing inflammation.

Spontaneous resolution does occur in many patients with postoperative discitis and vertebral osteomyelitis. Intermittent antibiotic therapy obscures the diagnosis of postoperative vertebral osteomyelitis. Turnbull described a patient who developed postoperative staphylococcal lumbar vertebral osteomyelitis three years after successful surgery for a herniated disc. The patient required three operations before a psoas abscess was successfully treated.[79]

Epidural Abscess

Epidural abscess after decompression is rare but should be considered in a patient with increasing neurological symptoms and signs in the early postoperative period. It may be difficult to differentiate from an expanding hematoma in the absence of systemic evidence of infection.

MRI can localize the site of infection and provide more information than CT regarding the extent of abscess involvement and the degree of cord compromise.

Decompression and aggressive antibiotic management are the cornerstones of therapy. Epidural abscess often arises in association with vertebral osteomyelitis and is an indication for early decompression.

Meningeal Cyst/Pseudomeningocele

Meningeal cysts rarely cause early recurrent radiculopathy after disc excision and are reported in fewer than 1% of patients. Incidental durotomy during disc excision does not compromise the later results if the dural leak is recognized and closed; durotomy that is unrecognized or that is incompletely repaired can produce a slowly expanding mass. Nerve roots can become trapped in the meningeal cyst and cause pain. Physical examination occasionally reveals soft tissue bulging, that may or may not be recognized as fluctuant but often increases when the patient stands. Myelography and MRI are important diagnostic studies to identify meningeal cysts. Removal of the meningeal cyst requires careful dissection around the cyst and identification of the dural opening. The cyst should be opened to avoid injury to involved nerve roots prior to excision. Closure can be accomplished by closing the dura with or without duraplasty.

MIDTERM FAILURES (WEEKS TO MONTHS)

Herniated Intervertebral Disc

There are many explanations for persistent pain caused by disc herniation. An inadequate discectomy produces pain because of continued nerve root irritation. Patients do not report any pain-free interval and sometimes awaken from surgery complaining of their pre-operative pain. Recurrent intervertebral disc herniation at the previously decompressed level may also occur. Patients with this problem often have a pain-free interval of more than six months. The patient with a herniated disc that ruptures at a different level usually benefits from a repeat operation. Patients may describe persistent severe pain and paresthesias in a radicular distribution after unsuccessful lumbar disc surgery. The pain is superimposed on an area of residual numbness that is constant and described as either burning or ice cold. It is often more distressing than the original disc herniation pain. These patients with pain of nerve injury or deafferentation sometimes respond to spinal cord stimulation (SCS).[44,55]

Recurrent Disc Fragment

The incidence of recurrent rupture after laminectomy has been reported to range from a low rate of 0.26% for ruptures that occur within the first six weeks after surgery (on the same side and level) to a rate of 18% for recurrences that take place at any time or any level after the initial operation. Recurrent disc herniation may occur on the same side and at the same level as the prior operation, on the opposite side at the same level, or at an entirely new level. A compilation of 268 cases revealed 43% of failures were at the same level and 22% were at a different level.[24] Vigorous disc space evacuation does not prevent recurrent disc herniation. In some cases, the patient is pain free for years after surgery, and then back and sciatic pain suddenly return. MRI with gadolinium-DTPA (Gd-DTPA) and CT myelography can confirm a diagnosis of disc herniation but may be difficult to interpret because of postoperative changes. Physical examination reveals signs of disc herniation with positive tension signs. Once the diagnosis is established and nonsurgical treatment fails, surgery is indicated for intractable pain. Previous back surgery does not preclude an excellent result; some patients feel better after the second operation than after the first. Frymoyer and associates have shown that the outcome from surgery after recurrent disc herniation and after primary disc excision is identical.[25]

Ikko and associates analyzed the spine one week postoperatively and described soft tissue mass composed of blood and early scar tissue on the posterior aspect of the disc space which is always present in both symptomatic and asymptomatic patients.[84] Teplick and Haskin reviewed 750 patients with persistent postoperative symptoms and found that recurrent disc problems can be distinguished from epidural fibrosis.[76,77] Fibrosis is characterized by thecal sac retraction toward the soft tissue lesion, a location above or below the disc space, an indistinct border, and a shape that conforms to rather than compresses the dural sac.

Scar tissue is generally less dense than recurrent disc fragments. In contrast, recurrent disc compresses rather than conforms to the sac, has a sharp border, and has a density of 90 to 120 Hounsfield units(Hu). Postoperative CT appearance normalizes over time with a decrease of hyperdense fibrotic material. On CT it is difficult to distinguish symptomatic patients from asymptomatic patients.

Battered-Root Syndrome/Perineural Scarring

Perineural scarring is a common occurrence after spinal decompression although clinical failure from perineural scarring occurs in only 1% to 2% of patients who undergo disc excision.[25] Nerve root scarring may be caused by excessive bleeding, conjoined nerve roots, and the use of cottonoid patties. The immediate postoperative course is generally benign but may be associated with incomplete resolution of sciatica, sometimes accompanied by an increased sensory or even motor deficit. Sciatica and back pain gradually increase over three to six months. A variety of surgical therapies have been advocated, including scar removal with membrane interposition, radical decompression, longitudinal sectioning of scar over nerve root, spinal fusion, and electrical stimulator implantation.[6]

Epidural Scarring

Scar tissue around the dura and nerve roots can cause recurrent sciatica. Prevention is essential because of the lack of effective surgical therapy for epidural fibrosis. In this difficult patient population, the differentiation of recurrent disc herniation from scar is critical because re-operation on scar often produces a poor surgical result and additional scarring. CT with intravenous contrast, which has an accuracy rate of 67% to 100% in distinguishing scar tissue from disc, is technically demanding, involves a large contrast load, and includes only single-plane imaging. Intravenous contrast increases the diagnostic accuracy of CT from 43% to 74%, which makes differentiating between recurrent herniated disc fragments and postsurgical scar tissue more likely.[11,72] Recurrent disc fragments are avascular and enhance only at the periphery, whereas postsurgical scar tissue demonstrates uniform enhancement after infusion of intravenous contrast material. The peripheral enhancement observed in recurrent disc herniation is thought to be to the result of a thin layer of surgical scar tissue or vascularity in the annulus fibrosus or epidural venous plexus. Firoozonia studied 143 patients with persistent symptoms, 52 of whom subsequently underwent re-exploration.[19] Noncontrast CT established the diagnosis (scar or disc) in 31 patients, and the diagnosis was confirmed at surgery. A correct diagnosis was made for 12 patients by intravenous contrast enhancement. It is worth noting that 33% of the patients in this study did not demonstrate enhancement of scar and 29% failed to show enhancement of the disc margins. In contrast, Schubiger and Valvanis reported nearly homogeneous enhancement of all surgical scars and the margins of all recurrent disc herniations.[69] CT following myelography may be a useful adjunct to routine myelographic films, although CT should not be used as the sole diagnostic test for recurrent herniations.

MRI allows differentiation of recurrent disc herniation from epidural scar. MRI has 100% sensitivity, 71% specificity, and 89% accuracy in distinguishing recurrent disc herniation from epidural scar. Bundschuh evaluated 20 patients with MRI, 14 of whom underwent exploration.[9] MRI diagnosis was confirmed in 12 patients at surgery. Eight of nine of these patients also had CT findings confirmed at surgery.

Epidural fibrosis can be differentiated from disc material by signal intensity and the configuration and margination of the extradural mass on unenhanced MRI scans. Recurrent disc herniations are seen at or near the disc space, exhibit mass effect, and, on T1-weighted images are slightly hyperintense compared to fibrosis. Free fragments are hyperintense on T2-weighted images. Unenhanced epidural scar that lacks mass effect is not contiguous with the disc space and is hypo- or isointense on T1-weighted images. On T2-weighted images, fibrotic scar has higher signal intensity than disc material or annulus. Sotiropolous compared the diagnostic accuracy of contrast CT to unenhanced MRI in 25 patients and found that unenhanced MRI is equivalent to contrast-enhanced CT for distinguishing scar from disc.[45] Anterior epidural scars are slightly hypo- to isointense relative to intervertebral disc on T-weighted images. Anterior epidural scars show increased signal on T2-weighted images. Scar generally conforms to the dural margin, with retraction of the thecal sac toward the scar. Lateral and posterior scar exhibits similar characteristics, but not as consistently. Increased signal intensity at the operative sites is often noted laterally, posteriorly, and within the paraspinal musculature, whereas low signal intensity on T2-weighted images is not unusual for lateral and posterior scar.

Herniated discs, except free fragments, are often in contiguity with the parent disc space. Small protruded discs are low in signal intensity on T2-weighted images. Larger protruded, extruded, and free fragments can show central high intensity on T2-weighted images, which creates a problem in differentiating the herniated material from scar tissue and the high-signal-intensity CSF. A rim of low signal intensity surrounds these larger disc herniations, allowing for good contrast between the CSF and the herniated material. This low signal intensity may reflect the remnants of the outer annular fibers and the posterior longitudinal ligament.

MRI with intravenous Gd-DTPA administration is the most accurate technique for distinguishing scar from disc. Hueftle and associates analyzed the role of Gd-enhanced MRI in the differentiation of scar tissue from disc.[34] Enhanced MRI was able to predict operative findings with 100% accuracy in 30 patients evaluated with MRI before and after administration of 0.1 mmol/kg Gd. Hueftle and associates reported uniform scar enhancement on early postcontrast T1-weighted images, whereas recurrent discs exhibited peripheral enhancement on delayed postcontrast images.

Injection of Gd-DTPA consistently enhances anterior epidural scar irrespective of the time since surgery. The following three components are necessary for contrast enhancement of any tissue: vascular supply, route for contrast material out of the vasculature, and some amount of interstitial space to sequester the contrast. Disc material does not enhance on early postinjection images because of its avascular nature. Disc material may enhance on delayed images (greater than 30 minutes after injection) because of diffusion of contrast into the disc from adjacent vascularized tissue. In cases with a mixture of scar and disc material, scar will enhance and the disc material will not enhance on early postinjection images. Problems can occur when the volume of nonenhancing herniated disc is small relative to the volume of enhancing scar, where partial volume averaging might obscure the disc. The disc material will enhance if sufficient time elapses for contrast material to diffuse into the disc material from the surrounding vascular scar. It is important to obtain both sagittal and axial T1-weighted images before and after contrast. Patients should not be moved between the pre- and postcontrast scans to assure precise comparison between the same regions of interest. Postinjection images should be completed within 20 minutes of contrast administration. In one study of 44 patients at 50 re-operated levels, 96% accuracy was reported in differentiating scar from disc with pre-and postcontrast MRI in the postoperative lumbar spine.[67]

Whereas limited data is available on the use of contrast in the immediate postoperative period, enhancement is visible in the epidural space within the first four days of surgery. Pathological changes are difficult to differentiate from the tremendous changes that normally occur after any surgical procedure. This creates a problem in identifying enhancement.

Careful hemostasis and gentle handling of the neural tissue will decrease scar tissue formation, and the use of fat grafts at the time of the initial surgery can diminish scarring. A free or pedicled fat graft is superior to materials such as Gelfoam. Free fat grafts should be less than 5 mm in thickness to prevent cauda equina compression and to enhance graft vascularization.

Arachnoiditis

Although arachnoiditis was originally described as a complication of infection, we prefer the term *chronic adhesive arachnoiditis,* derived from the descriptions of Horsley and Stookey.[40]

The Imaging Diagnosis of Arachnoiditis
Much confusion exists over what constitutes *arachnoiditis.* Some radiologists have used the term to describe minor inflammatory changes that occur with the injection of any intrathecal agent. Arachnoiditis is characterized by partial or complete block of spinal fluid flow; narrowing of the subarachnoid space; obliteration of nerve root sheaths; apparent thickening or clumping of nerve roots; irregular distribution of contrast agents, with loculation being common; formation of cysts; and immobility of oil-based contrast agents. Myelography remains the standard method for diagnosing the problem because MRI can be misinterpreted.

The Clinical Syndromes of Arachnoiditis
Most patients diagnosed with arachnoiditis have low back and lower extremity symptoms; recurrent symptoms are often similar to those that occurred originally.

A neurogenic claudication syndrome has been diagnosed in some patients who complain of leg weakness and burning pain that is affected by sitting or standing. Bowel or bladder dysfunction is common in these patients. The burning character of the pain, associated with hyperpathia and claudication, suggests arachnoiditis but cannot be differentiated from other forms of spinal stenosis.

Causes of Arachnoiditis
Any agent injected into the lumbar subarachnoid space has the potential to cause arachnoiditis. Oil-based agents were used for years with minimal problems. Whereas early water-soluble contrast agents were extremely noxious, improvements to these agents have reduced the potential for inflammation. Little evidence is available that the use of the modern clinical contrast materials causes a significant incidence of arachnoiditis. Traumatic or repeated myelography, particularly with multiple surgeries, may affect the incidence of arachnoiditis.[40]

All authors stress the fact that the new syndrome of chronic adhesive arachnoiditis is quite different from the rapidly progressive arachnoiditis that complicates infection. The patients are stable, neurological deterioration occurs but is rare, and pain is the predominant issue.

Diagnosis and Treatment of Arachnoiditis
The diagnosis of arachnoiditis usually occurs in the course of repeat myelography. In our experience, clear-cut abnormalities that would otherwise be candidates for reparative surgery should be treated even if arachnoiditis is diagnosed. The arachnoiditis will not detract from the potential success of reparative surgery. Direct surgery on the arachnoiditis should not be considered unless the patient has a progressive neurological deficit. Surgery to correct arachnoiditis is a delicate and dangerous operation, and the surgeon must be very familiar with this highly technical procedure. Pain relief occurs in fewer than half of the patients, and the risk of a substantial new neurological deficit is high.

Alternatives to Direct Therapy
SCS is the most effective therapy to relieve the pain in those patients with arachnoiditis and FBSS who are not candidates for any other procedure. Brain stimulation and intrathecal narcotic pumps have both successfully reduced pain in severely disabled patients. The use of chronic oral narcotic administration is undergoing investigation in a select group of patients. Improved myelographic techniques, the newest water-soluble agents, and improved surgical techniques may all contribute to reduce the incidence of this difficult complication.

Spinal Stenosis

Multiple operations can produce both axial and radicular pain in the patient with spinal stenosis. The etiology may be progression of degenerative disease, previous inadequate decompression, or overgrowth of a previous posterior fusion. Spinal stenosis and scar often co-exist. Bony compression is an indication for laminectomy; in the presence of substantial scar tissue, however, pain relief may be minimal.

LONG-TERM FAILURES (MONTHS TO YEARS)

Instability is defined as abnormal or excessive movement of one vertebra on another, which may cause pain. The patient's intrinsic back disease or excessively wide bilateral laminectomies may be responsible for the instability. Patients complain predominantly of back pain, and physical examination is often unremarkable. Relative flexion/sagittal plane translation of more than 8% of the AP diameter of the vertebral body or a relative flexion/sagittal plan rotation of more than 9% or degrees between adjacent segments are the most commonly cited radiographic guidelines for instability of the lumbar spine.[88] Spinal fusion should be considered for symptomatic patients with evidence of instability.

The incidence of postdecompression spondylolisthesis ranges from 2% to 10%, whereas the incidence of progressive slippage after decompressive laminectomy in patients with pre-operative degenerative spondylolisthesis is even higher. The factors that contribute to postdecompression slippage include patients younger than 40 years of age with normal disc heights, and patients who have undergone extensive surgery. The extent of surgery is an important contributor in the development of postoperative instability. Discectomy at the time of laminectomy may cause additional instability. Complete laminectomy and bilateral facetectomies will also create spinal instability.

Symptoms sufficient to require later stabilization occur in only 3% of patients following simple discectomy. It is possible to excise 50% of both facets or 100% of one facet without significantly altering the stiffness of human intervertebral segments. After extensive spinal decompression, accentuation of pre-existent deformity occasionally occurs but is often asymptomatic. Radical facetectomy for degenerative spondylolisthesis always produces increased deformity but is frequently asymptomatic. Greater disc space height at the time of decompression, the absence of osteophytes, discectomy at the time of decompression, and a younger age may predispose the patient to later deformity. Presence of any or all of these factors can indicate the need for fusion at the time of decompression. Younger patients who undergo multilevel decompressive laminectomies for congenital or mixed spinal stenosis commonly develop a new deformity after the laminectomy.

Pseudarthrosis of Prior Fusion

Pseudarthrosis is a complication that may stem from technical faults by the surgeon or from biological deficiency of the patient. The incidence of pseudarthrosis depends on the number of levels fused, the techniques involved, and whether the patient smokes. The overall rate of pseudarthrosis is higher in two-level compared to one-level fusion, with the lumbosacral junction presenting a special challenge. The variety of therapeutic options for FBSS emphasizes the lack of a uniform method of treatment. The majority of conditions producing low back or sciatic pain is nonlethal and can be successfully managed without further surgery. Nonsurgical therapy can be effective and involves minimal risk and cost. Recognition of the "failed back" as a syndrome has resulted in the development of algorithms for its management. Treatment options include physiological, behavioral, and rehabilitative measures and a number of surgical procedures. The literature on the treatment of FBSS and its results encompasses many different outcome measures, obtained in a number of ways, at variable follow-up intervals. Lack of uniformity in treatment and outcome measures makes comparison of therapies difficult.

Treatment of the FBSS should include surgery for only a small minority of patients. In reported series on re-operation, success has been defined most commonly by patient self-reports of pain relief and satisfaction with treatment results. Fifty percent estimated that relief of pain is a common criterion for "success." Return to work is an outcome measure that is given particular emphasis by rehabilitation programs. Analgesic requirements are commonly considered, as are the ability to engage in activities of daily living, preservation of strength, sensation, and bladder and bowel function.

The source of follow-up information is of fundamental importance in interpreting outcomes. Reports from physicians' and surgeons' offices and hospital records commonly overestimate results and are substantially more favorable than patient interviews by disinterested third parties. Reports of outcome of re-operation and behavioral/rehabilitation programs have, with few exceptions, been based upon the former. Third-party interview is the most objective evaluation mechanism for obtaining follow-up of pain therapies.

TREATMENT OPTIONS

Nonsurgical Treatment

Certain general principles should be followed in treating FBSS, irrespective of the pathological process.

Rehabilitation is an important component in the management of FBSS patients, and programs specializing in this are proliferating. The ultimate goal of rehabilitation is restoration of the patient to a functional status. Psychiatric and psychosocial comorbidities must be identified and treated. The effect of economic issues must be addressed. Psychological dysfunction affects the patient's ability to cope as well as the rehabilitation process. Detrimental pain behaviors can be modified by appropriate therapies, and it is important to use these psychotherapeutic techniques within the context of an overall program.

The psychological needs of each patient must be identified and treated specifically because stereotyped programs are generally of little value. Professional assessment of patients' physical therapy needs and an individualized regimen of graduated exercise are essential. Formal evaluation and treatment sessions allow the patient to understand the techniques and rationale for physical therapy. Patients with FBSS must be urged to translate the short-term pain relief resulting from effective application of therapies into increased productive activity.

In some cases, hospitalization in a multidisciplinary pain treatment program may be necessary. Abuse of medications, including narcotics and benzodiazepines, must be curtailed. Pain management centers focus on increasing the quality of life and physical function in spite of residual pain that maximal therapy cannot relieve. The pain treatment center also educates the patient about physical and nonphysical factors in chronic pain and the realistic expectations from therapy.

Patients initially require therapy to stretch muscles back to a functional length; they also need coordinated muscle activity with intensive physical reconditioning to improve strength and endurance. Some patients require specific therapy to address myofascial pain and careful instruction in body biomechanics to prevent further insults.

The concept of productive rehabilitation or work hardening with worksite-style conditioning has been both practical and popular. Work-hardening programs specify when patients are fit to return to work and what practical work restrictions are necessary. Patients should gain the physical capacity and confidence to do their jobs and to lead more normal lives once they have completed the program.

Surgical Treatment/Re-Operation

The physician is obliged to rule out a persistent surgical problem as part of the surgical history. Surgery should be viewed as part of a continuum of care rather than as the sole event leading to functional restoration of the patient.

An ongoing complaint of pain in the absence of defined pathology is not an indication for an operative procedure. The majority of patients are not surgical candidates; they should be protected from ineffective surgical procedures and treated with measures to improve back function. Surgery should only be considered if the patient suffers from either compression and/or instability, particularly if the disease is progressive or associated with major neurological deficits. Stereotyped procedures applied without considering the physical and psychological components of each patient are virtually guaranteed to fail. Patients with spondylotic disease characterized by disc herniation, canal and foraminal stenosis, and instability benefit the most from surgery. Radicular pain, back pain related to activity and relieved by rest, improvement with stabilization, and neurogenic claudication will improve with surgical intervention.

The first re-operations on the lumbar spine were reported less than 20 years after the original description of lumbar disc surgery. A variety of procedures have been reported, with a wide range of "success" rates. The reported success rate for re-operation for FBSS has varied from 12% to 100%. Loss of neurological function is rare after re-operation. The presence of positive tension sign, focal and correlative neurological deficit, and a positive confirmatory radiographic study are strong indications that mechanical nerve-root compression will be found at surgery. Surgical results under these circumstances are generally excellent provided that complications are avoided. It is important to recognize the limitations and benefits of interventional therapy. Appropriate and definitive decompression and/or stabilization procedures should be done in conjunction with an intensive low back rehabilitation effort in patients with pathology amenable to surgery. The residual effects of abnormalities already treated definitively (e.g., disc herniation causing root injury before its removal) from untreated and iatrogenic abnormalities are sometimes difficult to distinguish when a patient needs re-operation. Repeat surgery may be the only way to relieve the patient's pain if a correctable lesion exists. Another operation will not help and may have an adverse effect if such a lesion is not present. Patients with pathology amenable to surgical intervention should be offered re-operation, usually decompression or stabilization.

The initial decision to operate is most important; once recurrent pain occurs after surgery, the potential for relief is limited at best. It is no longer acceptable to consider exploratory surgery of the lower back when objective criteria are not met. The residual effects of abnormalities already treated definitively (e.g., disc herniation causing root injury before its removal) may be difficult to differentiate from untreated and iatrogenic abnormalities in patients considered for re-operation.

If the surgeon is convinced that a disc protrusion was originally present, surgery may be necessary to exclude persistent root compression from retained disc fragments or unrelieved lateral recess stenosis. Statistics from several studies show that 57% to 66% of patients with persistent symptoms after lumbar spine surgery suffered from root compression within the lateral recess. These series failed to account for patients in whom adequate central and foraminal decompression did not relieve low back pain.

Prior to re-operation, the surgeon should review the contrast studies to be certain of the location of the original disc injury. Fragments that are lateral or in the axilla of the nerve root are often overlooked. Repeat surgery is relatively easy within days of the first operation but is more difficult several weeks later, when adhesions are present. We prefer to extend the bone removal above and below the original laminotomy, which increases the exposure and allows identification of normal structures prior to removing epidural scar at the original operative site. A foraminotomy is necessary to expose the axilla of the root, and a portion of the facet joint must be removed to obtain lateral exposure. Tactile exploration using a blunt nerve hook of Olivecrona to palpate in all directions is also important. An experienced surgeon can often sense the presence of a fragment by the absence of root or dural pulsations or by a sense of fullness at the end of the nerve hook. The root must be completely mobilized and retracted to confirm the presence of a disc fragment.

A complete laminectomy may have to be considered to adequately expose the surgical site if canal stenosis is present. Osseous compression most often occurs in the lateral recess but may occur at the pedicle or in the foramen. Dural erythema can frequently be identified at the site of compression after bone removal.

Careful repeat exposure is mandatory, since dural tears, anomalous nerve roots, and other abnormalities may be overlooked or not recorded in the operative note. The patient will do well if definite correctable pathology is found at early re-operation. The prognosis is guarded, however, if no pathology is found and surgical indications were marginal at the beginning.

Decompressive surgery is indicated when the patient's complaints of pain are compatible with demonstrated compression. The other problem for which surgery is generally indicated is overt, serious instability. Whereas the patient may be temporarily relieved by bracing, nothing will correct the problem except stabilization. Spinal fusion is used to stabilize segments that have been damaged to such a degree that normal physiological forces will cause damage to neural structures or progressive loss of biomechanical integrity.

Loss of stability may occur following operative decompression and destabilization of a spinal motion segment. *Stability* is a mechanical term that is often used without a clear or precise definition. Clinical instability does not necessarily indicate mechanical instability. Patients with clinical instability have abnormal symptomatic motion, whereas patients with mechanical instability do not necessarily have these symptoms. Patients with symptomatic instability are able to function, although minor changes in motion may precipitate severe symptomatic back and/or leg pain. Symptoms and signs that may be indicative of clinical instability include low back pain exacerbated with standing and lifting and relieved by lying down. A sudden catch when extending from the flexed to the straight posture and a feeling of disconnection in the lumbar spine accentuated by motion are helpful in identifying instability. Lumbar bracing may provide some relief in these patients. Clinical instability is frequently present in patients who have had previous surgeries for back disorders.

Patients who respond well to bracing can be treated satisfactorily with fusion of the involved segments. Objective criteria that suggest local instability exists include demonstrated motion on flexion/extension films; progressive spinal deformity in any direction; and spondylolisthesis, particularly if there is progressive significant facet arthropathy and traction spurs. Surgical destruction of zygapophyseal joints is another indication, as is demonstrated pseudarthrosis. Following an attempted fusion, signs of instability in the lumbar spin from L1 to L5 include greater than 3 mm of transitory motion and greater than 10 degrees of angulatory motion compared to aft levels. The transitory limit at the lumbosacral junction is 4 mm, and the angular limit is 20 mm. Values that exceed these limits often indicate instability. MacNab analyzed the causes of nerve root involvement and showed that traction osteophytes indicate instability of a motion segment.[47] Careful exploration of the integrity of the zygapophyseal joints, the status of the pars interarticularis, and the articular processes is necessary before the spine is fused.

North and associates conducted a retrospective review of their experiences with re-operation on the lumbosacral spine in an effort to identify patient characteristics and treatment methods associated with the most successful outcomes.[56] Surgical techniques and strategies for repeat operation included decompression with aggressive removal of extruded disc and hypertrophic scar, generous lateral decompression, and foraminotomy (but not facetectomy, except in cases of spondylolysis). Spondylolysis, spondylolisthesis, or gross instability on dynamic flexion/extension films was corrected with intertransverse and facet fusion of autologous bone graft. The operative procedures in this study included discectomy (24%), foraminotomy (50%), laminectomy (80%), excision and/or lysis of epidural scar (28%), and fusion (27%, including repair of pseudarthrosis in 4%). One hundred and two patients were interviewed an average of 5.05 years postoperatively by disinterested third parties. North and associates describe 34% of the surgeries as successful, defined as a 50% reduction in pain lasting at least 2 years or until last follow-up. Twenty-one patients disabled before surgery returned to work postoperatively; 15 who worked pre-operatively became disabled and/or retired. Patients reported loss of neurological function (strength, sensation, bowel and bladder control) more often than improvement in daily activities. A majority reduced or eliminated their intake of analgesics after re-operation.

Outcome was better for younger and female patients. Favorable outcome was associated with a history of good results from prior surgeries, a small number of prior operations, the absence of epidural scar requiring surgical lysis, employment before surgery, and the predominance of radicular (as opposed to axial) pain. No relationship between outcome and inclusion of a fusion in the operative procedure was found.

Ablative Procedures

Ablation of the involved primary afferent neurons is expected to provide pain relief whether pain originates in a joint, disc, or ligament as a nociceptive mechanism or as abnormal activity in an injured peripheral nerve, root, or dorsal root ganglion. After nerve injury, activity signaling pain may originate in neuromas or in dorsal root ganglia. Large myelinated afferents, which do not normally conduct pain sensation, may transmit postinjury hyperalgesia. Primary afferent ablation should address all of these mechanisms.

Dorsal rhizotomy may reduce persistent radicular pain after lumbosacral surgery.[59] More proximal radiofrequency thermocoagulation of the primary spinal nerve trunk and ganglion has been described. Uematsu and associates described percutaneous spinal rhizotomy to relieve nociceptive pain in the affected limbs.[80] This procedure can result in a motor and sensory deficit if performed at a functioning root level. Dorsal rhizotomy does not interrupt all afferent input, because numerous ventral root afferents with cell bodies in the dorsal root ganglia exist, and these convey pain from peripheral receptors even after dorsal rhizotomy. Dorsal root ganglionectomy has also not been effective for FBSS. One study of 13 patients reported no "successes" in the mean follow-up period of 5.5 years.[59]

Percutaneous radiofrequency lumbar facet denervation (medical branch posterior primary ramus neurotomy) is a simple peripheral ablative procedure for patients with mechanical low back syndrome. North and associates report that facet denervations are successful on a long-term basis in just less than one half of

the patients interviewed.[59] This result compares favorably with that of re-operation, with the advantage that the morbidity of facet denervation is negligible. Failure of prior disc surgery suggests that significant symptomatic disc disease is absent at the initial procedure. Failure can also result from poor clinical selection of patients who may be nonspecifically refractory to any treatment.

The problem may lie in the pathophysiology of pain following nerve injury and deafferentation. The effectiveness of ablative procedures to relieve pain may be limited by a number of anatomical and physiological changes occurring after primary afferent ablation. Nerve fibers sprout into denervated areas in the peripheral nervous system. After dorsal rhizotomy, intact axons from dorsal roots above and below the lesion form new central synapses in the dorsal horn. Dorsal horn recordings show confirmatory receptive field expansion and abnormal bursting activity. Single unit recordings during thalamic electrode implantation to treat the pain from deafferentation show abnormal bursting activity and soniatotopic map reorganization.[88]

Attempts to screen patients and to improve outcome for these procedures have used diagnostic paravertebral nerve root blocks pre-operatively. Nerve root blocks can be misleading and do not reliably predict the results of ablative or decompressive procedures. Nerve blocks distal to painful root or peripheral nerve lesions may provide temporary relief. These nonspecific results may reflect the systemic effects of lidocaine but are probably related to a central mechanism that interrupts pain sensation after blockade of major afferent input to the painful segment. Permanent interruption of the same input does not necessarily afford lasting relief.

Many fusion patients experience minimal postoperative pain following posterolateral fusion of the transverse processes and facet joints. Rees suggests that the early postoperative absence of pain results from denervation of the facet joints during the fusion.[88] Percutaneous procedures to denervate the facet joints were devised, using a modified tenotomy knife with posterior ramus section, that yielded a 99% success rate; the success rate was associated with a 20% incidence of subcutaneous hematomas. Fluoroscopically guided temperature-controlled radiofrequency thermocoagulation of the articular nerve branches has since been added to percutaneous procedures. Low-voltage stimulation at the proper site reproduces the patient's pain without eliciting a motor response. One study of low-voltage stimulation showed significant improvement in 88 of 100 unoperated patients with low back pain and/or sciatica with no motor weakness.[88]

Percutaneous lumbar facet denervation is a simple ablative procedure for patients with mechanical low back pain. Patients with prior lumbar surgery respond less well to facet injections or denervations than do unoperated patients. In our experience, previously operated and unoperated patients show minimal differences in response to nerve blocks and no difference in response to denervations.[55] Coagulation can produce a motor or sensory deficit if the electrode is placed too close to the primary spinal root or articular ramus (below the intertransverse ligament). Deafferentation procedures are irreversible and have the potential to alter the substrate for alternative procedures such as electrical stimulation devices. Ganglionectomy destroys primary afferents that ascend in the dorsal columns, which may render SCS ineffective.

Dorsal Column/Spinal Cord Stimulation

In 1965, Shealy and associates introduced electrical stimulation of the spinal cord to treat patients with intractable, chronic pain.[41] Before 1980, surgeons used arachnoid, subdural, or intradural electrode systems, with a laminectomy required for permanent placement of the electrode. Contemporary programmable systems with multiple electrodes are more reliable, and clinical outcome is significantly better than the older single-channel devices. SCS provides an effective reversible technique for the management of chronic intractable pain, and FBSS has been the most common indication for this procedure. The modern epidural electrodes avoid much of the morbidity associated with the earlier systems that included problems with SCF leakage and lead migration. The most frequent complications of the electrode systems are technical or equipment-related. Infection is infrequent but does occur in about 5% of procedures;[41] epidural electrode placement has eliminated spinal fluid leakage and arachnoid scarring.

SCS should only be considered for patients who have exhausted standard surgical therapy and in whom inoperable arachnoid fibrosis and/or nerve root injury are the major pathological conditions. Percutaneous placement of electrodes involves potential morbidity and discomfort to the patient comparable to diagnostic nerve blocks, myelography, and denervation procedures. The two types of epidural electrodes in use are a narrow silastic strip containing four electrode discs and a single or multicontact insulated wire electrode. The electrode is tunneled into the dorsal epidural space by percutaneous or semipercutaneous techniques with the patient under local anesthesia and with mild intravenous sedation. Intra-operative stimulation must produce reproducible paresthesias covering the area of the patient's pain. All electrodes are inserted through a Touhy-style needle placed in the dorsal epidural space. A two to seven day period of trial stimulation using percutaneous extension wires

and an external pulse generator is recommended to determine the optimal parameters for pain relief. The surgeon can then calculate when the patient receives worthwhile stimulation-induced analgesia and which electrode poles deliver optimal analgesia.

After successful trial stimulation, a second operation is necessary to implant the lead. A passively driven radiofrequency-coupled receiver is placed in a subcutaneous pocket, with the battery and adjustable pulse generator contained in a unit equipped with a detachable antenna disc. The fully implantable pulse generator is a recent innovation to the implant system. Programmable multicontact devices that permit noninvasive selection of stimulating anodes and cathodes facilitate selection of an effective stimulation combination. Correspondence of stimulation paresthesias with the topography of the pain is important for the patient to obtain pain relief.

Researchers have attempted to understand the physiological and pharmacological mechanisms involved in the analgesic effects of SCS. Linderoth and associates showed that SCS caused an increase in extracellular gamma-aminobutyric acid (GABA) in the dorsal horn of rats. Stimulation affects the firing pattern of neurons, and increased GABA concentration reduces the release of excitatory amino acids in the dorsal horn.

Kumar and associates analyzed the effects of SCS on 114 patients with FBSS. Long-term pain relief was reported in 52 patients and failure in 49 patients, after follow-up periods that averaged five years. Thirteen patients did not receive permanent implants because of failure during the trial stimulation period. No significant differences were found in the success rates of males and females to SCS, although better results in women patients have been reported previously in the literature. North and associates followed 50 patients with SCS implants for five years postoperatively.[58] The outcome was considered successful in 53% of patients after two years, whereas 47% of patients called the implant a success after five years. An important benefit of SCS is the significant reduction in drug usage reported by most patients.

Patients with radicular pain have better results from SCS and re-operation for FBSS than patients with axial (low back) pain. Technical improvements in SCS have increased the physician's ability to treat axial pain; axial pain is mechanical or nociceptive rather than neuropathic, for which SCS is a less effective procedure. Although the original physiological rationale for dorsal column stimulation (based on the gate-control theory of spinal cord pain processing) has come into question, the technique satisfactorily relieves pain in selected patients.

A prospective, randomized study is necessary even though SCS has good results in patients with a history of problems with pain management. The natural history of neural compression and/or instability or pseudarthrosis managed conservatively with pain relieving techniques such as SCS is unknown. The conditions of many of these re-operated patients may have deteriorated postoperatively, but their deterioration may have been worse without surgery. Long states that, "effective use requires a thorough understanding of the pain states to be treated, appreciation of the comorbidities that accompany chronic pain, an infrastructure to support the patient and the surgeon, and a dedication to lifelong care for the patient with the implant."[41]

Deep Brain Stimulation

Deep brain stimulation (DBS) provides an effective, reversible, nondestructive technique for the surgical management in selected patients with intractable nociceptive and/or central deafferentation pain states, including FBSS. The two principal DBS sites are the periaqueductal/periventricular gray region of the midbrain and caudal thalamus, and the ventroposterior medial/ventroposterior lateral thalamic somatosensory relay nuclei including the posterior limb of the internal capsule. The mechanisms, pathways, and neurotransmitters involved in stimulation-produced analgesia remain an area of active investigation and have been effective in some patients with low back or lower extremity pain that is refractory to peripheral nerve section or SCS. Research has shown that the periaqueductal/periventricular gray area is the most effective stimulation site. In three studies of patients with DBS implants, 58 (72%) had the system internalized and 42 of these (72%) experienced substantial long-term pain relief. Although severe complications are rare, greater risks are associated with deep brain stimulation than with other neuromodulatory modalities.[88]

Intraspinal Narcotics

Intraspinal narcotic therapy has been reported in a small series of FBSS patients with encouraging results. None have extended follow-up or disinterested third-party assessment, making comparison with other therapies difficult. Chronic subarachnoid narcotic infusion in patients with arachnoiditis, with a demonstrated propensity to react adversely, is problematic.

REHABILITATION PROGRAMS AND FBSS

Because rehabilitation is an important part of the management of FBSS, rehabilitation programs specializing in this area are proliferating. Patients who completed such programs have high rates of reported functional improvement and return to work, although pain rat-

ings are not reduced. These programs complement surgical management for selected patients, but the roles of these different therapies awaits prospective study.

SUMMARY

Because FBSS comprises a wide range of primary pathologies, the determination of precise treatments and outcomes is difficult. It is difficult to assess treatment options or outcomes accurately until clarifications with subsets of diagnoses are achieved. The FBSS diagnosis is too broad to be meaningful and should be eliminated.

The overall goal in the management of the patient with FBSS is to maximize quality of life, using a treatment program that is highly effective yet poses the smallest amount of risk. The diagnosis and management of FBSS often requires sophisticated diagnostic imaging and multidisciplinary input. Many patients are best served by a comprehensive pain treatment program. The cornerstone of any successful program for patients with FBSS is accurate diagnosis, allowing precisely targeted therapy. The inherent complexity of these cases necessitates a diagnostic and therapeutic protocol that is precise and cost-efficient.

The initial decision for surgery must be based on valid criteria and a clear anatomical diagnosis, with imaging studies that confirm the clinical diagnosis rather than provide the primary indication for operation. The best solution for recurrent symptoms after spine surgery is a preventive one that avoids inappropriate surgery. Criteria for surgical intervention must be strictly applied, and postoperative emphasis on rehabilitation must be maintained. The patient with persistent or recurrent symptoms forces the surgeon to reassess the original indications for surgery. With the lack of strong indications for surgical intervention, together with psychosocial issues, the possibility exists that repeat surgery will not solve the problem. The treating physician has to determine the cause of the pain through history, physical examination, and confirmatory studies, even with clear indications for the initial surgery. If the second operation is well founded, the probability of success is high and approaches the success rate of the primary procedure.

The surgical treatment options for FBSS include re-operation, but this applies to few patients. Ablative procedures, with the exception of facet neurotomy, have a low yield and high morbidity. Reversible, minimally invasive treatments such as SCS have a more favorable benefit-risk ratio. In the assessment of FBSS, the goals and expectations of both the patient and the physician must be clear. Expectations of surgical procedures are often unrealistic and beyond what could be expected from any form of therapy. Recognition of the patient's needs, goals, and expectations will provide a more successful outcome. Prospective comparisons of treatment methods and continued research into the pathological basis of pain in FBSS should lead to better selection criteria and more effective therapy.

REFERENCES

■

1. Barrios C, Ahmed M, Arrotegui JI, et al: Clinical factors predicting outcome after surgery for herniated lumbar disc: an epidemiological multivariate analysis. **J Spinal Disord** 3:205-9, 1990.
2. Berns DH, Blaser SI, Modic MT: Magnetic resonance imaging of the spine. **Clin Orthop** 244:78-100, 1989.
3. Bircher M, Tasker T, Crawshaw C, et al: Discitis following lumbar surgery. **Spine** 13:98-102, 1988.
4. Bobman SA, Atlas SW, Listerud J, et al: Postoperative lumbar spine: contrast-enhanced chemical shift MR imaging. **Radiology** 179:557-62, 1991.
5. Bogduk N, Long DM: Percutaneous lumbar medial branch neurotomy: a modification of facet denervation. **Spine** 5:193-200, 1980.
6. Braun IF, Hoffman JC Jr, David PC: Contrast enhancement in CT differentiation between recurrent disc herniation and postoperative scar: prospective study. **AJR** 145:785-90, 1985.
7. Brodsky AE, Kovalsky ES, Khalil MA: Correlation of radiologic assessment of lumbar spine fusions with surgical exploration. **Spine** 16:S261-65, 1991.
8. Brown H, Pont M: Diseases of the lumbar spine: ten years of surgical treatment. **J Neurosurg** 20:410, 1963.
9. Bundschuh CV, Stein L, Slusser JH, et al: Distinguishing between scar and recurrent herniated disc in postoperative patients: value of contrast-enhanced CT and MR imaging. **AJNR** 11:949-58, 1990.
10. Burton CV: Causes of failure of surgery on the lumbar spine: ten-year follow-up. **Mt Sinai J Med** 58:183-87, 1991.
11. Burton CV, Kirkaidy WW, Yong HK, et al: Causes of failure of surgery on the lumbar spine. **Clin Orthop** 157:191-99, 1981.
12. Crock HV: Anterior lumbar interbody fusion: indications for its use and notes on surgical technique. **Clin Orthop** 165:157-63, 1982.
13. Dauch W: Infection of the intervertebral space following conventional and microsurgical operation on the herniated lumbar intervertebral disc. **Acta Netirochir** 82:43-49, 1986.
14. DePaima A, Rothman R: The nature of pseudoarthrosis. **Clin Orthop** 59:113, 1968.
15. Esses SI, Moro JK: The value of facet joint blocks in patient selection for lumbar fusion. **Spine** 18:185-90, 1993.
16. Fager CA, Freidberg SR: Analysis of failures and poor results of lumbar spine surgery. **Spine** 5:87-94, 1980.
17. Fairbank J, Park W, McCall I: Apophyseal injection of local anesthetic as a diagnostic aid in primary low-back pain syndromes. **Spine** 6:598-605, 1981.
18. Finnegan W, Fentin J, Marvel J, et al: Results of surgical intervention in the symptomatic multioperated back patient. **J Bone Joint Surg** 61:1077-82, 1979.
19. Firooznia H, Krischeff II, Rafii M, et al: Lumbar spine after surgery: examination with intravenous contrast enhanced CT. **Radiology** 163:221-26, 1987.
20. Ford L, Key L: Postoperative infection of the intervertebral disc space. **Sotith Med J** 48:1295, 1955.
21. Fouquet B, Goupille P, Jattiot F: Discitis after lumbar disc surgery. **Spine** 17:356-58, 1992.
22. Fraser R, Osti O, Vernon-Roberts B: Discitis after discography. **J Bone Joint Surg** 69B:26-35, 1987.
23. Frymoyer JW, Cats-Barit BW: Predictors of low back pain disability. **Clin Orthop** 221:89-98, 1987.
24. Frymoyer JW, Cats-Barfl BW: An overview of the incidences and costs of low back pain. **Orthop Clin North Am** 22:263-71, 1991.
25. Frymoyer JW, Matteri RE, Hanley EN, et al: Failed lumbar disc surgery requiring second operation: a longterm follow-up study. **Spine** 3:7-11, 1978.
26. Frymoyer JW, Nelson RM, Spangfort E, et al: Clinical tests applicable to the study of chronic low-back disability. **Spine** 16:681-82, 1991.
27. Frymoyer JW, Rosen JC, Clements J, et al: Psychologic factors in low-back-pain disability. **Clin Orthop** 195:178-84, 1985.
28. Gieseking H: Lokalisierte Spondylitis nach operiertern Bandscheibenvorfall. **Zenti-albi Chir** 76:1470, 1951.
29. Greenwood J, McGuire T, Kimball F: A study of causes of failure in the herniated disc operation: an analysis of 67 repeated cases. **J Neurosurg** 9:15-, 1952.
30. Grenier N, Vital J, Greselle J, et al: CT discography in the evaluation of the postoperative lumbar spine. **Neuroradiology** 30:232-38, 1988.
31. Guyer RD, Collier RR, Ohnmeiss DD, et al: Extraosseous spinal lesions mimicking disc disease. **Spine** 13:328-31, 1988.
32. Howe J, JW F: The effects of questionnaire design on the determination of end results in lumbar spinal surgery. **Spine** 10:804-5, 1985.
33. Hudgins W: The role of microdiscectomy. **Orthop Clin North Am** 14:589-603, 1983.
34. Hueftle MG, Modic MT, Ross JS, et al: Lumbar spine: postoperative MR imaging with GD-DTPA. **Radiology** 167:817-24, 1988.
35. Ikko E, Lahde S, Koivukangas J, et al: Computed tomography after lumbar disc surgery. **Acta Radiol** 29:179, 1988.
36. Kahn T, Roosen N, Messing A, et al: Follow-up studies with GD-DTPA enhanced MR imaging of the asymptomatic postdiscectomy lumbar spine. **Radiology** 177:233, 1990.
37. Kern C: Delayed death following disc surgery. **Texas State Med J** 50:158, 1954.
38. Kopecky K, Gilmor R, Scott J, et al: Pitfalls of computed tomography in diagnosis of discitis. **Neuroradiology** 27:57-66, 1985.
39. Krempen JF, Smith BS: Nerve root injection: a method for evaluating the etiology of sciatica. **J Bone Joint Surg** 56A:1435-44, 1974.

40. Long D: Chronic adhesive spinal arachnoiditis: pathogenesis, prognosis, and treatment. **Neurosurg** 2:296, 1992.

41. Long DM: Stimulation of the peripheral nervous stem for pain control. **Clin Neurosurg** 31:323-43, 1983.

42. Long DM: Nonsurgical therapy for low back pain and sciatica. **Clin Neurosurg** 35:351-59, 1989.

43. Long DM: Failed back surgery syndrome. **Neurosurg Clin North Am** 2:899-919, 1991;.

44. Long DM: Decision making in lumbar disc disease. **Clin Neurosurg** 39:36-51, 1992.

45. Long DM, Filtzer DL, BenDebba M, et al: Clinical features of the feedback syndrome. **J Neurosurg** 69:61-71, 1988.

46. Love J, Rivers M: Spinal cord tumors simulating protruded intervertebral discs. **JAMA** 179:878, 1962.

47. MacNab I: Negative disc exploration: An analysis of the causes of nerve root involvement in 68 patients. **J Bone Joint Surg** 53A:891-903, 1971.

48. Mansour A, Nabos J, Taddonio R: Psoas abscess: thirty four years after pyogenic osteomyelitis of the spine. **Orthopedics** 2:26, 1979.

49. Mayfield F: Complications of laminectomy. **Clin Neurosurg** 23:435-39, 1976.

50. McCulloch J: **Principles of Microsurgery for Lumbar Disc Disease.** New York: Raven Press, 1989.

51. Milward F: Changes in the intervertebral discs following lumbar puncture. **Lancet** 2:183, 1936.

52. Mixter WJ, Barr JS: Rupture of the intervertebral disc with involvement of the spinal canal. **New Engl J Med** 211:210-15, 1934.

53. Nashold BJ, Hrubec A: *Lumbar Disc Disease: A Twenty-Year Clinical Follow-up Study.* St. Louis: Mosby, 1971.

54. Neill S: Computed tomography in failed back syndrome. **Radiography Today** 57:9-12, 1991.

55. North R, Zeidman S: Failed back surgery syndrome. **Cont Neurosurg** 16: 1, 1993.

56. North RB, Campbell JN, James CS, et al: Failed back surgery syndrome: 5-year follow-up in 102 patients undergoing repeated operation. **Neurosurgery** 28:685-91, 1991.

57. North RB, Cutchis PN, Epstein JA, et al: Spinal cord compression complicating subarachnoid infusion of morphine: case report and laboratory experience. **Neurosurgery** 29:778-84, 1991.

58. North RB, Ewend MG, Lawton MT, et al: Spinal cord stimulation for chronic, intractable pain: superiority of "multi-channel" devices. **Pain** 44:119-30, 1991.

59. North RB, Kidd DH, Campbell JN, et al: Dorsal root ganglionectomy for failed back surgery syndrome: a 5-year follow-up study. **J Neurosurg** 74:236-42, 1991.

60. Norton W: Chemonucleolysis versus surgical discectomy: comparison of costs and results in workers' compensation claimants. **Spine** 11:440-43, 1987.

61. Patrick BS: Extreme lateral ruptures of lumbar intervertebral discs. **Surg Neurol** 3:301-4, 1975.

62. Pilgaard S, Aarhus N: Discitis following removal of lumbar intervertebral disc. **J Bone Joint Surg [Am]** 51 A:713, 1969.

63. Ramirez L, Thisted R: Complication and demographic characteristics of patients undergoing lumbar discectomy in community hospitals. **Neurosurgery** 25:226-31, 1989.

64. Roberts M: Complications of lumbar disc surgery. **Spinal Surg** 2:13, 1988.

65. Ross JS: Magnetic resonance assessment of the postoperative spine: degenerative disc disease. **Radiol Clin North Am** 29:793-808, 1991.

66. Ross JS, Masaryk TJ, Modic MT, et al: MR imaging of lumbar arachnoiditis. **AJR** 149:1025-32, 1987.

67. Ross JS, Masaryk TJ, Schrader M, et al: MR imaging of the postoperative lumbar spine: assessment with gadopentetate dimeglumine. **AJR Am J Roentgenol** 155:867-72, 1990.

68. Scherbel A, Gardner W: Infections involving the intervertebral discs. Diagnosis and management. **JAMA** 174:370, 1960.

69. Schubiger O, Valvanis A: Postoperative lumbar CT: technique, results, and indications. **Am J Neuroradiol** 4:595-97, 1983.

70. Smith AS, Blaser SI: Infectious and inflammatory processes of the spine. **Radiol Clin North Am** 29:809-27, 1991.

71. Sorenson L, Mors O, Skorlund O: A prospective study of the importance of psychological and social factors for the outcome after surgery in patients with slipped lumbar disc operated on for the first time. **Acta Neurochir** 88:119, 1987.

72. Sotiropoulos S, Chafetz NI, Lang P, et al: Differentiation between postoperative scar and recurrent disc herniation: prospective comparison of MR, CT, and contrast enhanced CT. **AJNR** 10:639-43, 1989.

73. Spangfort E: The lumbar disc herniation: a computer aided analysis of 2,504 operations. **Acta Orthop Scand (Suppl)** 142:1-95, 1972.

74. Spengler DM, Freeman C, Westbrook R, et al: Low back pain following multiple lumbar spine procedures: failure of initial selection? **Spine** 5:356-60, 1980.

75. Sullivan C, Bickel W, Svien H: Infections of vertebral interspaces after operations on intervertebral discs. **JAMA** 166:1973, 1958.

76. Teplick JG, Haskin ME: Intravenous contrast-enhanced CT of the postoperative lumbar spine: improved identification of recurrent disc herniation, scar, arachnoiditis, and discitis. **AJR** 143:845-55, 1984.

77. Teplick JG, Haskin ME: Review: computed tomography of the postoperative lumbar spine. **AJR** 141: 865-84, 1983.

78. Thibodeau A: Closed space infection following removal of lumbar intervertebral disc. **J Bone Joint Surg [Am]** 5OA:400, 1968.

79. Turnbull F: Postoperative inflammatory disease of lumbar discs. **J Neurosurg** 10:469, 1953.

80. Uematsu S, Jankel WR, Edwin DH, et al: Quantification of thermal asymmetry: part 2. Application in low-back pain and sciatica. **J Neurosurg** 69:556-61, 1988.

81. Waddell G, Kummel EG, Lotto WN, et al: Failed lumbar disc surgery and repeat surgery following industrial injuries. **J Bone Joint Surg [Am]** 61:201-7, 1979.

82. Waddell G, Somerville D, Henderson L, et al: Objective clinical evaluation of physical impairment in chronic low back pain. **Spine** 17:617-28, 1992.

83. Walsh T, Weinstein J, Sprath K: Lumbar discography in normal subjects: a controlled prospective study. **J Bone Joint Surg [Am]** 72A:1081-88, 1990.

84. Weiss T, Treisch J, Krazner E: CT of the postoperative lumbar spine: the value of intravenous contrast. **Neuroradiology** 28:241-45, 1986.

85. White AH: Low back pain. **Instr Course Lect** 34:416-19, 1985.

86. Wiesel SW: The multiply operated lumbar spine. **Instr Course Lect** 34:68-77, 1985.

87. Wilkinson HA: Failed disc syndrome. **Am Fam Physician** 17:86-94, 1978.

88. Zeidman SM, Long DM: Failed back surgery syndrome. In Menenzes AH, Sonntag VKH, eds: **Principles of spinal surgery.** New York, 1996, McGraw-Hill, 657-79.

CHAPTER 13

Intradiscal Electrothermal Annuloplasty: The IDET Procedure

ROBERT F. HEARY, M.D.

INTRODUCTION

Intradiscal electrothermal (IDET) annuloplasty is a minimally invasive procedure for the treatment of degenerative disc disease. This procedure has been used in the lumbar spine of patients who have failed conservative treatment regimens and who might otherwise be candidates for a spinal fusion procedure. As this is a recently developed procedure, there is only relatively short-term follow-up data available, and as such, the procedure has not been widely accepted.

The IDET procedure was developed by specialists in physical medicine and rehabilitation, Drs. Jeffrey and Joel Saal. This procedure was developed to offer patients with chronic discogenic low back pain an option other than chronic pain management for spinal fusion.[18] Over the past five years, the IDET procedure has been performed by surgeons (neurological, orthopaedic) and nonsurgeons (physical medicine and rehabilitation, anesthesiology, radiology).

Chronic low back pain may be the result of degenerative disc disease of the lumbar spine (or discogenic back pain). Chronic low back pain may also be the result of disturbances of the sacroiliac joints, or the zygapophyseal facet joints, or it may be the result of infections and/or neoplasms in the spinal and extraspinal tissues. In addition, nonspinal causes of chronic low back pain may include systemic diseases, particularly those that occur in the retroperitoneal region. Also, psychological disturbances may manifest themselves as chronic low back pain. O'Neill and associates described the anatomical structures, which are potential sources of axial lumbar pain as including the intervertebral discs, the myofascial tissues, and the synovial joints.[15] The IDET procedure is specifically devised to treat degenerative disc disease resulting in chronic low back pain. The diagnosis of degenerative disc disease is, in itself difficult to accurately determine.

The clinical history, physical examination findings, and radiographic imaging studies necessary to diagnose lumbar degenerative disc disease are outlined in detail in this textbook in the chapter on discography. All proponents of the IDET procedure agree that if the diagnosis of degenerative lumbar disc disease is suggested by these criteria, then a provocative discogram is required prior to performance of an IDET procedure.

Lumbar discography was originally described by Lindblom in 1948.[11] In 1970, Crock described a pattern of abnormality that he termed "internal disc disruption". This term is clinically synonymous with what today is referred to as degenerative disc disease of the lumbar spine.[4] It is this entity that the IDET procedure is designed to treat. In 1987, Sachs and associates published the Dallas discogram description. This description included functional information as well as radiographic criteria for disc disease. In that description, concordant pain was defined as a reproduction of a patient's usual axial back pain when dye was injected into the intervertebral disc.[22] This has led to the term "provocative discography" in which the patient's clinical response, from a pain standpoint, to the injection of dye is a significant factor as to whether an intervertebral disc is thought to be the source of low back pain. The premise that degenerative disc disease of the lumbar spine may be successfully treated with intervention by either the IDET procedure or a spinal fusion has been the subject of some controversy. Furthermore, the use of provocative discography to accurately diagnose this condition has spurred additional controversy. Further details regarding this issue are described in the chapter 4 on discography.

The natural history of degenerative lumbar disc disease includes a loss of hydrostatic pressure, which leads to a buckling of the annular lamellae. This may lead to an increased focal segmental mobility as well as increased shear stress to the wall of the annulus. As the patient continues to load the degenerative disc, pain may be referred into the buttocks and leg either by stimulation of the dorsal root ganglion or from direct chemical irritation of the lumbar nerve roots.[18] Previously, if a patient with degenerative disc disease of the lumbar spine failed a conservative treatment regimen, the option of a spinal fusion procedure was entertained. Spinal fusion for the treatment of chronic low back pain resulting from degenerative disc disease has been variably successful.[5,18,23] Problems with spinal fusion procedures include the morbidity of the procedure, adjacent segment degeneration, the possibility of repeat surgery, and perioperative complications.[17] Other treatment options do exist for patients with chronic, unremitting, discogenic low back pain. Aggressive nonoperative care is indicated for all patients with this condition. Previously, patients who failed conservative therapy were offered either long-term pain management or a spinal fusion. The IDET procedure has been proposed as a minimally invasive procedure, which is intermediate between a long-term pain management program and a spinal fusion procedure.[17]

THE INDICATIONS FOR IDET

Patient selection criteria for the IDET procedure are similar to those used for spinal fusion for degenerative disc disease of the lumbar spine. Saal and Saal have published detailed inclusion criteria, which include unremitting, persistent low back pain for a minimum six-month period of time. An additional criterion is a failure of satisfactory improvement with a nonoperative care program that includes back education, activity modification, a progressive intensive exercise program, a trial of manual physical therapy, use of oral nonsteroidal anti-inflammatory drugs. Failure of an epidural steroid injection is another selection criterion.[17] These authors have described the failure of the conservative (nonoperative) treatment, as a minimum six-month period of comprehensively applied nonoperative care with the patient reporting persistent pain and disability, dissatisfaction with quality of life, and a desire to pursue alternative treatment options.[19] Physical examination should include a normal neurological exam with a negative straight leg raising sign. Magnetic resonance imaging (MRI) does not demonstrate a nerve root or spinal cord compression. A positive provocative discogram with concordant pain at low pressure, demonstrated at one or more levels, along with a painless control level, is an essential component of the diagnostic work-up.[17]

The importance of provocative discography cannot be understated. In an innovative study by Boden and associates, performed in 1990, patients with no symptoms related to the lumbar spine underwent MRI stud-

ies. These authors determined that approximately one third of clinically asymptomatic patients have an abnormal MRI, and as such, they determined that this study is overly sensitive.[2] Accordingly, additional study is required to establish the diagnosis of clinically relevant degenerative disc disease. Provocative discography has been touted as a useful tool for this purpose. Karasek and Bogduk have stated that inclusion criteria for surgery include the presence of concordant pain at the abnormal disc level, as well as a presence of a nonpainful control disc injection. In addition, they have described the importance of the presence of a radial fissure, which reaches at least the outer third of the annulus fibrosis, and an intact outer perimeter to the annulus fibrosis.[9] O'Neill and associates in 1999, described the importance of recognizing the potential impact of psychosocial factors in diagnosing and treating patients with spinal pain.[15]

Exclusion criteria for the IDET procedure would include inflammatory arthritides; non-spinal conditions, which could mimic lumbar pain; medical or metabolic disorders that would preclude follow-up participation; and prior surgery at the symptomatic level.[17,19] In the study published by Saal and Saal in 2000, all 62 patients undergoing the IDET procedure had been offered a spinal fusion and refused this procedure.[1] As previously stated, these indications for the IDET procedure are relatively strict and would be consistent with indications typically used by surgeons considering a spinal fusion procedure.

TECHNIQUE

The IDET procedure is performed via a standard disc puncture technique. This is a sterile procedure performed percutaneously with biplane fluoroscopy. A radiolucent table is frequently used. The patient may be positioned either prone or in a lateral position and the procedure is performed either in the operating room or in a fluoroscopy suite. Anesthesia will typically involve use of local anesthesia as well as possibly light intravenous sedation. Preferably reversible or short acting sedative drugs are used. General anesthesia is not used for fear of not detecting nerve root symptoms during the procedure. The disc is routinely entered immediately ventral to the superior articular process of the zygapophyseal facet joint.

Upon confirmation of needle placement utilizing biplane fluoroscopy, a 30-cm catheter with a 6-cm active resistant tip is placed through the localization needle (Figure 13-1).[15] The catheter is then navigated through the nucleus pulposus to the offending portion of the annulus.[19] Whereas the approach may be from either side, typically the approach is from the patient's less painful side.[9] Although the majority of researchers describe navigating the catheter along the

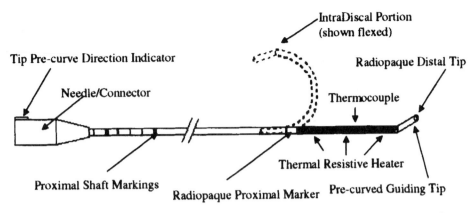

FIGURE 13-1 ■ Line drawing of the catheter utilized in the IDET procedure. The distal portion of the catheter is flexible and this is the only portion of the catheter that provides thermal energy during treatment.

inner portion of the annulus fibrosis, Karasek and Bogduk have described positioning the catheter between the lamellae of the annulus fibrosis.[9] Once appropriate positioning of the thermal resistive coil portion of the catheter is confirmed, the tip of the catheter is heated to a temperature between 85 to 90°C.[9,17,18] In the protocol described by Saal and Saal, heating is raised to 90°C over a 13-minute period of time and then maintained at 90°C. for a 4-minute period of time.[17] A single heating treatment is administered (Figure 13-2). After the procedure, the patient is transferred to a recovery area and is discharged home on the day of the procedure.

Saal and Saal have described extensive postoperative guidelines for care in the post-procedural period.

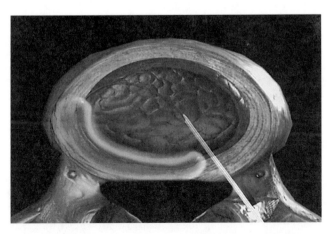

FIGURE 13-2 ■ Diagram of the usual position of the catheter during an IDET procedure. The flexible tip is in the typical position with the flexed catheter resting along the inner portion of the posterior wall of the annulus fibrosis. The markings surrounding the flexible tip of the catheter are an artist's rendition of the area exposed to thermal energy during the procedure.

This includes bracing for a six- to eight-week period of time with limited activity with respect to work, sitting, and driving. A gentle progressive exercise regimen is then enacted.[18] In the first month following the IDET, the patient is involved with walking and low intensity leg stretching exercises. In the second month, low intensity floor stabilization exercises are performed. In the third month, the intensity exercises slightly increase. The patient is advised to avoid tennis, running, or skiing until the fifth or sixth month postprocedure. There is a maximum of six weeks of physical therapy that begins during the second or third month.[17]

RESULTS

The most consistent criticism of the IDET procedure has involved a lack of long-term outcome results. The majority of short-term outcome results have been reported by investigators who were either the inventors/developers of the technique or investigators with consultant agreements. Nonetheless, longer-term outcome results are becoming increasingly available and are reviewed in the text that follows.

In 2000, Saal and Saal published outcome results with a mean follow-up period of 16 months.[17] The visual analog scale (VAS) and SF-36(short form 36) scales were used in these studies. The visual analog scale and SF-36 are outcome instruments which have been previously validated.[6] In the study by Saal and Saal, at a mean follow-up of 16 months, 62 patients were evaluated. Thirty patients had undergone a single level procedure and 32 patients had undergone multilevel procedures. The mean VAS improved 3.0. The mean SF-36 scores improved 20 points. Defining a positive improvement as a VAS improvement of greater than two points and an SF-36 improvement of greater than seven points, Saal and Saal documented improvement in VAS in 71% of their patients, in the

SF-36 physical function scale in 71% of their patients, and in the SF-36 bodily pain scale in 74% of their patients. Nineteen percent of patients did not demonstrate positive improvement on any scale.[17]

Karasek and Bogduk performed a study in which the included patients were those for whom their insurance companies had approved the procedure. The control group, which they described as "convenience" controls, was patients whose insurance companies refused payment for the procedure. With these obvious methodological flaws, they documented a greater than 50% reduction in pain in 60% of treated patients, with 23% of these patients being pain-free at a mean follow-up of three months.[9]

At the 2000 Annual Meeting of the North American Spine Society, Thompson and Eckel reported the results of a nationwide registry of multicenter outcomes. A total of 28 physicians participated and 259 patients were included. One hundred seventy patients (65%) responded to a survey six months following the procedure. Of these responders, 76% of patients self-reported a reduction in their pain at the six-months follow-up.[24]

In 2000, Liu and associates reported on 50 patients undergoing the IDET procedure with a mean duration of follow-up of eleven months. They defined a clinically favorable response as an improvement of VAS of greater than or equal to two points and found 60% of patients in the clinically favorable category. They also determined that the results were less favorable with time decreasing to 43% favorable at 12 months and 33% at 18 months (Factors that were predictive of success included: age less than forty, nonsmoker, female sex, duration of symptoms less than four years, less severe annular tears and catheter placement that was judged as perfect during the procedure.[12])

In 2000, Derby and associates published results for 32 patients with a mean twelve-month follow-up. These investigators found that 78% of patients stated the procedure had "met their expectations, or that they would undergo the same treatment for the same clinical outcome." They found (62.5% of patients had a favorable outcome, 25% showed no change, and 12.5% had a nonfavorable outcome.[5]) Interestingly, further analysis of Derby's results demonstrates that 41% of the patients with either no change or an unfavorable outcome were included in the 78% of patients who felt the procedure had met their expectations. In attempting to reconcile this discrepancy, it is difficult to understand how patients with severe pain, prior to the procedure, who either did not improve or worsened, would state that the procedure had met their expectations or that they would undergo the same procedure for the same outcome.

Wetzel and associates presented the preliminary results of the first multicenter, prospective, cohort study trial of the IDET procedure at the North American Spine Society Meeting in 2000. In this review, a total of 78 patients were in the original intent to treat group. Eight withdrew, leaving 70 patients in the study cohort. There were five treatment failures, of which four went on to spinal fusion procedures. These researchers found an apparent benefit of increased social functioning and less work impairment as a result of pain, which suggested a positive therapeutic effect from the IDET procedure. A mean duration of follow-up was not described; however, only 20 of the 70 patients had one-year follow-ups.[25]

The first follow-up study of the IDET procedure with two-year follow-up was presented by Saal and Saal at the 2000 North American Spine Society Annual Meeting. In this study population, 55 patients with a mean age of forty-one years were reviewed. Mean preoperative symptoms had been present for 60 months prior to the procedure. Twenty-seven patients underwent single level treatment and 28 patients underwent multilevel treatment. At two-year follow-up, these authors found a mean VAS change of 3.2, a mean SF-36 physical function change of 20 points, and a mean SF-36 bodily pain change of 17.8 points. All of these changes were statistically significant. Improvement in the SF-36 scale of at least seven points was demonstrated in 71% of patients for physical function and in 74% of patients for bodily pain. Eleven percent of patients did not improve on either SF-36 subscale. (Saal and Saal concluded that in a cohort of patients with chronic, unremitting low back pain of discogenic origin, who had failed to improve with aggressive nonoperative care, a statistically significant and clinically meaningful improvement on the SF-36 and VAS scores can be achieved with a minimum two-year follow-up after the IDET procedure.[19])

THE SCIENCE BEHIND IDET

In 1998, Saal and Saal presented at the North American Spine Society Annual Meeting in San Francisco, CA. In this presentation, they proposed that collagen is modified and nociceptive pain receptors were damaged by the IDET procedure. They postulated this as the mechanism of action for the IDET procedure.[21] Subsequent journal articles and presentations referenced this presentation as the proposed mechanism of action of the IDET.[5-9,12,23-25] Despite an extensive review of peer-reviewed journal articles, proof of the modulation of collagen and destruction of nociceptors is not available. It appears that the proponents of the IDET procedure are in near uniform agreement that collagen modification and destruction of nociceptors is the mechanism of action of the IDET. Remarkably, the only references made to support this concept refer to the oral presentation made at the North American Spine

Society in 1998. The data to support the assertions from that 1998 presentation have never been published in a peer-reviewed journal format by any investigators.

In a peer-reviewed article in 2000, Saal and Saal stated that "it is the authors' hypothesis that collagen modification resulted in a biomechanical alteration of the functional spinal segment."[20] Furthermore, in that same article, Saal and Saal stated "in the author's opinion, the granulation tissue and nerve in growth that occurs in disrupted discs should not recur after thermal treatment. Animal studies are currently underway to examine these issues."[20] Finally, Saal and Saal stated "it is unlikely, therefore, that the long-term effect produced by thermal treatment of the discs at the temperature used in this study, would harm the treated segment beyond the known consequences of the degenerative cascade."[20] Despite the lack of scientific support for this hypothesis , the IDET procedure is being utilized in the clinical setting.

THE EFFECTS OF THERMAL ENERGY ON TISSUES

The impetus for the development of the IDET procedure came from prior experience among orthopaedic surgeons using thermal energy in the treatment of glenohumeral joint capsules of the shoulder. Theoretically, thermal energy applied to the glenohumeral joint capsule allowed for modification of this capsule with improvement in function of the shoulder joint. Numerous peer-reviewed journal articles on the thermal effects on tissues have been published. Hayashi and associates examined glenohumeral joint capsule tissue in cadavers. They found that at temperatures greater than 65°C consistent shrinkage of the specimens and histologic alteration characterized by hyalinization of the collagen occurred.[7] Similarly, Obrzut and associates used a sheep model. In their study, glenohumeral joint capsules were placed in a 37°C bath and treated with radiofrequency energy at five distinct temperatures (60°C, 65°C, 70°C, 75°C, and 80°C). Tissue shrinkage was significant at 80°C, with 14% shortening demonstrated. Tissue shrinkage was not significant below 65°C. At a distance of 1.5 mm from the radiofrequency probe, none of the five tested temperatures was able to demonstrate a tissue temperature of 45°C.[14] Naseef and associates performed a study on the effects of heating bovine knee capsules. They found that thermal shrinkage of the knee capsules correlated with denaturation of collagen fibers and depended on both the temperature of the heating element and the duration of time to which the tissue was exposed to the heat.[13] In 2000, Arnoczky and Askan, attempted to determine the clinical implications of thermal modification of connective tissues.

Specifically, they attempted to determine the biological fate of the shrunken collagen tissues after thermal energy. Temperatures required to shrink collagen (greater than 65° C) were also found to destroy cellular viability. As a result, the thermally modified tissues are devitalized and must undergo a biological remodeling. Their theories as to how the biological repair response may help clinically include the following:

1. Maintenance of the initial capsular shrinkage.
2. Secondary fibroplasia and resulting thickening of the joint capsule.
3. A loss of afferent sensory stimulation due to destruction of the sensory receptors.

They also postulated that a combination of these three factors may occur in order to provide clinical improvement.[1]

Pokharna and Phillips studied collagen crosslinks in human lumbar intervertebral discs. They found that alterations in the collagen crosslinks with aging and disc degeneration occurred. They hypothesized that these changes may contribute to the loss of disc integrity and play a role in the pathogenesis of the degenerative process.[16] Kleinstueck and associates presented a study at the 2000 North American Spine Society Meeting. In this study, they performed temperature mapping experiments on eight human cadaver specimens. A total of 320 measurements were made on eight lumbar intervertebral discs. A temperature of 65°C was able to be achieved only within 1 mm of the IDET thermal resistance coil used to heat the disc material. The annular thickness of these specimens was 12 mm. These authors determined that the maximum average temperature along the path of the catheter was 57.5°C and the mean temperature at the level of the posterior annulus of the disc ranged between 39 to 42°C. They concluded that except for a very limited margin around the catheter, which did not exceed 1 to 2 mm, the necessary temperature to induce shrinkage of collagen (65°C) was not measured within the disc. Furthermore, biomechanical testing of five human cadaver specimens treated with IDET demonstrated an increased motion in all five specimens following application of the heat.[10]

Saal and Saal, performed thermocouple measurements along the posterior annular wall following 15.5 minutes of *in vivo* heating with a maximum temperature of 90°C. They found the temperature immediately adjacent to the catheter to be 75°C. At the center of the annulus, the temperature reached 60°C, and at the outer annular wall, 42°C was reached. In the epidural space, temperatures reached 38°C.[18] Whereas this demonstrated that temperatures in the epidural space were certainly safe, the majority of the posterior annulus fibrosis did not achieve a temperature adequate to modulate collagen. The preponderance of published data involving thermal energy to intervertebral disc tissue demonstrates that a temperature of 65°C or greater is necessary in order to shrink collagen. Review of this available scientific data does not show evidence that a significant percentage of intervertebral discs exposed to the IDET thermal resistive coil would achieve a temperature adequate to cause modulation of collagen.

A second postulated mechanism of action of the IDET procedure involves destruction of nociceptive pain fibers. Cavanaugh and associates used a silver impregnation technique to analyze the intervertebral discs and posterior longitudinal ligaments of New Zealand white rabbits. They determined that nerves measuring 1 to 3 microns were present around the entire periphery of the discs. There were no encapsulated nerve endings seen within the annulus of the discs, whereas occasional encapsulated endings were seen on the annular surface and the posterior longitudinal ligament.[3] For the IDET procedure to effectively damage these nociceptive pain fibers, the temperature at the outer annular wall would need to be sufficient to destroy these nerve endings. The temperature mapping studies of both Kleinstueck and associates, and Saal and Saal demonstrate that posterior annulus temperatures range between 39 to 42°C.[10,18] Kleinstueck and associates stated that temperatures sufficient to ablate nerves in the clinically relevant area of the posterior annulus were not achieved.[10] Whereas the hypothesis that collagen shrinkage and/or modulation, as well as nerve ending damage of nociceptive fibers, is the mechanism of action for the IDET procedure, the preponderance of published scientific data does not support this conclusion. Definitive proof of the mechanism of action by which the IDET procedure may beneficially affect the intervertebral disc is not available.

COMPLICATIONS

By all reports, the complication rates of the IDET procedure are very low. In a follow-up study of 62 patients with 16-month follow-up, Saal and Saal reported no new radicular pain, no neurological deficits and no adverse events. No patient's condition was worsened by the procedure.[17] Anecdotal reports have surfaced on a number of complications related to the IDET procedure. There have been reports of bacterial discitis, thermal nerve root injury, and catheter breakage as a result of kinking. The most serious and devastating complication has been a report of the development of cauda equina syndrome following the IDET procedure. In this report, a catheter was misplaced within the spinal canal resulting in an acute cauda equina syndrome, and after six months, no clinical improvement had occurred.[8]

Persistent back pain may result following the IDET procedure and this may be either just a treatment failure or the result of an inflammatory (nonbacterial) discitis. In addition, following the IDET procedure, radiculopathy may occur, which is usually transient, and may be the result of inaccurate needle placement or a direct nerve root injury. The exact incidence of these minor transient complications has not been accurately reported to date. Of significant concern, the inventors of this procedure, Drs. Saal and Saal, in the abstract of their presentation at the 2000 North American Spine Society Meeting, stated "the long-term consequences of intradiscal treatment with this catheter are not known currently."[20]

CRITICISMS OF THE IDET PROCEDURE

The IDET procedure has been subjected to numerous criticisms. The lack of adequate long-term follow-up data is a substantial concern for any invasive procedure. Furthermore, the mechanism of action of the IDET procedure is unclear. As has been previously discussed, although modulation of collagen and destruction of nociceptive pain receptors have been postulated mechanisms, no peer-reviewed journal article has demonstrated proof of these hypotheses. In addition, there is a lack of animal data on the IDET procedure. With respect to human experimentation, there is no prospective randomized data available that compares the IDET procedure with a second group of patients having a similar post-procedural therapy course. Likewise, there are no controlled studies with reasonable control populations. Karasek and Bogduk published a "controlled" trial of the IDET procedure. This study had dramatic methodological flaws in that the patients placed in the control group were a "convenience" control sample. The convenience controls were patients who were denied coverage of the procedure by their insurance companies and, thus, these patients were denied the procedure. Obviously, these patients may have very significant bias in their outcome results. In fact, none of the patients in the control treatment group completed further follow-up.[9]

Another major criticism of the IDET procedure involves the potential for investigator bias in evaluation of this procedure. Drs. Saal and Saal are the developers and inventors of the technique. These two investigators are also the only group to publish two-year follow-up data. Furthermore, hypotheses generated on the mechanism of action have routinely been attributed to these investigators whereas peer-reviewed publication of this information has never been published. In addition to the developers of the technique, numerous other investigators have financial consultant agreements with the company that has marketed this device (Oratec Interventions, Inc., Menlo Park, CA).

As with essentially any advances in procedure-oriented medicine, the initial work and follow-up has been performed by the developers of the technique. Subsequent data provided by consultants is ordinarily the next step and this has also been published. The next step in the determination of the efficacy of the IDET procedure will include independent studies, animal experimentation studies, and controlled studies. These data have not yet been published in a peer-reviewed format.

CONCLUSIONS

The IDET procedure is increasingly being performed in the United States. Both surgeons and non-surgeons perform this procedure. It is imperative that all spine surgeons familiarize themselves with the science, the indications, and the technique of the IDET procedure. The decision whether to perform an IDET procedure should be made following a review of the available basic science and clinical data by the individual practitioner.

A very limited amount of data has been published in peer-reviewed journals for analysis of the IDET procedure. Numerous presentations have been made at various spine society meetings that allow for review of only published abstracts. Whereas many authors describe a favorable experience with the IDET procedure, review of the available published literature reveals many caveats raised by the same authors. Saal and Saal have stated "further study is necessary to define the mechanisms and reasons for clinical improvement."[17] These same authors have suggested that the positive results of their patient population should be validated in placebo controlled randomized trials, which compare IDET with alternative therapies.[17] Similarly, Wetzel and associates noted that the specific mechanism of action remains imprecise and incompletely delineated.[25] O'Neill and associates noted that there has been little research undertaken investigating the efficacy of intradiscal therapies, and, consequently, there is little published evidence supporting their use.[15] Saal and Saal have also commented that studies are currently underway to evaluate the mechanism of action, the placebo effect, and the biomechanical changes, that occur in the intervertebral disc following the IDET procedure.[18] Singh stated that issues that require further classification include the exact mechanism of action, the reasons for failure, the optimal treatment parameters, the long-term outcome results, and the possibility of disc deterioration beyond the natural progression of disc degeneration.[23] Finally, Karasek and Bogduk have stated that until

other authors can achieve results equivalent to their study, intradiscal electrothermy should not be considered ready for wholesale use in the public.[9]

The decision to perform the IDET procedure rests on the individual physician. A review of the mechanism of action of the IDET procedure shows that the science behind this procedure is at best questionable, and at worst, incorrect. The potential for bias among the early investigators is clear. Early results estimating a 60% to 76% clinical improvement rate are encouraging. It is not clear whether patients subjected to the extensive post-procedural therapy regimen of the IDET procedure would do as well clinically if this exercise regimen alone, without the actual thermal energy applied to the disc, was used.

The IDET procedure lacks animal experimentation data. The IDET procedure lacks peer-reviewed journal evidence for its mechanism of action. The IDET procedure lacks any randomized, well-controlled studies to demonstrate its efficacy. Until these important scientific questions are answered, the IDET procedure should be considered an experimental procedure. As with any newer, therapeutic, invasive procedures, if the long-term results, as well as controlled studies, demonstrate the efficacy of this procedure, then and only then, should the IDET procedure become a part of the armamentarium of spine surgeons treating patients.

REFERENCES

1. Arnoczy SP, Aksan A: Thermal modification of connective tissues: basic science considerations and clinical implications. **J Am Acad Orthop Surg** 8:305-13, 2000.
2. Boden SD, Davis DO, Dina TS, et al: Abnormal magnetic-resonance scans of the lumbar spine in asymptomatic subjects: a prospective investigation. **J Bone Joint Surg** 72A:403-8, 1990.
3. Cavanaugh JM, Kallakuri S, Ozaktay AC: Innervation of the rabbit lumbar intervertebral disc and posterior longitudinal ligament. **Spine** 20:2080-85, 1995.
4. Crock HV: A reappraisal of intervertebral disc lesions. **Med J Australia** 1:983-89, 1970.
5. Derby R, Eek B, Chen Y, et al: Intradiscal electrothermal annuloplasty (IDET): A novel approach for treating chronic discogenic back pain. **Neuromodulation** 3:82-88, 2000.
6. Deyo RA, Battie M, Beurskens AJ, et al: Outcome measures for low back pain research. A proposal for standardized use. **Spine** 23:2003-13, 1998.
7. Hayashi K, Thabit G III, Massa KL, et al: The effects of thermal heating on the length and histologic properties of the glenohumeral joint capsule. **Am J Sports Med** 25:107-12, 1997.
8. Hsia AW, Isaac K, Katz JS: Cauda equina syndrome from intradiscal electrothermal therapy. **Neurology** 55:320, 2000.

9. Karasek M, Bogduk N: Twelve-month follow-up of a controlled trial of intradiscal thermal annuloplasty for back pain due to internal disc disruption. **Spine** 25:2601-07, 2000.

10. Kleinstueck F, Diederich C, Naw W, et al: The IDET procedure: temperature distributions and biomechanical effects on human lumbar disk. Presented at the **15**[th] **Annual Meeting of the North American Spine Society**, New Orleans, Louisiana, October 25-28, 2000.

11. Lindblom K: Diagnostic puncture of intervertebral discs in sciatica. **Acta Orthop Scand** 17:231-39, 1948.

12. Liu B, Manos RE, Criscitiello AA, et al: Clinical factors associated with favorable outcomes using intradiscal electrothermal modulation (IDET). **Presented at the 15**[th] **annual meeting of the North American Spine Society**, New Orleans, Louisiana, 2000.

13. Naseef GS III, Foster TE, Trauner K, et al: The thermal properties of bovine joint capsule. The basic science of laser- and radiofrequency- induced capsular shrinkage. **Am J Sports Med** 25:670-74, 1997.

14. Obrzut SL, Hecht P, Hayashi K, et al: The effect of radiofrequency energy on the length and temperature properties of the glenohumeral joint capsule. **Arthroscopy** 14:395-400, 1998.

15. O'Neill C, Derby R, Kenderes L: Precision injection techniques for diagnosis and treatment of lumbar disc disease. **Seminars in Spine Surgery** 11:104-18, 1999.

16. Pokharna HK, Phillips FM: Collagen crosslinks in human lumbar intervertebral disc aging. **Spine** 23:1645-48, 1998.

17. Saal JA, Saal JS: Intradiscal electrothermal treatment for chronic discogenic low back pain: a prospective outcome study with minimum 1-year follow-up. **Spine** 25:2622-27, 2000.

18. Saal JA, Saal JS: Intradiscal electrothermal therapy for the treatment of chronic discogenic low back pain. **Operative Techniques in Orthopaedics** 10:271-81, 2000.

19. Saal JA, Saal JS: Intradiscal electrothermal treatment (IDET) for chronic discogenic low back pain with two year follow-up. Presented at the **15**[th] **annual meeting of the North American Spine Society**, New Orleans, Louisiana, 2000.

20. Saal JS, Saal JA: Management of chronic discogenic low back pain with a thermal intradiscal catheter. **Spine** 25:382-88, 2000.

21. Saal JA, Saal JS: Thermal characteristics of lumbar disc: evaluation of a novel approach to targeted intradiscal thermal therapy. Presented at the **13**[th] **annual meeting of the North American Spine Society**, San Francisco, 1998.

22. Sachs BL, Vanharanta H, Spivey MA, et al: Dallas discogram description—a new classification of CT/discography in low-back disorders. **Spine** 12:287-94, 1987.

23. Singh V: Intradiscal electrothermal therapy: a preliminary report. **Pain Physician** 3:367-373, 2000.

24. Thompson K, Eckel T: IDET [TM] Nationwide registry preliminary results: 6 month follow-up data on 170. Presented at the **15**[th] **annual meeting of the North American Spine Society**, New Orleans, Louisiana, 2000.

25. Wetzel FT, Andersson GBJ, Peloza JH, et al: Intradiskal electrothermal annuloplasty (IDET) to treat discogenic low back pain: preliminary results of a multi-center prospective cohort study. Presented at the **15**[th] **annual meeting of the North American Spine Society**, New Orleans, Louisiana, 2000.

CHAPTER 14

Spinal Cord Stimulation

■

RICHARD B. NORTH, M.D.

INTRODUCTION

Over 25 years ago, electrical stimulation of the spinal cord using implanted electrodes was introduced as a reversible technique of the management of chronic, intractable pain.[93] As a reversible alternative to ablative procedures, this prototypical "neuroaugmentative" procedure was appealing, but the indications for neurosurgical intervention for chronic, benign pain were not widely understood at that time. As the behavioral and psychological issues in pain management have become more widely appreciated, and as programs specializing in chronic pain have proliferated, the process of patient selection has been refined considerably. At the same time, there have been major improvements in implantable spinal cord stimulation devices, which have significantly enhanced clinical results.[75,80]

MECHANISMS OF PAIN RELIEF BY SPINAL CORD STIMULATION

The original rationale for the treatment of pain by implanted electrical stimulation devices was provided by the "gate theory" published by Melzack and Wall.[67] The gate theory postulated that central transmission of pain was governed by a mechanism in the dorsal horn of the spinal cord that responded to an excess of small fiber activity over large fiber activity in the peripheral nervous system. In a mixed population of nerve fibers, the large fibers are more susceptible than the small fibers to recruitment by an externally applied electrical field. This suggests that at a critical stimulation amplitude, large fibers might be recruited selectively, closing the spinal "gate." Electrical stimulation of peripheral nerves might accomplish this by orthodromic conduction along sensory fibers. In a mixed peripheral nerve, this could occur at the expense of unwanted motor effects, at amplitudes close to perceptual threshold.

Alternatively, electrical stimulation over the dorsal columns of the spinal cord might take advantage of spatial segregation of sensory and motor pathways. Antidromic conduction along the dorsal columns, and through collateral processes of primary afferents into the dorsal horn, could achieve the same effect over a wide area.

The gate theory has been the subject of considerable controversy, and there are pathological conditions in which experimental evidence directly contradicts it; for example, hyperalgesia can be signaled by large fibers.[14, 72] In these circumstances, however, relief of pain by spinal cord stimulation (SCS) can be explained in terms of a frequency-related conduction block, at branch points of primary afferents into dorsal horn and dorsal column fibers.[13] In fact, we have found that patients have a clear preference for a minimum pulse repetition rate of 25 per second, given a free choice of rate adjustments.[80] There are other possible mechanisms, of course, that might be frequency dependent, such as those involving dorsal horn interneurons or descending fibers.[25,32,55] Some effects of SCS, particularly those pertinent to the treatment of peripheral vascular disease, appear to be mediated by the sympathetic nervous system.[57]

The electrical fields produced within the spinal cord by SCS have been modeled by computerized finite element techniques.[16,33,99] These models have yielded voltage and current profiles in agreement with in vitro measurements made in cadaver and primate spinal cord.[88] They predict that the longitudinal position of an electrode array is critical to achieving the desired segmental effect, and that maximal selectivity for longitudinally oriented midline fibers, as opposed to dorsal root fibers, is achieved with bipolar midline stimulation, with contact separated by approximately 6 to 8 mm. This modeling is complemented by anatomical findings that the entering dorsal root fibers are relatively superficial within a few segments of their entry into the spinal cord.[26] Furthermore, the mean diameter of ascending fibers in the fasciculus gracilis decreases as they ascend.[81] In aggregate, these findings are consistent with clinical experience that the position and spacing of SCS electrodes are critical, and that advancing electrodes cephalad in an attempt to achieve broader effects may only elicit excessive local segmental effects.[46]

Careful psychophysical study methods applied to SCS patients have shown subtle decrements in normal nociceptive sensation; acute pain thresholds are not affected to a degree that might lead to undesirable effects such as Charcot joint production.[54,63,76] This is consistent with the reported efficacy of SCS for neuropathic as opposed to nociceptive pain. Phenomena observed clinically, such as prolonged latency and persistence of pain relief described by many SCS patients, remain to be explained.[75,76] Changes in the cerebrospinal fluid content of neurotransmitters and their metabolites have been observed; but pharmacologic manipulations, such as naloxone administration, have no effect on the relief of pain by SCS.[31,56] A relevant animal model of chronic neuropathic pain showing apparent relief by SCS has been developed only recently.[68]

Clinical Applications

The criteria for treatment of chronic, benign pain with implanted devices in general, and SCS in particular, have been developed as follows.

IMPLANTED DEVICES FOR INTRACTABLE PAIN

General Indications

1. An objective basis for the complaint of pain (i.e., a specific diagnosis) has been established. In failed back surgery syndrome, for example, there should be an abnormality on diagnostic imaging, such as postsurgical scar, or an objective neurological finding, consistent with the patient's distribution of reported pain. It should be borne in mind, of course, that these abnormalities may be epiphenomena that are not necessarily associated with pain. Furthermore, they may be iatrogenic, and the patient's original surgery, as judged by original records, may not have been indicated.[61]
2. Alternative treatments have been exhausted or are unacceptable by comparison. Again, considering the failed back surgery syndrome as an example, re-operation in general involves greater potential risk and often lower yield.[74,79]
3. Psychological clearance has been obtained to rule out significant drug habituation problems, major

psychiatric diagnoses, or significant personality disorders, and to address issues of secondary gain.[58] Formal psychological testing may be useful in this regard; it has been reported to be most effective in a negative sense, identifying a subset of patients who are poor candidates for SCS.[17]
4. Technically, the procedure's efficacy should be demonstrated by a therapeutic trial with a temporary electrode. In most patients, radicular pain is more easily treated than axial pain, and neuropathic pain is more responsive to SCS than is nociceptive pain. These and other general considerations are subject to testing in specific individuals by percutaneous, temporary electrode trials.

Specific Indications for Spinal Cord Stimulation

Failed back surgery syndrome has been the most common indication for spinal cord stimulator implantation in our experience, and in the United States' experience in general.[74] This condition is also known as *lumbar postlaminectomy syndrome*, a straightforward descriptive diagnosis, and *arachnoiditis*, a misnomer, because arachnoid fibrosis is in fact the underlying pathology, and there is not active inflammatory process in chronically symptomatic patients. Because achieving overlap of the low back by stimulation paresthesias is technically difficult, often requiring complex arrays of electrodes and systematic psychophysical testing, patients with a chief complaint of low back pain are suboptimal candidates.[47] In fact, axial low back pain is commonly mechanical or nociceptive; as such, it may not respond as well to SCS as does pain associated with nerve injury or deafferentation.[89] Having selected patients in whom low back pain was not the chief complaint, we have observed minimal associations between the percentage of low back pain and the treatment outcome.[74,80] In patients with low back and sciatic pain, it has been reported that unilateral lower extremity pain is more easily treated but we have not observed this.[43,65,80,84,85,100]

Peripheral vascular disease has been the most commonly reported application of SCS in Europe in recent years.[9] It is unique among applications of SCS for intractable pain, in that there are measurable changes in lower extremity perfusion, and not simply subjective reports of pain relief in response to treatment.[38] In patients in whom revascularization procedures are not feasible, and in whom lower extremity pain is intractable to a degree that may lead to amputation, SCS may offer not only pain control, but also improved limb salvage.[2]

It was observed serendipitously in 1984 that angina pectoris responds to SCS; specific clinical treatment protocols followed.[2,70,90] Exercise tolerance increases and electrocardiographic changes such as ST segment depression are reduced in ambulatory patients as well as in the laboratory. Myocardial metabolism improves, as reflected by lactate production and extraction. Myocardial oxygen consumption is reduced, and coronary sinus blood flow decreases.[18,62] Biologically useful pain signaling myocardial infarction apparently is not compromised by SCS.[1] Sympathetically mediated effects appear to be important.[30] Cerebral blood flow has been reported to improve with SCS, as well.[35]

Spinal cord injury patients with well-circumscribed segmental pain at the level of injury often respond very well to SCS. In our 20-year published experience, the rate of successful percutaneous trials for this condition was over 90%.[80] The same patients are generally good candidates for dorsal root entry zone lesions; this alternative, however, requires a laminectomy and intradural exposure that may make it an unattractive alternative in some patients. Postcordotomy dysesthesias are another iatrogenic form of spinal cord injury pain, often superimposed upon the original pain problem, leading to cordotomy; this syndrome also responds to SCS, in many cases. Pain associated with spinal cord lesions of other causes, such as multiple sclerosis, frequently responds; this must be distinguished from reports of improvement in neurological function, however, which have been controversial.[4,97] These applications require further investigation.

Peripheral nerve injury or neuralgia, causalgia, and so-called *reflex sympathetic dystrophy* respond well to SCS in many cases.[5] In our 20-year experience, the rate of successful percutaneous trials was lower than for other conditions, to a statistically significant degree.[80] This may not be clinically significant, however. Most patients nevertheless responded and proceeded to permanent implantation, following a simple percutaneous trial.

Postamputation syndromes, specifically phantom limb pain, respond to SCS in most cases.[42] Stump neuroma pain is usually responsive; it may properly be considered as one of the peripheral nerve injury syndromes mentioned previously but often coexists with or is difficult to distinguish from phantom pain.

PERCUTANEOUS ELECTRODE TRIALS

The earliest SCS electrodes required a laminectomy to introduce a planar electrode structure into the spinal canal. As it became apparent that not all patients achieved pain relief from SCS no matter how careful the selection process, and with recognition of the importance of electrode placement to technical success, percutaneous techniques for temporary electrode placement were developed.[27,34,36] In the late 1970s, these were adapted for use with chronically implanted systems.[76,107] Figures 14-1 and 14-2 illustrate percutaneous dorsal epidural electrode placement.

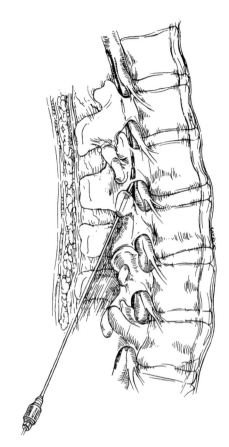

FIGURE 14-1 ■ A shallow angle of approach facilitates percutaneous dorsal epidural electrode placement through a modified Tuohy needle.

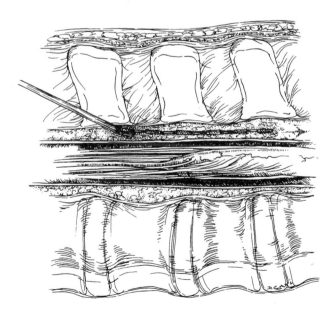

FIGURE 14-2 ■ A linear array of electrodes placed percutaneously is advanced in the dorsal epidural space.

A temporary, percutaneous electrode may be placed under local anesthesia without any need for sedation or premedication that might compromise the patient participation in the procedure. Because achieving overlap of the distribution of the patient's pain by stimulation paresthesias is the primary technical goal of the procedure, the freedom to longitudinally map the spinal epidural space over multiple segments is a major advantage of the percutaneous approach.[46,75] Temporary electrode placement, which may be time consuming in the naïve patient, may be performed in the fluoroscopy suite, avoiding the time constraints and expense of using an operating room. With the temporary electrode in position, the patient can use a temporary stimulation device under ordinary, ambulatory conditions, so that its effects may be judged away from the time pressures of the operating, and so that the patient may become familiar with the device's controls. During this test phase, measurements of stimulation current thresholds in individual patients can be made, and if a fully implanted device powered by a primary cell is under consideration, its longevity can be estimated. When the patient returns to the operating room for permanent electrode implantation, the procedure is expedited by this prior experience.

A temporary electrode may be placed in such a way as to allow its subsequent conversion for use with a chronic implant. This requires use of a percutaneous extension cable, tunneled subcutaneously. Accordingly, such an electrode must be placed in an operating room, as opposed as to a fluoroscopy room. Furthermore, its removal or conversion to a permanent implant requires a return to the operating room. This may unduly influence the patient and the physician, who have made a major investment of time and potential morbidity in the temporary electrode, to convert it to a permanent system. A strictly temporary percutaneous electrode, which may be withdrawn at the bedside, involves no such commitment. Furthermore, temporary percutaneous extensions have been associated with an increased rate of infection.[40,46]

The criteria for proceeding from a temporary to a permanent implant have varied widely and arbitrarily. Some authors have required as much as 70% to 75% reported relief and others as little as 30%.[6,20,52,65] Percutaneous trials as long as two months, and as short as single-stage implantation with only intra-operative testing, have been reported.[29,66] In some series (single-stage implants), all patients are implanted, whereas in others, as few as 40% to 47% of patients screened with temporary electrodes have gone on to receive permanently implanted devices.[19,95] As summarized in Table 14-1, however, it is not clear that any of these protocols substantially influences long-term success rates. It is clear, however, that a significant number of patients are long-term clinical failures, so there is a role for any

protocol that identifies and excludes such patients with high specificity, even if its sensitivity is arguable. Failure to achieve or maintain a clinically adequate response with a technically adequate temporary implant would seem to fulfill this criterion.

Accordingly, the author routinely considers a percutaneous trial successful and offers the patient a permanent implant when the patient reports a minimum of 50% pain relief while demonstrating improved activity and appropriate (i.e., improved or discontinued) use of analgesics, commensurate with reported relief of pain, over a period of at least two to three days. When the result is equivocal, the trial is extended. The potential morbidity of infection and epidural scarring (compromising permanent device implantation) must be balanced against the potential yield of a prolonged trial.

Spinal Cord Stimulation Devices

The earliest SCS electrodes were two-dimensional plates or arrays, which necessitated a laminectomy for direct placement in the dorsal epidural, endodural, or subarachnoid space.[11,71,100] There were several problems with this approach. First, it required a spinal surgical procedure simply to test patients before implantation of a permanent device. This introduced unnecessary morbidity and patient discomfort that could interfere with interpretation of the pain-relieving effects of SCS during a trial period. A laminectomy offers only limited access to the spinal canal for longitudinal exploration to map potential electrode positions. Assuming that patient selection and electrode placement have been optimized, however, laminectomy electrodes offer potential advantages. The electrodes may be secured directly to the dura to resist migration, and following encapsulation in scar tissue, the shape of laminectomy electrode arrays further resists migration.

Migration or malposition requiring surgical revision was a common problem with early percutaneously placed single electrodes.[76] This has been ameliorated by improvements in anchoring techniques to resist migration of the implant and by the introduction of linear arrays of electrodes individual contacts of which cannot migrate with respect to one another. The ability to select anode and cathode positions from multiple contacts allows compensation for minor changes as the patient shifts from the prone position, in which the device is implanted, to the erect or supine position, in which the device will be used. In aggregate, these improvements have reduced the need for surgical revision of electrode position to the extent that there may no longer be a significant difference in migration rates of percutaneous and laminectomy electrodes.[80] If a two-dimensional array is to be created by inserting multiple columns percutaneously, however, the potential for one column to migrate with respect to the other remains; this is eliminated by a fixed laminectomy array.[49] An additional potential advantage of laminectomy electrodes is their insulated backing that protects against potentially uncomfortable recruitment of small fibers located dorsal to the electrodes, for example, in the ligamentum flavum.

Implanted pulse generators used for spinal cord stimulation have evolved along with electrodes; programmable devices allow noninvasive selection of stimulating anodes and cathodes from contemporary electrode arrays. These systems allow adjustment under ordinary conditions of activity and posture, for optimal effect. As the patient gains experience with the system, and as more critical psychophysical testing becomes possible, this allows ongoing readjustments. These programmable, multicontact systems require surgical revision significantly less often than do older single channel systems, and their clinical results are significantly better.[75,80]

"Totally implanted" pulse generators for SCS have been available for a decade. An external programming device remains necessary for control of these systems, and the patient is required to carry a magnet to turn the device on and off and/or to control the amplitude within programmed limits. Like implanted cardiac pacemakers, they are powered by lithium primary cells; however, the energy required for SCS commonly exceeds that required for cardiac pacing by one or two orders of magnitude. Careful attention to individual patients' requirements is necessary to avoid frequent surgical replacement; pulse amplitude, pulse width, pulse repetition rate (frequency), electrode impedance or load (determined by size and number of active contacts), and duty cycle (hours of use per day) all are important. Externally powered, radio-frequency-coupled systems contain no life-limiting components. Adjustment is not compromised because of potential cell depletion, and the expense and potential morbidity of inevitable pulse generator replacement are avoided.

Clinical Results

The rates of success reported in the literature on SCS have varied widely, as summarized in Table 14-1. Results commonly are reported in terms of the number of permanent implants performed, and not upon the number of patients screened with temporary electrodes (which may or may not be specified). In some series, with rates of permanent implantation as low as 40%, adjustment for this would be very important; in other series, with rates of permanent implantation exceeding 75%, adjustment for this would be minor.[19,80] For other neurosurgical procedures for pain relief, success rates usually are reported in terms of the number of patients who undergo the definitive procedure and not the number who undergo test procedures such as myelography or diagnostic nerve blocks, the morbidity of which is similar to that of temporary percutaneous electrode placement. Neuro-augmentative techniques such as SCS and drug delivery system implantation have the inherent advantage of a low morbidity trial or test phase that emulates the definite procedure.

In addition to ratings of pain and its relief, criteria for success should include ongoing medication requirements, activities of daily living, changes in neurological function, work status, and overall health care costs.[6,80] Another important aspect of outcome assessment is the source of follow-up data. Interview by a clinically uninvolved third party, of course, has been reported to yield different results from physicians' office records and hospital charts, and third party interview results are reported increasingly in the literature on SCS.[11,28,40,43,59,73-76,80,91,98]

Computerized Methods of Stimulator Control

The implantation of arrays of electrodes, supported by programmable electronics, has improved technical results (overlap of pain by paresthesias) and clinical results of SCS. The number of possible anode and cathode assignments for a multicontact array, however, grows disproportionately as the number of contacts increases. Furthermore, at each electrode combination tested, it may be necessary to study a range of pulse parameters, in particular amplitude. Comparison between different electrode configurations is most appropriately made at identical subjective stimulus intensities.[47] The range of amplitudes from first perception to discomfort threshold may be considered as a scale, along which the amplitude at which the painful area is first stimulated may be scaled. In addition, if axial low back pain is to be targeted, precise control of the physiological midline is required, and thresholds for bilateral stimulation should be defined precisely.[3,48] Careful quantitative study of these parameters generates a large volume of data, best managed by computer.[3,47,77,78] Given suitable means of control, the patient can interact directly with a computer to accomplish this adjustment task.[77,78] Systems that control the implanted stimulator directly allow study of novel pulse sequences and modulation schemes; these may offer advantages over the monotonic pulse sequences in use for the past 25 years.

CONCLUSIONS

Spinal cord stimulation has become a relatively easily implemented, reversible technique for the management of chronic, intractable pain in properly selected

TABLE 14-1 ■ Rates of Success for SCS

Author, year	Implanted	Screened	Failed backs	Range	Mean	Results (≥50% relief)	FBSS Results (%)	Third Party Follow-up
	Number			**Follow-up**		**"Exc/good" (%)**		
Bel, et al, 1991[6]	14		14		2y	60	60	
Blond, et al, 1991[7]	58	59	59	12–72 mo	37 mo	89.5	89.5	
Blume et al, 1983[8]	20		20	Up to 3y		70	70	
Broseta et al, 1982[10]	11			3–20 mo	13 mo	64		
Burton, 1975[11]	75	0	55		1y	59		Yes (mfr.)
Burton, 1978[12]	198		186			43		
Clark, 1979[15]	13		6			54	67	
De la Porte, Van de Kelft, 1983[19]	36	94	36	3–96 mo	36 mo	60		
De la Porte, Van de Kelft, 1993[20]	64	78	78	1–7y	4y	55	55	
de Vera et al, 1990[22]	110	124	18			75		
Demirel et al, 1984[21]	33	48	11	2–5y		18		
Devulder et al, 1990[23]	45		23			78		
Devulder et al, 1991[24]	69		43	Up to 8 y		55		
Erickson, Long, 1983[28]	70	10		Up to 10y		15–20		Yes (60)
Hoppenstein, 1975[34]	27		12			58	64	
Hunt, et al, 1975[37]	13		5	9 mo–4y		15–31	20–60	
Kälin, Winkelmuller, 1990[39]			77			88	88	
Koeze, et al, 1987[40]	26	0	5		28 mo	46–62		Yes
Krainick/Thoden, 1989[41]	91	126	5	Up to 5 y		18		
Kumar et al, 1986[44]	60		54	6–60 mo		62		
Kumar et al, 1991[43]	94	121	56	6 mo–10 y	40 mo	66		Yes
Law, 1983[45]	81					36–80		
Leclercq, Russo, 1981[50]	20		20	1–>24 mo		50	50	
LeDoux, Langford, 1993[51]	26	32	32	Up to 5 y		76 @ 1 yr.	76 @ 1 yr.	
LeRoy, 1981[53]	49		49	1–63 mo	30.7 mo	60		No
Long, Erickson, 1975[59]	69		54	12–35 mo		18		Yes
Long , et al, 1981[60]	31		24	4–7 y		73 @ 3 yrs.		Yes
McCarron, Racz, 1987[64]	22			3–24 mo		68		
Meglio, et al, 1989[66]	64	109	19				23	No
Meilman, et al, 1989[65]	12	20	20	Up to 3.5 y		60	60	
Mittal, et al, 1987[69]	26	31	21			46		
Nielson, et al, 1975[73]	130	221	79	1–>35 mo		49	46	Yes
North, et al, 1991[74]	50	54	50		5.0 y	47	47	Yes
North, et al, 1993[80]	171	205	153	2–20 y	7.1 y	52		Yes
Pineda, 1975[82]	76		56			43	43	
Racz, et al, 1989[83]	26	0	18	12–42.7 mo		65		No
Ray, et al. 1982[84]	78		50	3–64 mo	19.4 mo	49		
Richardson, et al, 1979[86]	22	36	12	1–3 y		56		
Richardson, Shatin, 1991[85]	136		136		45 mo	67	67	Yes (mfr)
Robb/Robb, 1990[87]	79	65	22	6 mo–5 y		72	69	
Sánchez-Ledesma, et al, 1989[89]	33	49	0		5.5 y	57		
Shatin, et al, 1986[91]	116			0.9–13.3 mo		74 @ 6 mo		Yes (mfr)
Shealy, 1975[92]	80	0		7 mo		25	15–45	No
Shelden, et al, 1975[94]	27		3				67	
Siegfried, 1982[95]	89	191	75	1–8 y	4 y	37		
Simpson, 1991[96]	56	24	7	2 wk–9 y	29 mo	47		
Spiegelmann, Friedman, 1991[98]	30	43	18	3–33 mo	13 mo	60		Yes
Sweet, Wepsic, 1974[100]	98	100	33			21–42	15–45	
Urban, Nashold, 1978[101]	7	20	9			86		
Vogel, et al, 1986[102]	27	50	29	>3 yr		18.6		No
Waisbrod et al, 1985[103]	16		16	6–30 mo	16 mo	75		No
Winkelmuller, 1981[104]	71	94	56	4 mo–7 y			69	
Young, Shende, 1976[106]	27		17	16–51 mo		66≤50%		
Young, 1978[105]	51	14	25	12–67 mo	38 mo	65≤50%		

FBSS, failed back surgery syndrome; mfr., device manufacturer.

The literature on SCS exhibits a variety of follow-up intervals and methods, temporary electrode screening methods, and criteria for "success." Comparisons among studies or meta-analyses are difficult. An "excellent" or "good" result commonly signifies at least 50% reported relief of pain; but this is only one of many important outcome measures.

patients. The development of percutaneous placement of electrode arrays, and of programmable implanted electronics that allow noninvasive assignment of anode and cathode positions, have been major technical advances. These have significantly reduced the need for surgical revisions of implanted hardware, and they have substantially improved clinical results.

REFERENCES

1. Anderson C, Hole P, Ochoj H: Does pain relief with spinal cord stimulation for angina conceal myocardia infarction? **Br Heart J** 71:419-21, 1994.
2. Augustinsson LE, Carlsson CA, Holm J, et al: Epidural electrical stimulation in severe limb ischemia: evidence of pain relief, increased blood flow and a possible limb-saving effect. **Ann Surg** 202:104-11, 1985.
3. Barolat G, Massaro F, He J, et al: Mapping of sensory responses to epidural stimulation of the intraspinal neural structures in man. **J Neurosurg** 78:233-39, 1993.
4. Barolat G, Myklebust JB, Wenninger W: Effects of spinal cord stimulation on spasticity and spasms secondary to myelopathy. **Appl Neurophys** 5:29-44, 1988.
5. Barolat G, Schwartzman R, Woo R: Epidural spinal cord stimulation in the management of reflex sympathetic dystrophy. **Stereotactic Functional Neurosurg** 53:29-39, 1989.
6. Bel S, Bauer BL: Dorsal column stimulation (DCS): Cost to benefit analysis. **Acta Neuroshir** 52(suppl):121-23, 1991.
7. Blond S, Armignies P, Parker F, et al: Sciatalges chroniques par désafférentation sensitive aprés chirurgie de la hernie discale lombaire: aspets cliniques et thérapeutiques. **Neuroshirurgie** 37:86-95, 1991.
8. Blume H, Richardson R, Rojas C: Epidural nerve stimulation of the lower spinal cord and cauda equina for the relief of intractable pain in failed back surgery. **Appl Neurophysiol** 45:456-60, 1982.
9. Broseta J, Barbera J, De Vera J, et al: Spinal cord stimulation in peripheral arterial disease. **J Neurosurg** 64:71-80, 1986.
10. Broseta J, Roldan P, Gonzales-Darder J, et al: Chronic epidural dorsal column stimulation in the treatment of causalgic pain. **Appl Neurophysiol** 45:190-94, 1982.
11. Burton C: Dorsal column stimulation: optimization of application. **Surg Neurol** 4:171-76, 1975.
12. Burton CV: Session on spinal cord stimulation: safety and clinical efficacy. **Neurosurgery** 1:164-65, 1977.
13. Campbell JN, Davis KD, Meyer RA, et al: The mechanism by which dorsal column stimulation affects pain: evidence for a new hypothesis. **Pain** 5:S228, 1990.
14. Campbell JN, Meyer RA: Primary afferents and hyperalgesia, in Yaksh TL (ed.): **Spinal Afferent Processing**. New York: Plenum, 1986.
15. Clark K: Electrical stimulation of the nervous system for control of pain: University of Texas Southwestern Medical School experience. **Surg Neurol** 4:164-66, 1975.
16. Coburn B, Sin W: A theoretical study of epidural electrical stimulation of the spinal cord. Part I: Finite element analysis of stimulus fields. **Biomed Eng** 32:971-77, 1985.
17. Daniel M, Long C, Hutcherson M, et al: Psychological factors and outcome of electrode implantation for chronic pain. **Neurosurgery** 17(5):773-77, 1985.
18. de Jongste MJL, Haaksma J, Hautvast RWM, et al: Effects of spinal cord stimulation on myocardial ischaemia during daily life in patients with severe coronary artery disease: a prospective ambulatory electrocardiographic study. **Br Heart J** 71:413-18, 1994.
19. De la Porte C, Siegfried J: Lumbosacral spinal fibrosis (spinal arachnoiditis): its diagnosis and treatment by spinal cord stimulation. **Spine** 8(6):593-603, 1983.
20. De la Porte C, Van de Kelft E: Spinal cord stimulation in failed back surgery syndrome. **Pain** 52:55-61, 1993.
21. Demirel T, Braun W, Reimers CD: Results of spinal cord stimulation in patients suffering from chronic pain after a two year observation period. **Neurochirurgia** 27:47-50, 1984.
22. de Vera JA, Rodriguez JL, Dominguez M: Spinal cord stimulation for chronic pain mainly in PVD, vasospastic disorders of the upper limbs and failed back surgery. **Pain** (Suppl. 5):S81, 1990.
23. Devulder J, De Colvenaer L, Rolly G, et al: Spinal cord stimulation and the relief of chronic non-malignant pain in 45 patients. **Pain** 5:S236, 1990.
24. Devulder J, DeColvenaer L, Rolly G, et al: Spinal cord stimulation in chronic pain therapy. **Clin J Pain** 6:51-56, 1991.
25. Duggan AW, Foong FW: Bicuculline and spinal inhibition produced by dorsal column stimulation in the cat. **Pain** 22:249-59, 1985.
26. Dyck PJ, Lais A, Karnes J, et al: Peripheral axotomy induces neurofilament decrease, atrophy, demyelination and degeneration of root and fasciculus gracilis fibers. **Br Res** 340:19-36, 1985.
27. Erickson DL: Percutaneous trial of stimulation for patient selection for implantable stimulating devices. J Neurosurg 43:440-44, 1975.
28. Erickson DL, Long DM: Ten-year follow-up of dorsal column stimulation, in Bonica JJ (ed.): **Advances in Pain Research and Therapy**. New York: Raven Press, 1983.
29. Feler C, Kaufman S: Spinal cord stimulation: one state? **Acta Neurochir** 117:91, 1992.
30. Foreman RD: The neurological basis for cardiac pain, in Zucker IH, Gilmore JP (eds.): **Reflex Control of the Circulation**. Boston: CRC Press, 1991.
31. Freeman TB, Campbell JN, Long DM: Naloxone does not affect pain relief induced by electrical stimulation in man. **Pain** 17:189-95, 1983.
32. Handwerker HO, Iggo A, Zimmerman M: Segmental and supraspinal actions on dorsal horn neurons responding to noxious and non-noxious skin stimuli. **Pain** 1:147-65, 1975.
33. Holsheimer J, Struijk JJ: How do geometric factors influence epidural spinal cord stimulation? A quantitative analysis by computer modeling. **Stereotact Funct Neurosurg** 56:234-49, 1991.
34. Hoppenstein R: Electrical stimulation of the ventral and dorsal columns of the spinal cord for relief of chronic intractable pain: Preliminary report. **Surg Neurol** 4:187-94, 1975.

35. Hosobuchi Y: Electrical stimulation of the cervical spinal cord increases cerebral blood flow in humans. **Appl Neurophysiol** 48:372-76, 1985.

36. Hosobuchi Y, Adams JE, Weinstein PR: Preliminary percutaneous dorsal column stimulation prior to permanent implantation. **J Neurosurg** 37:242-45, 1972.

37. Hunt WE, Goodman JH, Bingham WG: Stimulation of the dorsal spinal cord for treatment of intractable pain; a preliminary report. **Surg Neurol** 4:153-56, 1975.

38. Jacobs JHMJ, Slaaf DW, Reneman RS: Dorsal column stimulation in critical limb ischemia. **Vasc Med Rev** 1:215-20, 1990.

39. Kälin M-T, Winkelmuller W: Chronic pain after multiple lumbar discectomies-significance of intermittent spinal cord stimulation. **Pain** 5:S241, 1990.

40. Koeze TH, Williams AC, Reiman S: Spinal cord stimulation and the relief of chronic pain. **J Neurolo Neurosurg Psych** 50:1424-9, 1987.

41. Krainick JU, Thoden U: Dorsal column stimulation, in Wall PD, Melzack R (eds.): **Textbook of Pain**. New York: Churchill Livingstone, 1989.

42. Krainick JU, Thoden U, Riechert T: Pain reduction in amputees by long-term spinal cord stimulation: long-term follow-up study over 5 years. **J Neurosurg** 52:346-50, 1980.

43. Kumar K, Nath R, Wyant GM: Treatment of chronic pain by epidural spinal cord stimulation: a 10-year experience. **J Neurosurg** 75:402-07, 1991.

44. Kumar K, Wyant GM, Ekong CEU: Epidural spinal cord stimulation for relief of chronic pain. **The Pain Clinic** 1(2):91-99, 1986.

45. Law J: Results of treatment of pain by percutaneous multicontact stimulation of the spinal cord, Presented by the American Pain Society meeting, Chicago, November 11-13, 1983.

46. Law J: Spinal stimulation: statistical superiority of monophasic stimulation of narrowly separated, longitudinal bipoles having rostral cathodes. **Appl Neurophys** 46:129-37, 1983.

47. Law JD: A new method for targeting a spinal stimulator: quantitatively paired comparisons. **Appl Neurophys** 50:436, 1987.

48. Law JD: Targeting a spinal stimulator to treat the "failed back surgery syndrome." **Appl Neurophys** 50:437-38, 1987.

49. Law JD, Kirkpatrick AF: Pain management update: spinal cord stimulation. **Am J Pain Manage** 2:34-42, 1991.

50. Leclercq T, Russo E: La stimulation epidurale dans le traitement del doleurs chroniques. **Neurochirurgie** 27:125-28, 1981.

51. LeDoux MS, Langford KH: Spinal cord stimulation for the failed back syndrome. **Spine** 18:191-94, 1993.

52. Leibrock L, Meilman P, Cuka D, et al: Spinal cord stimulation in the treatment of chronic low back and lower extremity pain syndrome. **Nebraska Med J** 69(6): 180-83, 1984.

53. LeRoy PL: Stimulation of the spinal cord by bio-compatible electric current in the human. **Appl Neurophysiol** 44:187-93, 1981.

54. Lindblom U, Meyerson BA: Influence on touch, vibration and cutaneous pain of dorsal column stimulation in man. **Pain** 1:257-70, 1975.

55. Lindblom U, Tapper N, Wiesenfeld Z: The effect of dorsal column stimulation on the nociceptive response of dorsal horn cells and its relevance for pain suppression. **Pain** 4:133-34, 1997.

56. Linderoth B: Effects of spinal cord stimulation on basic neurophysiological mechanisms. **Abst 1st Meeting Internat Neuromodulation Society**. Rome, 1992:2.

57. Linderoth B, Fedorcsak I, Meyerson BA: Peripheral vasodilation after spinal cord stimulation: animal studies of putative effector mechanisms. **Neurosurgery** 28:187-95, 1991.

58. Long DM: A review of psychological considerations in the neurosurgical management of chronic pain: a neurosurgeon's perspective. **Neurosurg Q** 1:185-95, 1991.

59. Long DM, Erickson DE: Stimulation of the posterior columns of the spinal cord for relief of intractable pain. **Surg Neurol** 4:134-41, 1975.

60. Long DM, Erickson D, Campbell J, et al: Electrical stimulation of the spinal cord and peripheral nerves for pain control. **Appl Neurophysiol** 44:207-17, 1981.

61. Long DM, Filtzer DL, BenDebba M, et al: Clinical features of the failed-back syndrome. **J Neurosurg** 69:61-71, 1988.

62. Mannheimer C, Eliasson T, Andersson B: Effects of spinal cord stimulation in angina pectoris induced by pacing and possible mechanisms of action. **Br Med J** 307:477-80, 1993.

63. Marchand S, Bushnell MC, Molina-Negro P, et al: The effects of dorsal column stimulation on measures of clinical and experimental pain in man. **Pain** 45:249-57, 1991.

64. McCarron RF, Racz G: Percutaneous dorsal column stimulator implantation for chronic pain control. Presented at North American Spine Society meeting. Banff, Alberta, Canada, June 25-28, 1987.

65. Meilman PW, Leibrock LG, Leong FTL: Outcome of implanted spinal cord stimulation in the treatment of chronic pain: arachnoiditis versus single nerve root injury and mononeuropathy. **Clin J Pain** 5:189-93, 1989.

66. Meglio M, Cioni B, Rossi GF: Spinal cord stimulation in management of chronic pain. A 9-year experience. **J Neurosurg** 70:519-24, 1989.

67. Melzack P, Wall PD: Pain mechanisms: a new theory. Science 150(3699):971-78, 1965.

68. Meyerson BA, Herregodts P, Linderoth B: Enhanced flexor in the mononeuropathic rat is attenuated by spinal cord stimulation. **Act Neurochir** 117:88, 1992.

69. Mittal B, Thomas DGT, Walton P, et al: Dorsal column stimulation (DCS) in chronic pain: report of 31 cases. **Ann Roy Coll Surg** 69(3):104-09, 1987.

70. Murphy DF, Giles KE: Intractable angina pectoris: management with dorsal column stimulation (case report). **Med J Aust** 146:260, 1987.

71. Nashold B, Somjen G, Friedman H: Paresthesias and EEG potentials evoked by stimulation of the dorsal funiculi in man. **Exp Neurol** 36(2):273-87, 1972.

72. Nathan PW: The gate-control theory of pain: a critical review. **Brain** 99:123-58, 1976.

73. Nielson KD, Adams JE, Hosobuchi Y: Experience with dorsal column stimulation for relief of chronic intractable pain. **Surg Neurol** 4:148-52, 1975.
74. North RB, Ewend MG, Lawton MT, et al: Failed back surgery syndrome: five-year follow-up after spinal cord stimulator implantation. **Neurosurgery** 28:692-99, 1991.
75. North RB, Ewend MG, Lawton MT, et al: Spinal cord stimulation for chronic, intractable pain: superiority of "multichannel" devices. **Pain** 44:119-30, 1991.
76. North RB, Fischell TA, Long DM: Chronic stimulation via percutaneously inserted epidural electrodes. **Neurosurgery** 1:215-18, 1977.
77. North RB, Fowler KR, Nigrin DA, et al: Patient-interactive, computer-controlled neurological stimulation system: clinical efficacy in spinal cord stimulation. **J Neurosurg** 76:689-95, 1992.
78. North RB, Nigrin DA, Fowler KR, et al: Automated 'pain drawing' analysis by computer-controlled, patient-interactive neurological stimulation system. **Pain** 50:51-58, 1992.
79. North RB, Kidd DH, Lee MS, et al: Spinal cord stimulation versus reoperation for the failed back surgery syndrome: a prospective, randomized study design. **Stereotact Funct Neurosurg** 1994..
80. North RB, Kidd DH, Zahurak M, et al: Spinal cord stimulation for chronic, intractable pain: two decades' experience. **Neurosurgery** 32:384-95, 1993.
81. Ohnishi A, O'Brien PC, Okazaki H, et al: Morphometry of myelinated fibers of fasciculus gracilis of man. **Neurol Sci** 27:163-72, 1976.
82. Pineda A: Dorsal column stimulation and its prospects. **Surg Neurol** 4:157-63, 1975.
83. Racz GB, McCarron RF, Talboys P: Percutaneous dorsal column stimulator for chronic pain control. **Spine** 14(1):1-4, 1989.
84. Ray DC, Burton CV, Lifson A: Neurostimulation as used in a large clinical practice. **Appl Neurophysiol** 45:160-206, 1982.
85. Richardson DE, Shatin D: Results of spinal cord stimulation for pain control: long-term collaborative study. Presented at American Pain Society, New Orleans, Poster #91240, November 8-10, 1991:56.
86. Richardson RR, Siqueira EB, Cerullo LJ: Spinal epidural neurostimulation for treatment of acute and chronic intractable pain: initial and long term results. **Neurosurgery** 5(3):344-48, 1979.
87. Robb LG, Robb MP: Practical considerations in spinal cord stimulation. **Pain** 5:S234, 1990.
88. Sances A, Swiontek TJ, Larson SJ, et al: Innovations in neurologic implant systems. **Med Instrum** 9(5):213-16, 1975.
89. Sánchez-Ledesma MJ, Garcia-March G, Diaz-Cascajo P, et al: Spinal cord stimulation in deafferentation pain. **Stereotact Funct Neurosurg** 53:40-55, 1989.
90. Sandric S, Meglio M, Bellocci F, et al: Clinical and electrocardiographic improvement of ischaemic heart disease after spinal cord stimulation. **Acta Neurochir Suppl** 33:543-46, 1984.
91. Shatin D, Mullett K, Hults G: Totally implantable spinal cord stimulation for chronic pain: design and efficacy. **Pace** 9:577-83, 1986.
92. Shealy CN: Dorsal column stimulation: optimization of application. **Surg Neurol** 4:142-45, 1975.
93. Shealy CN, Mortimer JT, Reswick JB: Electrical inhibition of pain by stimulation of the dorsal columns: preliminary clinical report. **Anesth Analg** 46:489-91, 1967.
94. Shelden CH, Paul F, Jacques DB, et al: Electrical stimulation of the nervous system. **Surg Neurol** 4:127-32, 1975.
95. Siegfried J, Lazorthes Y: Long-term follow-up of dorsal column stimulation for chronic pain syndrome after multiple lumbar operations. **Appl Neurophys** 45:201-04, 1982.
96. Simpson BA: Spinal cord stimulation in 60 cases of intractable pain. **J Neurol Neurosurg Psychiat** 54:196-99, 1991.
97. Simpson BA: Spinal cord stimulation. **Pain Rev** 1:199-230, 1994.
98. Spiegelmann R, Friedman WA: Spinal cord stimulation: a contemporary series. **Neurosurgery** 28:65-71, 1991.
99. Struijk JJ, Holsheimer J, Boom HBK: Excitation of dorsal root fibers in spinal cord stimulation: a theoretical study. **IEEE Trans Biomed Eng** 40:632-39, 1993.
100. Sweet W, Wepisc J: Stimulation of the posterior columns of the spinal cord for pain control. **Clin Neurosur** 21:278-310, 1974.
101. Urban BJ, Nashold B: Percutaneous epidural stimulation of the spinal cord for relief of pain: long term results. **J Neurosurg** 48:323-28, 1978.
102. Vogel HP, Heppner B, Humbs N, et al: Long-term effects of spinal cord stimulation in chronic pain syndromes. **J Neurol** 233:16-18, 1986.
103. Waisbrod H, Panhans C, Hansen D, et al: Direct nerve stimulation for painful peripheral neuropathies. **J Bone Joint Surg** 67(3):470-73, 1985.
104. Winkelmuller W: Experience with the control of low back pain by the dorsal column stimulation (DCS) system and by the peridural electrode system (Pisces), in Hosobuchi Y, Corbin T (eds.): **Indications for Spinal Cord Stimulation**. Amsterdam: Excerpta Medica, 1981.
105. Young RF: Evaluation of dorsal column stimulation in the treatment of chronic pain. **Neurosurgery** 3:373-79, 1978.
106. Young RF, Shende M: Dorsal column stimulation for relief of chronic intractable pain. **Surg Forum** 27:474-76, 1976.
107. Zumpano BJ, Saunders RL: Percutaneous epidural dorsal column stimulation. **J Neurosurg** 45:459-60, 1976.

Index